Nutrition
in
Pharmacy Practice

Nutrition in Pharmacy Practice

Ira Wolinsky and Louis Williams, Editors

American Pharmaceutical Association
Washington, D.C.

Acquiring Editor: Sandra J. Cannon
Managing Editor: Vicki Meade, Meade Communications
Assistant Editors: Mary De Angelo, Paula Novash, Kellie Burton, Martha Taggart
Layout Artist: Roy Barnhill
Graphics Support: Michele Danoff, Graphics by Design
Cover Design: Jim McDonald
Proofreaders: Amy Morgante, Mary De Angelo, Paula Novash
Indexing: Suzanne Peake

© 2002 by the American Pharmaceutical Association

Published by the American Pharmaceutical Association
2215 Constitution Avenue, N.W.
Washington, DC 20037-2985
www.aphanet.org

To comment on this book via e-mail, send your message to the publisher at
aphabooks@aphanet.org

        Library of Congress Cataloging-in-Publication Data

Nutrition in pharmacy practice / Ira Wolinsky and Louis Williams,
   editors.
       p. ; cm.
   Includes bibliographical references and index.
   ISBN 1-58212-023-4
   1. Drug-nutrient interactions. 2. Nutrition. 3. Dietary supplements. 4. Pharmacists.   I. Wolinsky, Ira. II. Williams, Louis,
1940-   .
   [DNLM: 1. Nutrition. 2. Diet Therapy. 3. Nutrition Disorders
--prevention & control. 4. Pharmacy--methods.   QU 145
N9744 2002]
RM302.4.N875 2002
615'.7045--dc21

2002011699

HOW TO ORDER THIS BOOK
Online: www.pharmacist.com
By phone: 800-878-0729 (from the United States and Canada)
VISA®, MasterCard®, and American Express® cards accepted.

Printed in Canada

Dedication

To Mary Ann, Daniella, David, Sandra, Indi, Bryan, and Marc.

Table of Contents

Preface

In preparing this volume two professional disciplines have intertwined: nutrition and pharmacy.

To function effectively as part of the modern health delivery team, the pharmacist should be knowledgeable in nutrition. Nutrition is an interdisciplinary, interprofessional field par excellence. It interacts and overlaps with all life science areas, including pharmacy. Very often the patient/consumer refers first to the pharmacist for nutritional advice. Therefore, the potential for pharmacists to give sound, accurate information about nutrition is enormous, and we hope this book will help them to do that.

We have assembled an excellent roster of authors with a wealth of clinical, research, and pharmacy experience. This book was written in response to the expressed needs of pharmacists as determined through a survey administered by the American Pharmaceutical Association. The topics covered were suggested by respondents to the survey.

Valuable input from our chapter authors has been incorporated in the organization of the book. If upon reading and using this volume you feel that anything important has been left out, please let us know your thoughts for future editions.

Ira Wolinsky, PhD
Louis Williams, PhD
July 8, 2002

Contributors

Melvin Baron, PharmD, MPA
Department of Pharmacy
School of Pharmacy
University of Southern California
Estelle Doheny Eye Institute
Los Angeles, California

Imad F. Btaiche, PharmD, BCNSP
Department of Pharmacy Services
College of Pharmacy
University of Michigan
Ann Arbor, Michigan

Louis J. Ciliberti, Jr., MS
Nutrition Program
School of Human Resources
University of Louisiana at Lafayette
Lafayette, Louisiana

Victoria DeVore, PharmD
Department of Clinical Sciences and
  Administration
College of Pharmacy
University of Houston
Houston, Texas

Grace Earl, PharmD
Department of Pharmacy Practice
Philadelphia College of Pharmacy
University of the Sciences in Philadelphia
Philadelphia, Pennsylvania

Kenneth Euler, PhD
Department of Pharmacological and
  Pharmaceutical Sciences
College of Pharmacy
University of Houston
Houston, Texas

Dorothy J. Klimis-Zacas, PhD
Department of Food Science and
  Human Nutrition
University of Maine
Orono, Maine

Grace M. Kuo, PharmD
Department of Family and
  Community Medicine
Baylor College of Medicine
Houston, Texas

Jennifer Malinowski, PharmD
Department of Pharmacy Practice
Nesbitt School of Pharmacy
Wilkes University
Wilkes-Barre, Pennsylvania

Sarah J. Miller, PharmD
Department of Pharmacy Practice
School of Pharmacy and Allied
  Health Sciences
University of Montana
Missoula, Montana

Lisa Nicholson, PhD, RD
Department of Food Science and Nutrition
California Polytechnic University
San Luis Obispo, California

Kelly P. Popa, RD, CSP
Department of Nutrition
Children's Hospital of Michigan
Detroit, Michigan

**Carol J. Rollins, PharmD, RD, BCNSP,
CNSD**
Department of Pharmacy Practice
College of Pharmacy
University of Arizona
Tucson, Arizona

May B. Saba, PharmD, BCNSP
Department of Pharmaceutical Services
Children's Hospital of Michigan and
  Wayne State University
Detroit, Michigan

Lynn Simpson, PharmD
Department of Clinical Sciences and
  Administration
College of Pharmacy
University of Houston
Houston, Texas

Debra Skaar, PharmD
Department of Experimental and
  Clinical Pharmacology
College of Pharmacy
University of Minnesota
Minneapolis, Minnesota

Robert E.C. Wildman, PhD, RD, LD
Nutrition Program
School of Human Resources
University of Louisiana at Lafayette
Lafayette, Louisiana

Louis Williams, PhD
Department of Pharmacological and
    Pharmaceutical Sciences
College of Pharmacy
University of Houston
Houston, Texas

Ira Wolinsky, PhD
Department of Human Development
University of Houston
Houston, Texas

Robin M. Zavod, PhD
Department of Pharmaceutical
    Sciences
Chicago College of Pharmacy
Midwestern University
Downers Grove, Illinois

CHAPTER 1

ESSENTIALS OF NUTRITION

Robin M. Zavod

No matter how old we are, how much money we have, or which diseases we are at risk of developing, nutritional status is at the core of our health and well-being. Nutrition is made up of a complex system of components, including fluids, macronutrients, vitamins, and trace minerals.

The nutrients we consume contain building blocks that are essential for growth and maturation. To prevent deficiency and help people get the nutrients they need, it's important to have guidelines for each age bracket. In recent years, study after study has identified exciting benefits of maintaining good nutrition, such as reducing the risk of cancer, osteoporosis, and coronary artery disease.

Health care practitioners can be more effective in promoting good health if they are familiar with the biochemical roles and responsibilities of each nutritional component and know about the physiological effects of deficiencies. Equally important is understanding how the components interact with one another, how disease states alter nutritional status, and how prescription medications contribute to nutrient deficiency.

This chapter introduces the major components of the human diet including carbohydrates, proteins, lipids, vitamins, and minerals. It also describes the biochemical processes associated with energy production, digestion, absorption, and transport. A section on nutrition throughout the life cycle points out specific issues at each developmental stage.

CARBOHYDRATES, LIPIDS, AND PROTEINS

Carbohydrates

Carbohydrates, such as glucose and glycogen, are the primary form of readily available energy in the body. They typically provide 50% to 60% of our dietary-based energy sources and are found as monosaccharides, di- and oligosaccharides, as well as polysaccharides. Each of these sugar homo- or heteropolymers vary in taste, texture, rate of digestion, and the degree to which they are absorbed from the gastrointestinal tract.

Important Definitions

❏ **Adequate Intake (AI),** determined if there is not enough scientific evidence available to calculate an EAR (see below), is based on observed or experimentally determined estimates of what appears to be an adequate intake for each specific age and gender group.

❏ **Daily Reference Value (DRV):** Dietary references for macronutrients considered energy-producing sources, including fat, saturated fat, cholesterol, carbohydrate (including fiber), protein, fiber, sodium, and potassium. The DRVs are derived from the values listed below, which describe the relative percentage of each macronutrient found in a healthy diet.

Fat:	30% of calories/energy intake
	(only a third of which should come from saturated fat)
Carbohydrate:	55% to 60% of calories/energy intake
Protein:	10% to 15% of calories/energy intake
Fiber:	11.5 grams per 1000 calories

❏ **Daily Values (DV):** A dietary reference found on food labels that combines DRVs and DRIs for children above the age of 4 and adults. The food label indicates the percent of a daily value that each food serving provides based on a 2000-calorie diet. This type of information allows a consumer to determine if a food product is high in fiber or low in fat, for example. The macronutrient information on the label does not apply to children under age 4. (The Food and Drug Administration [FDA] has established only protein DVs for children 2 to 4 years old.) Foods for children under age 2 do not carry information about calories associated with fat, saturated fat, unsaturated fat, polyunsaturated fat, monounsaturated fat, and cholesterol because infants' fat intake should not be restricted. When babies do not take in enough energy—much of it in the form of fat—the result can be failure to thrive.

❏ **Dietary Reference Intakes (DRI):** Reference values that can be used to assess diets for healthy populations. DRIs refer to at least three types of reference values: Estimated Average Requirement, Recommended Dietary Allowance, and Tolerable Upper Intake Level. Since the last version of the U.S. Recommended Daily Allowances (U.S. RDA) was released in 1989, new research on nutrient requirements, food components, and good health led to the development of DRIs.

❏ **Estimated Average Requirement (EAR):** The intake level estimated to meet the requirement defined by a specified indicator for 50% of people in a specific age and gender group. At this level of intake, the remaining 50% of the group would not have its needs met.

- ❑ **Reference Daily Intake (RDI):** Guidelines for dietary intake of vitamins, minerals, and protein. "Reference Daily Intake" replaces the term "U.S. Recommended Daily Allowance (U.S. RDA)," which used to apply to the values determined by the FDA for use on food labels. The name was changed because people tended to confuse "U.S. RDAs" with the "RDAs" (Recommended Dietary Allowances) determined by the National Academy of Sciences for various population groups.
- ❑ **Recommended Dietary Allowance (RDA):** The daily level of dietary intake sufficient to meet the needs of nearly everyone in a specific age and gender group. This list of nutrient allowances, published by the Food and Nutrition Board of the National Academy of Sciences, provides benchmarks of nutritional adequacy in the United States. The RDA values are gradually being replaced by DRIs, which reflect increased knowledge of nutrients and their role in preventing disease.
- ❑ **Tolerable Upper Intake Level (UL):** The maximum level of daily intake at which a nutrient is unlikely to pose adverse health risks for most people in a specific group.
- ❑ **U.S. Recommended Daily Allowances (U.S. RDA):** Established by the FDA in 1973 as a reference for use in nutrition labeling, this term has been replaced by "Recommended Daily Intake (RDI)."

The metabolically important polysaccharides include amylose and amylopectin (plant starches) and glycogen (animal starch).[1] Amylose is a long unbranched polymer of glucose that is found in 15% to 20% of the starchy foods that we consume. Glycogen and amylopectin, on the other hand, are highly branched polymers of glucose. Plant starches are typically stored in cells with rigid cellulose walls. We consume several types of these starches, but to digest them we must cook the foods that contain them to free the carbohydrates from these cells. When someone consumes more carbohydrates than the body requires, the carbohydrates are stored in the form of glycogen. In an average adult about 150 g of glycogen is stored in muscle and 90 g is stored in the liver.

A number of polysaccharides consumed are of no nutritional consequence because they are not cleaved into smaller units that can be absorbed. β-Glycans are basic cellulose polymers comprised of both sugars and non-carbohydrate moieties.[1] These polymers, typically found in oats and barley, are classified as "soluble fiber" because of their branched shape and size. Hemicelluloses are cellulose polymers that contain only carbohydrates. They are typically found in bran and whole grains and are generally considered insoluble fibers.

Oligosaccharides are smaller than polysaccharides in molecular weight. They are typically water soluble and sweet in taste, but not all are cleaved by digestive enzymes. As a result, some of these polymers serve as a fermentable

Nutrient and Health Claims

Manufacturers must follow specific regulations set by the Food and Drug Administration (FDA) when making nutrient content claims about their products. Several of the more common claims are defined in Table 1-1.

The health claims that manufacturers can report are also carefully regulated by the FDA under the Nutrition Labeling and Education Act (NLEA). Health claims differ from nutrient claims because they link the nutrient contents of one or more food products to a disease or health-related condition. They are also different from "structure/function" claims that describe how a nutrient might affect the structure or function of the body in ways other than disease risk reduction. The FDA is not involved in assigning these structure/function claims but requires that the manufacturer ensures that the claim is true. The 10 relationships between nutrient content and the risk of a disease or health-related condition that are allowed by the FDA under the NLEA are found in Table 1-2. In this type of reporting, manufacturers are explicitly forbidden to quantify any given product's effectiveness in risk reduction and can only use the words "may" or "might" to describe these relationships.

food source for intestinal flora. When people consume excessive amounts of raffinose (beets) or strachyose (legumes and squash), the intestinal flora flourish and produce gas and a bloated feeling.

Sucrose (cane sugar: glucose + fructose), lactose (milk sugar: glucose + galactose) and maltose (malt sugar: 2 glucose units linked in an α-1,4 linkage rather than the normal β-1,4 linkage) are the edible disaccharides used for energy.[1] Sucrose is readily hydrolyzed to its monosaccharide components in the presence of mild acid or the enzyme invertase. Lactose is produced in the mammary glands of most mammals and is not as soluble or as sweet as the other disaccharides. Maltose is a byproduct of starch polymer hydrolysis and is sweeter than its parent polymer.

The phosphorylated form of glucose is the primary sugar involved in carbohydrate metabolism and energy production. In a fasting state, the blood's concentration of glucose ranges from 70 mg/dL to 115 mg/dL. Fasting levels below 60 mg/dL are characteristic of hypoglycemia and levels above 125 mg/dL are characteristic of hyperglycemia. Glucose (grape sugar), fructose (a component of sucrose), and galactose (a component of lactose) are the monosaccharides associated with energy production. Glucose, both as a monomer and as part of the disaccharide sucrose, makes up a sizeable fraction of the total content of most fruits and vegetables. Fructose is the sweetest of the monosaccharides. As fruit ripens, fructose content increases because sucrose is hydrolyzed to glucose and fructose. Honey comes from the sucrose found in the nectar of flowers. This sucrose is hydrolyzed by bee invertase to glucose and fructose.

TABLE 1-1 Regulations for Nutrient Claims

Claim	Requirements
Free (no, without, zero, trivial source of, dietarily insignificant source of)	Product contains no amount of or "physiologically inconsequential" amounts of one or more of: fat, saturated fat, cholesterol, sugars, sodium and calories (e.g., calorie free = < 5 calories/serving; sugar or fat free = < 0.5 g/serving).
Reduced	One serving of a nutritionally altered product that contains at least 25% less of a given nutrient or calories than a reference product contains. This term may not be used with a reference product that meets the characteristics for "low."
Less (fewer)	One serving of a nutritionally altered or nonaltered product that contains at least 25% less of a given nutrient or calories than a given reference product.
Light	Two definitions: 1. One serving of a nutritionally altered product that contains at least 1/3 fewer calories or 1/2 the fat of a given reference product. 2. Sodium content of a low-calorie, low-fat food is decreased by 50%.
Low (little, few, low source of, small amount of)	Products can be consumed frequently without surpassing dietary guidelines for one or more of: total fat, saturated fat, cholesterol, sodium, and calories (e.g., low fat = < 3 g/serving; low saturated fat = < 1 g/serving; low sodium = < 140 mg/serving; very low sodium = < 35 mg/serving; low cholesterol = < 20 mg/serving or < 2 g saturated fat/serving). "Very low" is a claim that only refers to sodium content.
Lean and Extra Lean	Used to describe the fat content of meat, poultry, seafood, and game products Lean = < 10 g fat or < 4.5 g saturated fat or < 95 mg cholesterol/serving Extra Lean = < 5 g fat or < 2 g saturated fat or < 95 mg cholesterol/serving
High (rich in, excellent source of)	One serving contains > 20% of DV of any given nutrient.
Good Source	One serving contains 10%–19% of DV of any given nutrient.
More	One serving contains 10% more of DV of any given nutrient than the reference product does.

Lipids

Lipids are divided into two functional categories: those that are oxidized to become an energy source for the body (e.g., triglycerides) and those that are structural components of membranes, are involved in transporting fat, or serve as the building blocks for hormones (e.g., phospholipids, sphingolipids, glycolipids, and sterols such as cholesterol). Phospholipids are typically associated with the lipid bilayer structure of cellular membranes, whereas sphingolipids are present in brain and nervous tissue. Some lipids are biosynthesized in the body, whereas others come from the diet.

Dietary Fats

Not all that long ago, slathering butter on toast, topping baked potatoes with butter and sour cream, and eating deep-fried foods was considered

TABLE 1-2   Regulations for Health Claims

Nutrient-Disease Relationship	Rules for Use
Calcium + osteoporosis	Product must contain > 20% of calcium DV, have calcium content equivalent to phosphorous, and contain a form of calcium that is readily absorbed. Calcium content must be classified as "high." Target population must be identified and the need for exercise and healthy diet must also be stated.
Dietary fat + cancer	Product must meet "low" fat requirements; fish and game products must meet "extra lean" requirements.
Dietary saturated fat + cholesterol + coronary heart disease (CHD)	Product must meet "low saturated fat," "low cholesterol," and "low fat" requirements. Fish and game products must meet "extra lean" requirements. Claims must use "low saturated fat and cholesterol" and "coronary heart disease" or "heart disease."
Fiber-containing grain products + cancer	Product must be or contain a grain product, fruits, or vegetables and must meet "low saturated fat" requirements, and without fortification must be a "good source" of dietary fiber. Claim need not specify type of fiber.
Fruits, vegetables, and grain products that contain fiber + risk of CHD	Product must be or contain a grain product, fruits, or vegetables and must meet "low saturated fat," "low cholesterol," and "low fat" requirements and without fortification must contain 0.6 g soluble fiber per serving. Soluble fiber content must be listed.
Sodium + hypertension	Product must meet "low sodium" requirements. Must use "sodium" and "high blood pressure" in claim.
Fruits and vegetables + cancer	Fruits and vegetables must meet "low fat" requirements and without fortification be a "good source" of at least one of the following: dietary fiber, vitamin A, vitamin C. Claims must refrain from specifying any type of fatty acids.
Folic acid + neural tube defects	Supplements must contain sufficient folate, and food products must be naturally "good sources" of folate, but should not provide > 100% DV for vitamin A (as retinol) or vitamin D.
Dietary sugar alcohols + dental caries	Products must meet requirements for "sugar free." Pertains to products containing xylitol, sorbitol, mannitol, isomalt, lactitol, hydrogenated starch hydrolysates, erythritol, or hydrogenated glucose syrups. Fermentable sugar-containing products must not lower the pH of the mouth < 5.7. Products must state that consumption of foods high in sugars/starches between meals promotes tooth decay.
Soluble fiber + CHD	Products must meet requirements of "low saturated fat," "low cholesterol," and "low fat." Must state that fiber must be part of diet low in saturated fat and cholesterol. Product must contain sufficient soluble fiber (whole oat-containing foods must contain at least 0.75 g soluble fiber/serving; psyllium seed husk-containing foods must contain at least 1.7 g soluble fiber/serving).

normal. Only after several clinical studies correlated high-fat diets with an increased risk of heart disease, and certain studies showed that not all fats are the culprit, did we start paying closer attention to foods' fat content. In 1994, fat represented on average 34% of a person's intake of energy-producing foods.[2] The National Cholesterol Education Program recommends that fat should be no more than 30% of the total intake.[3]

Fats, chemical substances that contain fatty acids, are a highly concentrated source of energy for the body. The three primary types of fatty acids are saturated, monounsaturated (MFA), and two types of polyunsaturated (PUFA): omega-3 and omega-6. Saturated fats are typically found in animal-based products, whereas monounsaturated and polyunsaturated fats are found in foods of plant origin. *Trans* fatty acids are the products of partial hydrogenation of polyunsaturated fats and are typically solids at room temperature. There is limited evidence that these fatty acids not only increase low-density lipoprotein (LDL) cholesterol, but also decrease high-density lipoprotein (HDL) cholesterol, which makes them more atherogenic than saturated fatty acids.[4] *Cis*-monounsaturated fatty acids (e.g., oleic acid found in olive and canola oils and in nuts) may be associated with a cardioprotective effect, but there is some evidence that the observed lowering of LDL cholesterol is offset by a decrease in HDL cholesterol.[5]

Polyunsaturated and monounsaturated fats are not believed to promote the formation of the fatty deposits that can clog arteries. In fact, some evidence suggests that diets containing these types of fats have the ability to decrease the level of LDL cholesterol. Unfortunately, polyunsaturated fats (e.g., safflower and corn oils) also decrease the levels of HDL cholesterol. On a more positive note, products high in monounsaturated fats (e.g., olive and canola oils) tend to decrease LDL cholesterol with no effect on HDL cholesterol. Saturated fats (e.g., palmitic, lauric, and myristic acids) are the major cholesterol-elevating fatty acids in our diet.[6] It is recommended that saturated fats be limited to 8%–10% of the total intake.[7]

Why is it that Eskimo people have a diet rich in fat and cholesterol, yet are generally free of heart disease? The fish they consume (e.g., salmon and mackerel) contain high levels of omega-3 fatty acids (e.g., linolenic acid, an essential fatty acid), which lower LDL cholesterol and triglyceride levels.[8] Omega-3 fatty acids are also found in sardines, herring, anchovies, bluefish, and canola and soybean oils. An added benefit associated with these fatty acids is a decreased risk of thrombosis and lower blood pressure.[9] These effects are purported to be from two fatty acids derived from linolenic acid. Omega-6 fatty acids (e.g., linoleic acid, an essential fatty acid that is a component of corn, soybean, and safflower oils) have been shown to decrease levels of LDL cholesterol, but they also decrease levels of HDL cholesterol.

Cholesterol

The liver is responsible for producing all the cholesterol that the body needs. Cholesterol is used in the formation of cell membranes as well as brain and nerve tissue. The steroid hormones and bile acids are also derived from cholesterol. Even though we produce sufficient quantities to meet our needs, we consume many animal products that serve as a reservoir for cholesterol.

Cholesterol is absorbed from the gut and transported in the bloodstream as a complex with molecules of proteins and fats, called lipoproteins. Cholesterol is transported by both LDLs (most common) and HDLs. High levels of LDLs in the bloodstream can lead to fatty plaque deposits on arteries and

Guidelines for Healthy Eating

The U.S. Department of Health and Human Services and the U.S. Department of Agriculture publish dietary guidelines for people above the age of 2. There are seven of these guidelines, designed to promote healthy eating habits and reflect current knowledge about diet's impact on healthy living:

❑ Eat a variety of foods to get the energy (calories), protein, vitamins, minerals, and fiber you need for good health.

❑ Maintain a healthy weight to reduce your chances of having high blood pressure, heart disease, a stroke, certain cancers, and the most common kind of diabetes.

❑ Choose a diet low in fat, saturated fat, and cholesterol to reduce your risk of heart disease and certain types of cancer. Because fat contains more than twice the calories of an equal amount of carbohydrates or protein, a diet low in fat can help you maintain a healthy weight.

❑ Choose a diet with plenty of vegetables, fruits, and grain products that provide needed vitamins, minerals, fiber, and complex carbohydrates. They are generally lower in fat.

❑ Use sugars only in moderation. A diet with lots of sugars has too many calories and too few nutrients for most people and can contribute to tooth decay.

❑ Use salt and other forms of sodium only in moderation to help reduce your risk of high blood pressure.

❑ If you drink alcoholic beverages, do so in moderation. Alcoholic beverages supply calories, but little or no nutrients. Drinking alcohol is also the cause of many health problems and accidents and can lead to addiction.

Source: US Departments of Agriculture and Health and Human Services. *Nutrition and Your Health: Dietary Guidelines for Americans.* 4th ed. Washington, DC: US Government Printing Office; 1995. Home and Garden Bulletin No. 232.

can predispose a person to have a heart attack.[10] The mechanism behind this process involves LDL oxidation, specifically the peroxidation of the polyunsaturated fatty acids within LDL particles. Since LDLs don't hang on to their cholesterol well and are subject to this type of oxidation, they are called the "bad cholesterol." High levels of HDLs, on the other hand, do not cause plaque formation, but rather carry cholesterol to the liver for metabolism or excretion. A decreased level of HDL cholesterol, considered the "good cholesterol," is correlated with an increased risk of heart disease.[11] When patients have their cholesterol measured, the value reported is the total cholesterol present (mg/dL). This number should be kept below 200 mg/dL. The individual components should be analyzed as well to be sure they are in accordance with recommendations, as outlined in Chapter 9, page 347.

The Food Pyramid Promotes a Healthy Diet

The Food Guide Pyramid developed by the U.S. Department of Agriculture (see Figure 1-1) attempts to apply to daily living the seven principles in the sidebar on page 8. The pyramid, an outline of what to eat each day, is designed to help people choose foods for healthy living but is not intended to be prescriptive. It suggests that foods high in fat or cholesterol be consumed in moderation.

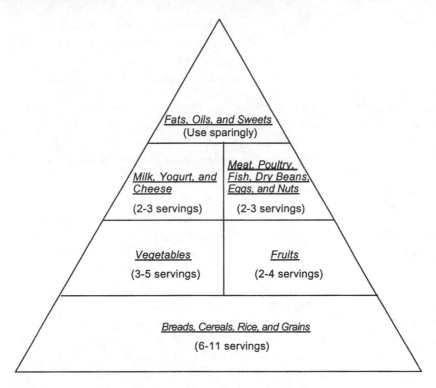

FIGURE 1-1   Food Guide Pyramid

Source: US Department of Agriculture. *The Food Guide Pyramid.* Hyattsville, Maryland: Human Nutrition Information Service; 1992. Home and Garden Bulletin No. 252.

People who want to maintain a healthy vegetarian diet can alter the pyramid as follows:

Milk, Yogurt and Cheeses	Dry Beans, Nuts, Seeds, Eggs, and Meat Substitutes
0-3 servings daily	2-3 servings daily
Examples:	Examples:
Milk, yogurt, cheese	Soymilk, tofu, or tempeh
If these products aren't eaten due to diet choice, then other calcium containing foods should be consumed.	Cooked dry beans or peas

Source: Vegetarian diets position of ADA. J Am Diet Assoc. 1997;97:1317-21.
Available at: http://www.eatright.org/adap1197.html. Accessed August 2, 2001.

Recommended Protein Consumption

The National Academy of Sciences recommends consuming the following number of grams of protein per day:

Adults: 0.8 g of mixed proteins/kg body weight/day.
Children older than 12 months: kg body weight × 2.2/day.
Pregnant women: 30 g/day more than is recommended for an adult, from the second month of pregnancy until the baby is born.
Lactating women: An additional 20 g/day above the recommendation for a nonpregnant adult, to allow for milk production.

Source: *Recommended Dietary Allowances*, 10th ed. Washington, DC: Food and Nutrition Board, National Research Council, National Academy of Sciences; National Academy Press: 1989:27.

Triglycerides

Fat can also be transported via triglycerides, otherwise known as triacylglycerols. Much of the body's store of fat is in the form of triglycerides, neutral compounds composed of glycerol that is esterified by three long chain fatty acids (typically different in length). The length of the fatty acids varies depending on the particular species. Triglycerides from cold-water creatures contain long, highly unsaturated fatty acids and are liquid even at low temperatures. Land-based animals have triglycerides composed of long, saturated fatty acids that are not readily subject to oxidation. As a result, this type of triglyceride is suitable for long-term storage, necessary in times of starvation or low food supply. Very-low-density lipoproteins (VLDLs) are responsible for transporting triglycerides in the body. People with high LDL cholesterol or low HDL cholesterol often have high triglyceride levels (> 200 mg/dL) and are at elevated risk for heart disease.[12]

Proteins

Whereas plants largely rely on carbohydrates for their structure, animals rely on proteins. Proteins are not only enzyme catalysts, but are also an integral part of cell structure and function. As catalysts, proteins control the rate of multiple biological processes and regulate hormone action. Proteins also have a role in transporting essential metabolites in the body.

Nine of these 20 amino acids (histidine, isoleucine, leucine, lysine, methionine, phenylalanine, threonine, tryptophan, and valine) either cannot be synthesized in the body or can't be synthesized at a sufficient rate to fully supply the body. These are classified as the essential amino acids. The rest are considered nonessential and can be biosynthesized independent of an individual's diet.

For several reasons, plant-based proteins are significantly more difficult to digest than animal-based proteins. Often encased in nondigestible cellulose, plant-based proteins are simply not available for digestion. In addition, some of these proteins are stored with enzymes that interfere with protein digestion. For example, soybeans contain trypsinase, an enzyme that inactivates trypsin, which is one of the major protein-digesting enzymes in the intestine. Food processing can also decrease the availability of certain amino acids. For vegetarians, it is important to prepare a mixture of food products to ensure that all the essential amino acids are consumed.

VITAMINS

Vitamin A

What do we really mean when we say "vitamin A"? This name generally describes compounds that have the same biological activity as retinol. Vitamin A is really a family of retinol isomers and oxidized derivatives of retinol, including retinol and retinoic acid.[13] The all-*trans* version, termed "synthetic vitamin A," has the greatest biological potency of all the vitamin A compounds and is 100% absorbed from the gastrointestinal (GI) tract.

Fifty percent of the vitamin A in the diet (whole milk, animal liver, eggs, and fortified foods including breakfast cereals, breads, and crackers) is in the form of esters of long chain fatty acids or retinol. The other 50% is found in the form of carotenoids (beta carotene), otherwise known as provitamin A. The carotenoids must undergo an enzyme-catalyzed cleavage reaction in the liver to become biologically active retinol. Several carotenoids (e.g., lycopene, lutein, and zeaxanthin) are not converted to retinol. Only one-third of carotenoids absorbed from the gastrointestinal tract actually become a biologically active form of vitamin A. Absorption of vitamin A is reduced in people who have abnormal fat digestion or absorption.[14]

Not all retinol isomers or derivatives have significant biological activity. The 11-*cis*-retinal is the only aldehyde derivative that reacts with the receptor protein opsin to form rhodopsin, the active element of visual pigment. This highly conjugated chromophore is able to absorb light from both the rods and cones of the retina, and through a series of chemical reactions, creates a neural signal that is sent to the brain. Patients often experience night blindness when the plasma concentration of retinal is less than 20 mcg/dL, which would cause the concentration within the retina to be low. In this scenario, opsin degrades, the rods deteriorate, and poor vision results.

Retinoic acid or vitamin A acid, the form of vitamin A found in all tissues except the retina, has several key biological functions. It is required for reproduction and embryonic development. A 25% increase in dose is recommended during pregnancy and lactation,[15] but caution is advised because vitamin A can accumulate to the point of being teratogenic.[16,17] Retinoic acid also inhibits proliferation of certain types of neoplastic cells and enhances immune function by mechanisms that are not entirely clear. There is limited evidence that vitamin A has a role in enhancing lymphocyte function.

Although a number of clinical studies, including the Carotene and Retinol Efficacy Trial, have examined beta carotene as a chemopreventative agent for lung cancer, these studies have been stopped due to an increased lung cancer incidence in the patient populations receiving beta carotene.[18]

The role of vitamin A in the growth and differentiation of epithelial cells is better understood and is especially important in mucous-secreting and keratinizing tissues. Vitamin A helps to maintain the linings of the eye as well as the lining of the respiratory, intestinal, and urinary tracts and plays an integral role in maintaining the integrity of the skin.[19] Retinoids are commonly dispensed to reverse changes that can occur in the epithelium of the respiratory tract, mammary gland, bladder, and skin. Although the synthetic retinoids (isotretinoin: Roaccutane or Accutane) are very effective treatments for acne, psoriasis, and other skin disorders, they should be reserved for severe cases because prolonged use can cause toxicity.[20]

The carotenoids have an additional purported biological role as antioxidants. They are not classical antioxidants in that they are not chain-breaking antioxidants and they do not promote peroxide decomposition.[21] It has been shown in the laboratory that carotenoids have some antioxidant effect in systems that contain singlet oxygen. However, they have not been documented as a consistently effective antioxidant in humans.[22,23] Patients who smoke are advised to steer clear of beta carotene supplementation (20 mg/day) due to the increased incidence of lung cancer observed in studies. Because the literature indicates that the carotenoids could theoretically play a role as an antioxidant but the clinical evidence does not bear this out, the Institute of Medicine has advised that the general public avoid beta carotene supplementation for the time being.[24]

Vitamin A deficiency rarely occurs in the United States and in Canada. Toddlers and preschool children have the highest risk of developing vitamin A deficiency, as well as children who live below the poverty level or who have inadequate health care. A subclinical form of vitamin A deficiency identified in the United States has been shown to cause an increased risk for respiratory and diarrheal infections.[19] Elsewhere in the world, vitamin A deficiency is a significant problem and is the leading cause of childhood blindness. In addition to blindness, the absence of vitamin A causes the skin to lose its normal secretory ability which can lead to skin irritation and infection.

Vitamin A, a fat-soluble vitamin, can cause hypervitaminosis A if consumed in excess, which may manifest itself as drying, hardening, and thickening of the skin, headache, fatigue, hair loss, loss of appetite, or liver damage. Among the many ways vitamin A may be listed on nutrition labels is 1 mcg of retinol, which is the same as 1 retinol equivalent (RE), which is equal to 33.3 vitamin A activity or 6 mcg beta carotene. Table 1-3 lists the Reference Daily Intakes for vitamin A and other key nutrients.

Vitamin D

Derived from cholesterol, vitamin D is biosynthesized in animals from its prohormone cholecalciferol (D_3), which is the product of solar ultraviolet

TABLE 1-3   Reference Daily Intakes (RDIs) or
Recommended Daily Allowances (RDAs)

Nutrient	Quantity
Vitamin A	800-1000 mcg retinol*
Vitamin D	200 IU
Vitamin E	8–10 mg d-α-tocopherol*
Vitamin C	60 mg
Thiamin (Vitamin B$_1$)	1.1–1.2 mg
Riboflavin (Vitamin B$_2$)	1.1–1.3 mg
Niacin (Vitamin B$_3$)	14–16 mg
Vitamin B$_6$	1.3–1.7 mg
Vitamin B$_{12}$	2.4 mcg
Folic Acid	0.4 mg
Pantothenic Acid	5 mg
Biotin	30 mcg
Calcium	1.0 g
Copper	2 mg
Iodine	150 mcg
Iron	18 mg
Magnesium	210–400 mg
Phosphorous	700 g
Zinc	12–15 mg

Note: These RDIs are based on 1989 revised Recommended
Dietary Allowances (RDAs).

* These vitamins are available in several forms.

irradiation of 7-dehydrocholesterol in the skin.[25,26] The biosynthesis of vitamin D is tightly regulated based on the serum concentrations of calcium, phosphate, parathyroid hormone, and active vitamin D.

Vitamin D must undergo activation via two oxidative metabolic transformations. The first oxidation to 25-hydroxycholecalciferol or 25(OH)D$_3$ (calcifediol: Calderol) occurs in the endoplasmic reticulum of the liver and is catalyzed by vitamin D 25-hydroxylase. This activation step is not influenced by plasma calcium concentrations. Calcifediol is the major circulating form (10 to 80 mcg/mL), as well as the primary storage form of vitamin D. In response to a hypocalcemic state and the secretion of parathyroid hormone, a second oxidation step is activated in the mitochondria of the kidney, catalyzed by vitamin D 1α-hydroxylase. The product of this reaction, 1,25-dihydroxycholecalciferol or 1,25(OH)$_2$D$_3$ (1,25-calcitriol, Rocaltrol, Calcijex) is the active form of vitamin D.

Classified as a hormone, vitamin D is responsible for maintaining plasma concentrations of both calcium and phosphate. Sterol-specific cytoplasmic receptor proteins (VDR; vitamin D receptor) mediate the biological action of vitamin D.[27] The active hormone is transported from the cytoplasm to the nucleus via the VDR and, as a result of the hormone's interaction with target genes, a variety of proteins are produced that stimulate the transport of calcium in each of the target tissues.[28] Active vitamin D works in concert with parathyroid hormone to enhance active intestinal absorption of calcium, to stimulate bone resorption, and to prohibit renal excretion of calcium.[27] If serum calcium or 1,25-calcitriol concentrations are elevated, then vitamin D 24-hydroxylase (in the renal mitochondria) is activated to oxidize $25(OH)D_3$ to inactive 24,25-dihydroxycholecalciferol, as well as to further oxidize active vitamin D to the inactive 1,24,25-trihydroxylated derivative.

Although vitamin D is endogenously biosynthesized, it is also consumed in the diet (milk, milk products, eggs, animal liver, fatty fish, fish oils, and fortified foods including milk and cereal). Older Americans (over age 50) are thought to have a greater risk of developing a deficiency either due to a decreased ability of the skin to convert the vitamin D precursor to its active form or a decrease in the ability of the kidney to activate vitamin D.[29] Also at risk for a vitamin D deficiency are people who are homebound, living in northern latitudes, or required to completely cover their bodies for religious reasons. A patient who suffers from fat malabsorption may also need vitamin D supplementation because it is fat soluble.

From a therapeutic perspective, vitamin D deficiency has been correlated with a greater incidence of hip fracture in postmenopausal women.[30] A limited association has been found between increased vitamin D intake and decreased bone loss in older women.[31] Vitamin D has shown promise as a protective agent against some cancers.[32] A correlation has been established between increased dairy intake and decreased colon cancer incidence, as well as between increased calcium and vitamin D intake and decreased colon cancer incidence.[33,34] Because vitamin D supplements have not been shown unequivocally to prevent cancer, vitamin D should not be considered a chemopreventative agent until appropriate clinical trials are conducted.

People are unlikely to ingest excessive amounts of dietary vitamin D unless they consume large volumes of cod liver oil. Hypervitaminosis D, characterized by nausea, vomiting, constipation, weight loss, poor appetite, and elevated plasma calcium levels, may result from over supplementation.[35] Elevated calcium levels can cause arrhythmias as well as calcinosis—deposits of calcium and phosphate in soft tissues.

Vitamin K

Vitamin K, originally named from $\underline{K}$oagulation Factor, is also a family of derivatives. There are plant-based derivatives (K_1, phylloquinone) and those that are synthesized by gram-positive bacteria located in the intestine (K_2, menaquinone, and K_3, menadione). Ninety percent of vitamin K stores in the liver (the major storage site) are menaquinones, suggesting that there is a more significant contribution via bacterial biosynthesis of this vitamin than that from the diet. Vitamin K is found in green leafy vegetables (major) and in dairy and pork products (minor). Dietary vitamin K is absorbed from the gastrointestinal tract with the help of bile salts and pancreatic juices.

Vitamin K plays an integral role in the coagulation cascade as a cofactor essential for activating several vitamin K-dependent coagulation factors (II, VII, IX, X). It also plays a role in calcium homeostasis via osteocalcin.

International Units

When multiple forms of the same vitamin have differing levels of biological activity (such as natural and synthetic versions), therapy is standardized according to units of activity rather than according to weight or volume. These units of activity are called international units (IU) because they adhere to an international agreement specifying the biological effect that is expected with a certain dose. For many substances there is no definite conversion between international units and units of weight or volume. Because consumers are used to seeing most vitamins and nutrients expressed in milligrams and micrograms on supplement labels, they are sometimes confused by the "IU" designation. Pharmacists should be prepared to explain it in clear layman's terms.

TABLE 1-4 Vitamin K Content in Multivitamins

Multivitamin Preparation	Micrograms Vitamin K
Centrum	25
Daily-Vite with Iron and Minerals	50
Decagen Tablets	25
Geritol Complete	25
Geritol Extend	80
Myadec	25
Preventamine Multivitamin Mineral Complex (w or w/o Iron)	60
Sigtab-M	25

Vitamin K deficiency is not a threat to adult health but can be a concern in newborns because they lack hepatic stores. Vitamin K prophylaxis was instituted in the 1950s to prevent the real, although small, risk of death or disability from vitamin K deficiency in the first 6 months of life via hemorrhagic disease.[36]

Therapeutically, vitamin K is used to reverse excessive anticoagulation, although the route of administration for optimal efficacy is under debate.[37] Patients should be aware that certain multivitamins (see Table 1-4) contain relatively large amounts of vitamin K, which could interfere with warfarin therapy should compliance with these vitamins vary.[38]

Vitamin E

Vitamin E, an essential fat-soluble vitamin, is the major antioxidant in cell membranes. It is found as a mixture of eight naturally occurring forms (tocopherols and tocotrienols), most with unique biological activities and potencies. The most common and active form of vitamin E, α-tocopherol, can be found in vegetable oils, mayonnaise, margarine, nuts, wheat germ, green leafy vegetables, and certain fortified foods (e.g., breakfast cereal).[39]

The actual amount consumed depends significantly on the method of processing, storing, and preparing of these foods. Most adults in North America do not get the recommended amount of vitamin E in their diet, as only 20% to 40% of what is ingested is actually absorbed. People on low-fat diets are even more likely to be deficient.

On labels for multivitamins and supplements, vitamin E content is expressed as vitamin E activity, such that 1 international unit (IU) is equivalent to 1 mg all-*rac*-α-tocopherol acetate, where all racemic α-tocopherol has 77% of the biological activity of RRR-α-tocopherol.[40]

Vitamin E has a variety of biological roles, including protecting several of the body's components against the damage caused by oxygen-based free radicals, stabilizing and maintaining the fluidity of membranes, and regulating protein synthesis and nucleic acid metabolism. Free radicals are formed as byproducts of normal metabolic processes as well as from the introduction of environmental chemicals into the body. Vitamin E can react with these oxygen-based radicals (e.g., singlet oxygen, hydroxyl and peroxyl radicals) and prevent the propagation reactions that normally perpetuate the formation of additional free radicals.[41] Ultimately, this translates into preventing peroxidation of polyunsaturated lipids found in the phospholipids of cellular membranes, as well as protecting proteins and nucleic acids from oxidative damage.[42] These protective processes are especially important in tissues subject to oxidative stress, including the nervous system, skeletal muscle, and red blood cells.[40]

Free radicals can interfere with numerous biological processes and may contribute to cardiovascular disease, certain cancers, and some central nervous system (CNS) disorders.[43] Vitamin E is thought to prevent or at least delay coronary heart disease by limiting the oxidation of LDL-cholesterol, a biomolecule that promotes coronary artery blockage.[44] Unfortunately, there is conflicting evidence that vitamin E has a beneficial effect in this disease state and it is clear that a patient must take supplements for at least 200 days to see even limited benefit. The HOPE study (Heart Outcomes Prevention Evaluation), which followed 10,000 people at high risk for stroke or heart attack, did not find significantly fewer cardiovascular incidents in the group taking vitamin E supplements as compared to the placebo group.[45] On the other hand, the CHAOS (Cambridge Heart Antioxidant Study) intervention trial showed a 77% decreased risk of heart attack in patients with coronary atherosclerosis who received 400 IU or 800 IU of vitamin E daily.[46]

Based on limited evidence, the chemoprotective effect of vitamin E has been extended to include cancer prevention. This stems from vitamin E's ability to prevent the formation of nitrosamines, highly reactive carcinogens formed in the stomach from nitrites in the diet, as well as its ability to enhance immune function.[47] Although several studies have tried to link vitamin E supplementation with a decreased incidence of cancer, the findings have been inconclusive. Limited evidence suggests that vitamin E supplementation helps decrease the incidence of prostate and breast cancers[48]; however, there is poor justification for using it as a cancer preventive agent.

Since vitamin E is absorbed along with fatty acids and triglycerides and this process requires some dietary fat and bile acids, it is not surprising that vitamin E deficiency could occur in people with fat malabsorption (Crohn's disease) or metabolism (β-lipoproteinemia) disorders and in premature infants with very low birthweight.[49,50] Deficiency of vitamin E is characterized by anemias and neurological problems due to poor nerve conduction. Vitamin E supplementation has not been correlated with any adverse health effects in the elderly, but long-term safety studies have not been completed.[51] Although vitamin E accumulates in adipose tissue, it is considered nontoxic. Because of its intrinsic anticoagulant activity there is some concern that elevated levels of vitamin E can lead to an increased risk of bleeding. Supplementation is contraindicated in patients with vitamin K deficiency and those receiving anticoagulant therapy.

Vitamin C

Vitamin C, or ascorbic acid, is one of the most widely used dietary supplements. It is a water-soluble vitamin that exists primarily in bodily fluids and not in fat tissue. Vitamin C is readily obtained in the diet in citrus fruits, cantaloupe, tomatoes, potatoes, leafy vegetables, papaya, sweet red peppers, and fortified foods. Foods high in vitamin C should not be soaked in water for extended periods and should be cooked in a microwave in the largest pieces possible to prevent loss of the vitamin via water. Properly stored frozen or canned foods can have a higher vitamin C content than fresh foods stored improperly in hot or humid conditions.[52]

Multivitamins and supplements are typically sold with vitamin C content measured in mg of ascorbic acid. Sodium ascorbate has the same biological activity as the free acid. Vitamin C is involved in diverse biological processes including biosynthesis of collagen, carnitine, steroid, and catecholamine; maintenance of capillary walls and blood vessels; and immune system function. Vitamin C is also required for efficient nonheme iron absorption. As an antioxidant, vitamin C is thought to interfere with the oxidation of LDL cholesterol and therefore reduce the risk of atherosclerosis. In addition, vitamin C interferes with cholesterol catabolism to bile acids and produces an increase in HDLs.[53,54] Clinical studies examining the influence of vitamin C levels on LDL and HDL levels have delivered mixed evidence about the influence vitamin C has on a given patient's lipid profile. There is even evidence against any direct correlation between vitamin C and lipid levels.

Because most of this vitamin is located in the serum, it is the primary scavenger of aqueous superoxide and hydroxyl free radicals. Alone, however, it is not a very effective chain-breaking antioxidant. The primary antioxidant role for vitamin C is in the recycling of nonreactive vitamin E radicals back to vitamin E. The resulting vitamin C radical is nontoxic and readily eliminated. Vitamin C interferes with the production of N-nitrosamines and other N-nitroso compounds from dietary nitrites and therefore prevents their reaction with endogenous amines. This is thought to be the chemical rationale for the reduced incidence of gastric cancers in people who consume foods high in vitamin C.[52]

Our immune systems normally use vitamin C in white blood cell production and in the proper functioning of T-cells and macrophages. Although it has been widely heralded as the "cure for the common cold," vitamin C has only been shown to decrease the severity and duration of a cold, with no effect on the incidence. [55,56]

Vitamin C deficiency results in scurvy, which is characterized by degeneration of the capillaries, bone, and connective tissues and results in bleeding gums, poor wound healing, and fatigue.[52] Chronic illness, prolonged fever, and infection increase the body's need for vitamin C. Limited supplementation may be warranted in smokers, in women taking oral contraceptives, corticosteroids, or aspirin, and in patients where decreased levels of vitamin C have been documented. Vitamin C toxicity, although limited, can manifest itself in the form of osmotic diarrhea, nephrolithiasis (formation of oxalate or cysteine stones), gout (formation of urate stones), or iron toxicity. In high concentrations, vitamin C can react with metals (e.g., Fe^{+3}) to become a powerful prooxidant and can then initiate or propagate the same free radical reactions that vitamin E prevents.[41,57] Because of these opposing roles as antioxidant and prooxidant, vitamin C supplementation is considered a dual-edged sword.

Thiamine (B₁)

The B vitamins are classified as "coenzymes" because they all are cofactors for enzymes that catalyze key biochemical reactions. Thiamine is a cofactor for several types of enzymes including pyruvate decarboxylase (catalyzes decarboxylation of α-keto acids) and the transketolase found in the hexose monophosphate shunt (allows for utilization of pentose sugars). As a result, thiamine has an essential role in converting carbohydrates into energy. Because patients on parenteral nutrition derive a substantial portion of their calories from dextrose, thiamine is important in this population.

Thiamine is found in the hull of rice grains, meats and fish, peas, beans, oatmeal, bran, and peanuts. Thiamine from the diet must undergo phosphorylation to the active form, thiamine pyrophosphate. Thiaminase, an enzyme that inactivates B_1, is found in blueberries and certain types of fish. Intestinal absorption of thiamine is limited to 8 to 15 mg/day. Only about 1 mg is degraded daily, so excessive supplementation is not necessary. This vitamin is readily excreted in the urine and has not been shown to cause toxicity when given orally.

Among people at risk for thiamine deficiency are alcoholics (decreased absorption and increased excretion of thiamine), those with a high carbohydrate intake, those suffering from malnutrition, heavy coffee drinkers, the chronically ill, and pregnant women. Early thiamine deficiency can manifest itself as anorexia, irritability, peripheral neuropathy, and tachycardia. Wet (cardiovascular-related) and dry (CNS- or encephalopathy-related) beriberi, as well as more extensive peripheral nervous system effects, are evidenced when thiamine deficiency is more advanced. Wet beriberi is characterized by an enlarged heart, peripheral edema, and high-output heart failure.[58] Psychological disturbances (depression, poor memory), Wernicke syndrome (acute vomiting, horizontal nystagmus, retinal hemorrhage, paralysis of eye muscles) and Korsakoff psychosis (retrograde and antigrade amnesia, confabulation) are all characteristic of dry beriberi. Treatment of an acute deficiency includes 50 to 100 mg intramuscularly or intravenously daily for a few days followed by 50 to 100 mg by mouth in divided doses until the patient is able to eat. If neurological deficits occur, then treatment includes 30 to 100 mg delivered parenterally until the patient is able to eat.[58]

Riboflavin (B$_2$)

Riboflavin is a constituent of two coenzymes, flavin adenine dinucleotide (FAD) and riboflavin phosphate (flavin mononucleotide [FMN]). Both are heavily involved in oxidative and reductive metabolic processes in the body as well as with the respiratory flavoproteins (e.g., xanthine oxidase).[58] Riboflavin is converted into these coenzymes via adenosine triphospate (ATP)-dependent phosphorylation reactions. It is considered an essential vitamin during times of growth (e.g., pregnancy, lactation, wound healing, surgery) and for maintaining vision, skin, nails, and hair.

Riboflavin is found in milk, eggs, meat, fish, organ meats, and whole grains and is synthesized by intestinal microorganisms as well. Riboflavin forms a complex with flavoproteins in the plasma and very little is stored. After riboflavin is converted to FMN by flavokinase, it is absorbed in the upper gastrointestinal tract. Patients taking riboflavin supplements should be alerted their urine may turn bright yellow.

Riboflavin deficiency alone is not common. When deficiency occurs, symptoms mimic those of other types of nutritional deficiencies, including sore throat, stomatitis, glossitis, corneal vascularization, genital dermatitis, magenta tongue, and photophobia.[58] Certain nutrients (e.g., iron, copper, zinc, saccharin, ascorbic acid) can form a complex with riboflavin and reduce its bioavailability. Several pharmacological agents prevent riboflavin from being converted to its active nucleotide form including chlorpromazine, imipramine, and amitryptyline. Excess consumption of ethanol can reduce the bioavailability from foods as well as hamper intestinal absorption. Breastfed babies may become deficient, as breast milk has low riboflavin content. Riboflavin deficiency can also result from boric acid poisoning because boric acid forms a complex with riboflavin and is then readily excreted.

Niacin (B$_3$)

Niacin, or nicotinic acid, is a component of four coenzymes: nicotinic mononucleotide (NMN), nicotinic acid mononucleotide (NAMN), nicotinamide adenine dinucleotide (NAD), and nicotinamide adenine dinucleotide phosphate

(NADP). NAD and NADP are involved as electron transfer agents in a wide variety of oxidative and reductive processes including lipid metabolism, tissue respiration, and glycogenolysis. Niacin also has a cholesterol-lowering effect in certain patient populations. Niacin is able to increase circulating HDL levels and decrease triglyceride, LDL, and total cholesterol levels. It is used therapeutically in treating hyperlipidemia (Types IV and V), but the flushing that can occur due to peripheral vasodilation when therapy is initiated can be difficult to manage.[59] (Note: 325 mg aspirin taken 30 to 60 minutes before a niacin dose or 81 mg chewable aspirin immediately beforehand may help decrease flushing.)

Niacin is synthesized from tryptophan in the body and is ingested in organ meats, lean meats, whole grains, legumes, and green vegetables. Nicotinic acid has been added to flour since 1939. Passive absorption of this vitamin occurs in the intestine, and low levels are stored in all tissues. Initially, niacin supplements should be taken in small doses to try minimizing flushing at the onset of therapy. The recommended doses of niacin for treating hypercholesterolemia range from 1.5 to 3 g/day, whereas doses of 3 g and higher are recommended for treating hypertriglyceridemia. Although this vitamin is available over the counter, patients who are using niacin to treat hypercholesterolemia or hypertriglyceridemia should be under a physician's care and should be carefully monitored.

Patients who are alcoholic, elderly, fad-dieters, cancer victims, or are recovering from an acute illness can become deficient in niacin. In addition, diets excessively high in corn are typically low in tryptophan, which can lead to deficiency. Cancer patients are predisposed to a niacin deficiency since tryptophan is shunted toward production of the neurotransmitter serotonin, which is ultimately used by the tumor. Patients with Hartnup's disease, in which intestinal and renal amino acid absorption is adversely affected, can have low levels of tryptophan and therefore be predisposed to niacin deficiency.[58]

The three D's of pellagra are the hallmarks of niacin deficiency: dermatitis, diarrhea, and dementia. First a sunburn-like skin rash appears; then symptoms progress to the gastrointestinal tract where the tongue becomes red and swollen, salivation increases, and diarrhea occurs. Mild CNS involvement is characterized by headache, dizziness, and poor memory. More severe cases of niacin deficiency can result in dementia and delusions. Typically this is observed in chronic alcoholics and in populations with protein calorie malnutrition.

Pyridoxine (B$_6$)

Vitamin B$_6$ is another water-soluble B vitamin with multiple forms: pyridoxine, pyridoxal, and pyridoxamine.[61] The active form of vitamin B$_6$ is pyridoxal-5'-phosphate. Vitamin B$_6$ is associated with more than 100 enzymatic processes involved in protein metabolism, red blood cell metabolism, and immune system function. It is a required cofactor in the conversion of the amino acid tryptophan to vitamin B$_3$ and is also involved in the synthesis of other vitamins. Vitamin B$_6$ is also a required cofactor in the biosynthesis or modification of several amino acids and in the biosynthesis of the neurotransmitters dopamine and serotonin.

Vitamin B_6 is involved in a wide variety of critical biological processes. Hemoglobin, found in red blood cells, carries oxygen to all tissues. Vitamin B_6 not only is involved in hemoglobin biosynthesis but it can also influence how much oxygen the hemoglobin can carry. White blood cells, the infection fighters, are produced by thymus, spleen, and lymph nodes. Vitamin B_6 maintains the integrity of these lymphoid organs and therefore has a direct effect on immune system integrity.[61] Glucose in the bloodstream is the fuel that cells consume in the presence of the hormone insulin. When blood glucose levels drop, vitamin B_6 is a coenzyme in reactions that convert carbohydrate stores into glucose for the body to use.[62]

Vitamin B_6 is found in meats, fortified cereals, lentils, nuts, and selected fruits and vegetables.[63] All phosphorylated forms of vitamin B_6 must undergo dephosphorylation by luminal phosphorylases prior to absorption, as only the unphosphorylated forms are absorbed via passive diffusion in the gut.[64]

Vitamin B_6 deficiency is relatively rare in the United States; its incidence is fairly easily correlated with poor diets. Populations at risk for vitamin B_6 deficiency include alcoholics, the elderly, asthmatic children taking theophylline, and people with a low-quality diet.[65] Symptoms, which range from glossitis and pellagra-like dermatitis to confusion, depression, and convulsions, sometimes can't be discerned from those of other nutritional deficiencies.[66] Vitamin B_6 deficiency can also stem from medication interactions. Isoniazid and penicillamine, for example, can interfere with vitamin B_6 activity. B_6 supplementation is used to treat seizures and acidosis in patients with an isoniazid overdose and a severe B_6 deficiency. The correlation between decreased vitamin B_6 levels and elevated concentrations of the naturally occurring amino acid homocysteine has been well documented, as has the correlation between high levels of homocysteine and an increased risk of heart disease and stroke.[67] Unfortunately there is no scientific evidence that B_6 supplementation will decrease levels of homocysteine and therefore decrease the risk of heart disease.

Controversies surround the question of whether vitamin B_6 is effective for treating several disease states. Although this vitamin is a coenzyme necessary for the biosynthesis of serotonin, B_6 supplementation has been found to have no therapeutic benefit in treating depression or migraine headaches, two conditions correlated with depressed levels of serotonin. As for the long-held belief that vitamin B_6 aids in treating carpal tunnel syndrome, there is no supporting clinical evidence. In fact, to prevent the documented neuropathy that has occurred in these patients due to excessive B_6 intake, a dosage of only 100 mg/day is recommended in carpal tunnel sufferers.[68] Another popular myth, which has failed to show scientific merit, is that vitamin B_6 diminishes the discomfort associated with premenstrual syndrome (PMS).[69]

It's important to note that because vitamin B_6 enhances the peripheral decarboxylation of L-dopa to dopamine, it decreases L-dopa's effectiveness in treating Parkinson's disease.

Cobalamin (B$_{12}$)

Vitamin B$_{12}$ (cyanocobalamin) is another B vitamin coenzyme essential for healthy nerve cells and red blood cells, and for DNA production. This vitamin is found in several forms including deoxyadenosylcobalamin, methylcobalamin, and hydroxycobalamin. Cyanocobalamin is used therapeutically and is found in the diet only in trace amounts. Each of these forms has a somewhat unique set of biological roles, whether as a cofactor for methyl transfer reactions or for radical generation.[70,71] The primary biological processes this vitamin affects are the breakdown of fatty acids, branched-chain amino acids, and cholesterol, as well as one-carbon metabolism.[71] As a cofactor in methyl transfer reactions, vitamin B$_{12}$ is essential for maintaining folate concentrations in the body and has an integral role in folate regeneration, transport, storage and metabolism. The enzymes associated with these processes are methionine synthase (methylcobalamine is the coenzyme for this enzyme) and methylmalonylCoA mutase (deoxyadenosylcobalamine is the coenzyme for this enzyme).[72]

Vitamin B$_{12}$ is found in several different protein sources, including fish, milk, eggs, meat, and poultry. Intestinal microorganisms also produce all forms of this vitamin. Although Vitamin B$_{12}$ is not present in any plant-based foods, an appropriate source for vegetarians is fortified cereals. When a protein source is ingested, the vitamin is scoured off of the protein on contact with gastric acid and pepsin. It is then bound to an intrinsic factor (IF) before it is absorbed. Absorption is hampered if the diet is high in foods containing vitamin C. Storage (typically a 3- to 6-year supply) is primarily in the liver.

People are unlikely to have a vitamin B$_{12}$ deficiency unless they have difficulty absorbing the vitamin or do not eat any animal or fortified products.[73] Conditions that might warrant supplementation include achlorhydria, thyrotoxicosis, hemorrhage, pregnancy, and malignancy. Characteristic symptoms of B$_{12}$ deficiency include weakness, loss of appetite, sore tongue or mouth, and neurological changes including numbness and/or tingling in the hands and/or feet.[74] Several of these signs can be confused with other nutritional deficiencies so a thorough evaluation is important.

Patients with pernicious anemia (which results from a failure of the gastric mucosa to secrete adequate intrinsic factor) will not absorb B$_{12}$ normally.[75] In this situation, B$_{12}$ must be administered monthly via intramuscular injection along with intrinsic factor. The slow absorption associated with intramuscular or subcutaneous administration is preferred, as large bolus doses lead to rapid excretion of the vitamin. Patients with a disorder of the stomach or small intestine (e.g., celiac disease, sprue) may develop enteritis and local inflammation, which can cause poor absorption of vitamin B$_{12}$.[76] Excess bacteria within the intestine can also decrease absorption. Pharmacological agents that can interfere with absorption include H$_2$ antagonists and proton pump inhibitors, which both decrease stomach acidity. Ethanol, bile acid sequestrants, aminoglycoside antibiotics, and the biguanide antihyperglycemic agents also interfere with B$_{12}$ absorption. Diseases that have an adverse effect on vitamin B absorption are listed in Table 1-5.

TABLE 1-5 Diseases with an Adverse Effect
on B Vitamin Absorption

Disease State	Nutrient Deficiency
Alcoholism	Folate, vitamin B_6
Atrophic gastritis	Vitamin B_6 and B_{12} (impaired absorption)
Liver dysfunction	Vitamin B_6
Gastric achloridia	Vitamin B_{12}

Because vitamin B_{12} is a cofactor in the regeneration of folic acid, B_{12} deficiency ultimately leads to folic acid deficiency. Supplementation with folic acid alone will correct the biochemical deficiency of folic acid, but it will not reverse the symptoms of B_{12} deficiency.[76]

Similar to vitamin B_6, vitamin B_{12} deficiency has been linked to elevated homocysteine levels and the corresponding increased risk of heart disease and stroke.[77] Unfortunately, there is no scientific evidence that B_{12} supplementation will decrease the levels of homocysteine and therefore decrease the risk of heart disease.

Folic Acid

Folic acid is another vitamin coenzyme used in the one-carbon transfer reactions in the biosynthesis of nucleic acids that make up DNA. It is also a coenzyme in the biosynthesis of several amino acids that are building blocks for proteins. Maintaining folic acid levels during times of rapid cell division and development, specifically during infancy and pregnancy, is absolutely essential. Folic acid is necessary for the formation of normal red blood cells and the prevention of anemia in both children and adults.[78]

Folic acid, in its inactive polyglutamate form, is found in several dietary sources including green vegetables, legumes, some citrus fruits, organ meats, and yeast. Since January 1998, flour and cereal grains have been fortified with folic acid to try to increase the levels of this vitamin in the general population.[79] Once folic acid is ingested, enzymes in the gut cleave off the polyglutamate linkage and the vitamin is converted to its active form (tetrahydrofolate) via two biosynthetic reductions. This activation requires the presence of vitamin C and NADPH (a reduced form of NADP, the active form of niacin). Tetrahydrofolate is then used in the biosynthesis of four different interchangeable one-carbon donors including N_5-methyl-tetrahydrofolate, the major storage form of activated folic acid. This one-carbon donor is stored in the liver, about 50% of which is in the form of a polyglutamate.

Folate deficiency is a potential problem in alcoholics, people on fad diets, pregnant women, and in people undergoing kidney dialysis or suffering from hemolytic anemia, cancer, or inflammatory disease.[80] Alcohol decreases folic acid absorption and enhances renal excretion. Several therapeutic agents, if taken simultaneously, impair folate absorption, including anticonvulsant agents, barbiturates, metformin, sulfasalazine, and triamterene.[81] Most signs and symptoms of folic acid deficiency are not overt, such as headaches, diarrhea, loss of appetite, weakness, and weight loss, and can be easily passed off as inconsequential. In women, the most prevalent problem associated with folate deficiency is the increased risk of birth defects, including neural tube defects and spontaneous abortion.[82,83] The Centers for Disease Control and Prevention recommends that all women of child-bearing age take folic acid supplements. Those not already taking folic acid supplements should start them at least 1 month before trying to become pregnant and should continue through the first trimester. A problem with this recommendation is that six out of nine prescription prenatal vitamin products do not deliver adequate amounts of folic acid.[84]

Anemia occurs when, for a variety of reasons—including folic acid deficiency—red blood cells are unable to carry sufficient oxygen. Although folic acid supplements can correct this type of anemia (often associated with reduced levels of vitamin B_{12}), they have no effect on the underlying B_{12} deficiency.

The correlation between decreased folic acid levels and elevated concentrations of homocysteine has been well documented, as has the correlation between high levels of homocysteine and an increased risk of heart disease and stroke.[85] Unfortunately, scientific evidence conflicts as to whether folic acid supplementation, which decreases the levels of homocysteine, affects the risk of heart disease. There is limited evidence suggesting that the risk of breast, colon, and pancreatic cancer is greater in people whose diet is deficient in folic acid.[86,87] Even though diet and disease cannot be directly correlated, it stands to reason that low levels of folic acid could result in DNA damage, ineffective DNA repair, or DNA that functions inappropriately, any of which could predispose a person to develop a cancerous condition.[88]

Cancer chemotherapy regimens tend to be toxic when they include methotrexate, an agent that inhibits the recycling of tetrahydrofolate-based one-carbon donors and therefore prevents the biosynthesis of DNA building blocks. In essence, methotrexate stunts tumor growth by depriving cancer cells of DNA. Unfortunately, methotrexate is not selective for cancer cells and therefore has an adverse effect on normal cells, as well. It has been suggested that folic acid supplementation may be able to control the side effects of methotrexate without decreasing its effectiveness.[88,89] Patients receiving methotrexate to treat noncancerous disease states—rheumatoid arthritis, lupus, psoriasis, asthma, and inflammatory bowel disease—often exhibit signs of folate deficiency and therefore are good candidates for folic acid supplementation.[90,91]

Pantothenic Acid

The active form of pantothenic acid, 4′-phosphopantetheine, is a precursor for coenzyme A, as well as a component of acyl carrier protein. Coenzyme A participates in biochemical processes that involve two-carbon (acetyl or acyl) transfers. Such processes include the oxidative metabolism of carbohydrates; gluconeogenesis; degradation of fatty acids; biosynthesis of sterols, steroid hormones, and porphyrins; and the post-translational modification of proteins and their corresponding building blocks.[58] The biosynthesis of fatty acids is an opposing biochemical role associated with the biological activity of acyl carrier protein.

Pantothenic acid, found in virtually every food, is especially abundant in organ meats. Since it is often found as a complex with proteins, the proteins must be hydrolyzed to allow release of this vitamin in its 4′-phosphopantetheine form. After dephosphorylation and conversion to panthothenic acid, it is absorbed in the intestine by both passive diffusion and active transport.[58] In the bloodstream it is taken up by erythrocytes, its primary means of transport. Pantothenic acid is taken into target tissues by active transport and is transformed into its coenzyme A form.

Although considered an essential nutrient, the amount of pantothenic acid that should be consumed daily has not been determined. For most adults 4 to 7 mg/day is considered reasonable, but in certain patient populations the amount consumed should be proportional to caloric intake.[58] Deficiency of this vitamin, which is very rare, causes impaired lipid biosynthesis and energy production.

Claims that pantothenic acid should be part of an "anti-stress" vitamin formulation or part of a supplement to prevent gray hair are not supported by scientific evidence.[92]

Biotin

Biotin, a natural component of egg yolks, exists in three forms: biocytin and the D- and L-sulfoxides. As a part of the B vitamin complex, this vitamin is a cofactor for enzymes that carboxylate four specific substrates involved in carbohydrate and fat metabolism: pyruvate, acetyl coenzyme A (CoA), propionyl CoA, and α-methylcrotonyl CoA.

Primarily produced by intestinal microorganisms, biotin is also found in organ meats, eggs, milk, and fish. Biotin deficiency is rare. Since it is associated with dietary protein in the form of biocytin, the protein must be hydrolyzed for biotin to be released. Intestinal biotinidase then converts biocytin into free biotin for absorption. Dietary biotin is absorbed in the small intestine, whereas that generated by intestinal flora is absorbed in the colon. Once in the bloodstream, biotin occurs predominantly in its free form. Biotin is stored in the liver.

Signs of a biotin deficiency include dermatitis, glossitis, muscle pain, anorexia, and electrocardiogram changes.[58] Patients with chronic inflammatory bowel disease may be predisposed to deficiency because of poor vitamin absorption. Those who need chronic parenteral nutrition should be given a vitamin formulation that contains biotin.

MINERALS

Calcium

Calcium is at the root of the statement heard from nearly every mother, "Drink your milk so you can have strong bones and teeth." This mineral not

Getting Enough Calcium

Following are the recommended amounts of elemental calcium consumption per day.

Newborns (0–6 months)	210 mg
Infants (6–12 months)	270 mg
Toddlers (1–3 years)	500 mg
Children (4–8 years)	800 mg
Teenagers (9–18 years)	1300 mg
Adults (19–50)	1200–1500 mg
Postmenopausal women not taking HRT*	up to 1500 mg
Postmenopausal women taking HRT*	1000 mg

* Hormone replacement therapy

Source: Reference 95.

only helps to build and maintain healthy teeth and bones, but it also helps maintain cardiovascular health (blood pressure, heartbeat, coagulation), control nerve transmission, regulate muscle growth and contraction, maintain cell membranes, and activate certain enzymes, such as lipase. Vitamin D is essential for facilitating calcium absorption. Approximately 1 kg of calcium—99% of which is found in the bone—is found in an average 70 kg adult.

The principal calcium salt in the crystalline lattice of teeth and bones is $Ca_{10}(PO_4)_6(OH)_2$. Plasma calcium levels are maintained by the interconnection of three hormones: parathyroid hormone, calcitonin, and vitamin D. As serum calcium concentrations fluctuate so do the plasma levels of these hormones. The normal plasma concentration of calcium is about 4.5 to 5.7 mEq/L, 50% of which is protein bound. The remainder of the calcium (46%) either forms a complex with the corresponding counter ions (e.g., chloride, carbonate) or exists in its free ionized form (4%). It is only the ionized form of calcium that is tightly hormonally regulated (plasma concentration varies less than 5%–10%).[93]

Consuming the right amount of calcium in childhood, adolescence, and early adulthood increases peak bone mineral density and may reduce the overall risk of osteoporosis. For people at low risk for developing osteoporosis who have adequate bone mineral density, consuming the recommended amounts of calcium is typically sufficient to prevent bone loss [94,95] (see sidebar above). Eating a well-balanced diet is often enough to meet a person's needs. Calcium is found in dairy products, tofu, beans, broccoli, green leafy vegetables, in the bones of sardines and salmon, and in several types of fortified foods.

Not all dietary calcium is absorbed equally. Calcium is poorly absorbed from foods high in oxalates, phytates, or phosphates, but foods high in lysine, arginine, vitamin D, and lactose enhance absorption. Patients who eat high-salt or high-protein diets excrete calcium more readily. Smoking and excess

TABLE 1-6 Percent of Elemental Calcium Content in Various Salts

Calcium Salt	% Calcium	mg elemental Ca per tablet
Calcium carbonate	40	
Tums (500 mg chewable)		200
Titrilac (1 g/5 mL suspension)		400 mg/5 mL
Alka-Mints (850 mg chewable)		340
Os-Cal 500 (1250 mg tablets)		500
Caltrate 600 (tablets)		600
Tricalcium phosphate	39	
Calcium chloride	27	
Tribasic calcium phosphate	23	
Posture (1565.2 mg tablets)		600
Calcium citrate	21	
Citrical (950 mg tablets)		200
Citrical Liquitab (2376 mg effervescent tabs)		500
Calcium lactate	13	
Generics (325 mg tablets)		42
Generics (650 mg tablets)		84
Calcium gluconate	9	
Neo-Calglucon (1.8 g/5 mL syrup)		115 mg/mL

caffeine consumption have been shown to decrease the absorption of calcium from both dietary sources and supplements.

There is some evidence that calcium supplements can reduce mild to moderate PMS symptoms.[96] In addition, epidemiological evidence correlates high calcium intake with a reduced risk of colorectal cancer.[97]

The actual amount of elemental calcium in the calcium salts available varies considerably. No one particular salt has been identified as an exceptional source of elemental calcium (see Table 1-6).[98,99] Because absorption of calcium from the gastrointestinal tract improves under acidic conditions (normally 25% to 40% of what was consumed is absorbed), medications that change the acidic environment of the stomach such as H_2 antagonists and proton pump inhibitors have an adverse effect on calcium absorption.[98,100] Total daily doses of elemental calcium over 500 mg should be spaced out over the day to improve absorption.[101] The more water-soluble salts, such as citrate, lactate, and gluconate, are more easily absorbed and less dependent on an acidic environment, which makes them appropriate alternatives for patients who produce low levels of acid. Although calcium citrate is the second most common supplement, it delivers a relatively low amount of elemental calcium by weight and should be taken with an empty stomach to improve absorption. Although calcium carbonate is poorly soluble, it is inexpensive and is the most concentrated calcium supplement, requiring that patients take only a few tablets per day with food or beverages such as citrus juice.

Patients should avoid calcium from supplements that include dolomite, oyster shell, and bone meal because they often contain unacceptable levels of lead or arsenic. In fact, calcium inhibits lead absorption, protecting teeth and bones from this toxic metal, so there is no reason to increase lead exposure via calcium supplements when there are alternatives.

Among complaints from patients starting on calcium supplements are bloating, gas, and constipation. (Evidence suggests that gastrointestinal tolerability for the citrate salt is poorer than for the carbonate salt.[101]) These side effects are normally temporary, subsiding as the body becomes accustomed to calcium supplementation. Taking supplements in divided doses throughout the day and gradually increasing from low to higher doses can help prevent or diminish these problems. Patients should be sure to drink plenty of water to reduce constipation.

Calcium absorption can inhibit the absorption of other minerals, such as iron. Calcium citrate, but not carbonate, enhances the absorption of aluminum and its deposition into tissues.[102] Too much zinc can hamper the absorption of calcium and vice versa. Pharmacological interactions with calcium must also be considered. Chronic use of corticosteroids, which inhibit calcium absorption, has been positively correlated with an increased incidence of bone fracture and osteoporosis. Although furosemide decreases serum calcium concentrations, the thiazide diuretics do the opposite. In addition, anticonvulsants, oral contraceptives, and cholestyramine have an adverse effect on calcium absorption.

Because bone is such a rich source of calcium, calcium deficiency is relatively uncommon. Malabsorption syndromes, hypoparathyroidism, vitamin D deficiency, impaired vitamin D activation, and long-term anticonvulsant therapy are a few conditions that can cause hypocalcemia. Calcium deficiency can cause muscle cramps, heart palpitations, brittle nails, hypertension, rheumatoid arthritis, tooth decay, convulsions, and limited neuropathy. Because increased protein intake increases the body's calcium requirement, people on high protein diets should consider calcium supplementation.

Iron

Iron, which is responsible for oxygenating red blood cells, is integral to the production of hemoglobin and the function of several enzymes. Iron is also involved in immune function and energy production. Functional iron, one of the two major forms, is found in hemoglobin, myoglobin and other heme enzymes, whereas stored iron is located primarily in hemoglobin, which contains 85% of the body's iron store.[103]

Non-heme iron is consumed from vegetables and whole grains. The heme form is found in meat, organ meats, and poultry.[104,105] Although the body absorbs only 10% of what is consumed, the heme form is absorbed most easily, especially in the presence of vitamin C, which increases absorption as much as 30%, and the B vitamins. Non-heme iron is best absorbed in the presence of meat and vitamin C, but in general is very poorly absorbed.[106]

Dietary iron is typically in the form of ferric hydroxide, which is solubilized and converted to ferric trichloride in the presence of gastric acid. Then, in the presence of vitamin C, it is converted to ferrous dichloride, which is more easily absorbed. Gastric acid as well as food components that form iron chelates facilitate iron absorption. The ferrous form of iron chelates with ascorbic acid and with sugars and amino acids in the diet to form low-molecular-weight complexes that are easily solubilized and absorbed. The ferric form of iron, found in the plasma, binds to apoferritin and becomes ferritin or hemosiderin, two storage forms of iron located in the intestinal mucosa, liver, spleen, and bone marrow.

Iron loss occurs at the rate of 0.5 to 1 mg/day, and loss is even higher during menstruation (15 to 20 mg/cycle), lactation (0.5 to 1.0 mg/day), and pregnancy (500 mg per term).[107] Disease states that limit iron absorption include peptic ulcers, diverticulitis, GI parasites, and ulcerative colitis. Pharmacological agents that interfere with iron absorption include salicylates, corticosteroids, and anti-inflammatory agents, all of which are GI irritants.[17] Antacids increase the pH of the stomach and some formulations chelate directly with iron to form insoluble precipitates. Fluoroquinolones and tetracyclines form a complex with this multivalent ion, causing these antibiotics to precipitate and rendering both the iron and the antibiotic completely ineffective. Excessive supplementation with zinc or vitamin E can also decrease iron absorption. Iron deficiency can be manifested in a variety of ways including split or spoon-shaped nails, fatigue, sore tongue, anemia, or headache.[108]

Iron supplements are available in either the ferrous or ferric form. Ferrous salts (succinate, lactate, fumarate, sulfate, glutamate, and gluconate) are absorbed three times better than the ferric salts (citrate, tartrate, pyrophosphate).[109] The percentage of elemental iron delivered varies with the type of iron salt: ferrous sulfate delivers 20%, ferrous gluconate 12% and ferrous fumarate 33%. Enteric coated tablets or delayed-release tablets delay absorption until they are past the duodenum, where iron absorption is poor. These formulations may be beneficial for people who experience gastric upset even if they are taking iron supplements that are considered easy on the stomach (fumarate and gluconate salts).[110]

Iron toxicity can occur in alcoholics (alcohol increases iron absorption) and in children who mistake the brown tablets for candy. Signs of toxicity include weak pulse, increased heart rate, drowsiness, and pale or clammy skin. A bluish discoloration of the fingernail beds, lips, and palms may accompany these signs. Desferal, an iron chelator, is used along with gastric lavage and sodium bicarbonate as a remedy for iron poisoning. Hemochromatosis, a rare disorder caused by a buildup of iron, causes bronze skin pigmentation, cirrhosis, diabetes, and heart disorders.[111]

Magnesium

Magnesium is required for normal bone formation, proper function of the CNS, protein biosynthesis, and carbohydrate metabolism. It is also a cofactor for several enzymes involved in metabolizing food components, regulating mitochondrial oxidative metabolism, and helping certain ion channels (including calcium channels) function properly.[112,113] Magnesium has an important role in nucleic acid biochemistry and in forming the second-messenger cyclic adenosine monophosphate (cAMP).[114] Classified as an electrolyte, magnesium interacts with a variety of hormones, second messengers, and growth factors as well as their respective receptors and signaling pathways.[112] The bone and intracellular compartment are the repositories of 99% of magnesium stored in the body, but only the 1% in the vascular space has any biological effect. However, two thirds of this 1% is bound to plasma proteins and is not biologically available.

Among the many foods that contain magnesium are whole grains, nuts, chocolate, peanuts, soybeans, legumes, green leafy vegetables, dairy products, and meats.[115] Only 30% of magnesium consumed in the diet is absorbed, and absorption is further decreased by high-fat meals, foods high in oxalic acid (e.g., spinach) and high levels of calcium, vitamin D, or protein. The amount of magnesium absorbed is inversely proportional to the amount consumed and excretion is primarily via the kidneys.[113] Magnesium supplements come in the form of oxide, gluconate, carbonate, and chloride salts and as amino acid complexes.

It has been proposed that magnesium supplements can help prevent depression, dizziness, heart disease, and high blood pressure. Along with vitamin B_6, magnesium is also thought to help dissolve calcium phosphate stones. There is evidence that treatment with magnesium after an acute myocardial infarction has a cardioprotective effect.[116]

Magnesium toxicity is a distinct possibility in the elderly, who tend to abuse magnesium-containing antacids and laxatives to relieve constipation, heartburn, or indigestion. Unfortunately, because symptoms of magnesium poisoning (e.g., irregular heartbeat, confusion, nausea, diarrhea, muscle weakness) can be easily mistaken for signs of stroke, they may go untreated. Patients on kidney dialysis are at risk for hypermagnesmia because their kidneys can no longer remove excess magnesium from the body.

Hypomagnesmia is characterized by anorexia, tremor, irritability, nervousness, confusion, seizures, and hyperactive reflexes.[117] Patients with alcoholism, diabetes, chronic diarrhea, chronic malabsorption, and renal disease may be at risk for magnesium deficiency.[118] Some concern has been raised that athletes on a calorie-restricted diet and those who engage in regular strenuous exercise may not consume enough magnesium to offset the loss of this electrolyte.[119] Loop diuretics and digitalis glycosides decrease tubular reabsorption of magnesium and can predispose patients to deficiency. Cisplatin, gentamicin, amphotericin, and cyclosporine cause increased kidney excretion of magnesium.[120]

Limited evidence suggests that giving magnesium supplements to patients with hypertension may help reduce blood pressure.[121] Results from the DASH (Dietary Approaches to Stop Hypertension) study indicate that diets high in magnesium, potassium, and calcium and low in fat and sodium could lower blood pressure.[122] The results from national surveys that evaluated the effect of nutritional factors on the risk of developing several disease states indicate that higher magnesium intake is correlated with decreased risk of coronary heart disease and stroke.[123,124]

Phosphorous

Phosphorous, along with calcium and magnesium, is an essential matrix component of teeth and bones. Kidney function, efficient use of vitamins, heart muscle contraction, and cell growth are additional biological processes linked to phosphorous. Serum calcium concentrations, as well as calcitonin and parathyroid hormone levels, maintain serum levels of phosphorous via phosphate concentrations.

Phosphorous is found in most foods, including carbonated beverages, asparagus, corn, dairy products, eggs, legumes, meats, poultry, and whole grains. Junk food diets deliver excessive amounts of phosphorous and can ultimately decrease the amount of calcium absorbed.

Hypophosphatemia is associated with metabolic problems that hamper CNS function, myocardial efficiency, and respiratory function. Whether patients should take supplements using sodium or potassium salts depends on their individual serum phosphorous levels.[125]

Potassium

Maintaining potassium levels is important for a healthy nervous system, a regular heart rhythm, and stable blood pressure. In conjunction with sodium, potassium also controls the water balance in the body.

Dietary sources of potassium include dairy foods, bananas, citrus fruits, cantaloupe, fish, legumes, meat, poultry, baked potato, and whole grains. Over-the-counter (OTC) potassium supplements do not deliver the same amount of elemental potassium as prescription supplements. For example, 250 mg of K-Dur (potassium chloride) delivers 130 mg of elemental potassium, whereas 250 mg of potassium gluconate in an OTC supplement delivers only 41.5 mg elemental potassium. Serum concentrations of potassium are altered by diuretics (loop and thiazide), severe burns, laxatives, severe diarrhea, and kidney disorders.

Results from the DASH study indicate that diets high in magnesium, potassium, and calcium and low in fat and sodium may lower blood pressures.[122] This study recommends a daily dose of 40-150 mEq of potassium.

Selenium

Selenium, a trace element, is classified as an essential antioxidant. Along with vitamin E and glutathione peroxidase, selenium protects the immune system from damage by oxygen-based free radicals. Selenium is an integral component of the immune system and is necessary for a functioning thyroid gland.[126] It also works in concert with vitamin E to maintain efficient heart function and is involved in producing antibodies.

The selenium content of meat and grains is determined largely by soil content, which can vary regionally.[127] Selenium is also found in nuts, chicken, dairy products, fish, garlic, organ meats, breads, and vegetables.

Selenium deficiency causes Keshan disease, characterized by an enlarged heart and poor cardiac function.[128] This disease is largely limited to areas within China where selenium content in the soil is poor. Also at risk for selenium deficiency are patients who rely exclusively on total parenteral nutrition (TPN)[129] or who suffer from intestinal disorders that cause malabsorption, such as Crohn's disease.

Limited evidence suggests that lower mortality rates from cancer (lung, colorectal, prostate) occur in populations with higher serum selenium levels.[130,131] The Supplementation en Vitamines et Mineraux Antixydants (SU.VI.MAX) Study is a prevention trial underway in France to help solidify the correlation between selenium status and development of cancer and other chronic diseases.[132] Right now, there is insufficient evidence about the link between selenium status and coronary artery disease or arthritis.[133] The ability of selenium to prevent damage from free radicals seems to relate to its ability to prevent glucose intolerance and complications associated with diabetes mellitus.[134] Selenium toxicity causes selenosis, a condition characterized by GI upset, hair loss, blotchy spots on nails, and nerve damage.[135]

Chromium

This trace element, intimately involved in glucose metabolism, maintains stable blood glucose levels by helping the body use insulin efficiently. Chromium also has a role in cholesterol, fat, and protein biosynthesis.

The average American diet is deficient because of poor chromium content in the soil and water. Chromium is commonly found in wine, beer, brown rice, sugar, cheese, meat, brewer's yeast, and whole grains. Canned foods may contain significant chromium content due to the mineral leaching from the can.[134] Only 1% to 2% of the chromium ingested is absorbed by the small intestine. Chromium can form complexes with several dietary components including amino acids, oxalates, phylates, and ascorbic acid. Depending on the complex formed, chromium absorption is either enhanced or diminished. Multivitamins that contain zinc and/or iron at pharmacologically relevant levels interfere with chromium absorption.[136] Chromium supplements are typically in the form of chloride picinolate or polynicotinate salts, all of which have excellent bioavailability.

Patients whose diabetes is poorly controlled excrete chromium, magnesium, and zinc at elevated rates.[134] Chromium deficiency is typically associated with glucose intolerance, hyperinsulinemia, and decreased receptor binding by insulin. Chromium is involved in phosphorylation reactions catalyzed by the β-subunits' tyrosine kinase activity,[137] which occur after insulin binds to its receptor. These reactions create the cellular signals necessary for proper glucose uptake by cells. Chromium also inhibits the enzyme tyrosine phosphatase, which stops the insulin receptor's response to the binding of insulin. By these two mechanisms, chromium plays a pivotal role in the body's use of glucose. Clinical studies to examine the effectiveness of chromium (400 mcg) in managing type II diabetes have shown improvement in fasting blood glucose values after 16 to 32 weeks of supplementation, as well as a decrease in glycosylated hemoglobin values after 4 months.[138,139]

Zinc

Zinc is a required component of hundreds of enzymes, including several metalloproteases (e.g. angiotensin converting enzyme). Found in all tissues, fluids, and organs (total body content is 1.4 to 2.3 g[134]), zinc has a role in protein and collagen biosynthesis and is important for the growth and function of the prostate gland and reproductive organs. This mineral also protects the liver from a variety of reactive chemicals and has a role in taste and smell perception. Insulin is stored as an inactive complex with zinc.

Sources of zinc include fish, legumes, meat, eggs, oysters, organ meats, soybeans, seeds, poultry, and whole grains. Zinc absorption is adversely affected by high-fiber foods and phytates.[140] The balance necessary for health benefit is tenuous, because ingesting more than 100 mg per day can depress the immune system. This problem is especially difficult to manage now that zinc gluconate has been purported to ward off colds.[141] Evidence for this claim has been questioned and it is recommended that products containing this ingredient be used on an acute basis only.

Zinc absorption occurs in the duodenum, and only about 30% of zinc that has been consumed is absorbed.[134] Zinc levels in the body can be depleted by chronic diarrhea, kidney disease, liver cirrhosis, diabetes, and high-fiber diets. Because zinc is primarily obtained from animal sources, vegetarians may be at risk for deficiency unless they eat a variety of legumes and nuts.[142] Excessive calcium consumption (more than 1400 mg/day) interferes with zinc absorption, as do iron and copper supplements. People with a zinc deficiency may have impaired wound healing, appetite loss, undesirable skin changes, and poor immune system function.[143]

Consuming too much zinc can lead to anemias, copper deficiency, and decreased levels of HDL cholesterol. Zinc supplements are used to treat the hypercuperemia associated with Wilson's disease.[144] The emetic effect of zinc in high doses limits the toxicity associated with accidental poisoning or excessive ingestion. Signs of toxicity include dehydration, poor muscle coordination, dizziness, and abdominal pain.[145]

DIGESTION, ABSORPTION, AND TRANSPORT OF NUTRIENTS

Carbohydrates

The three primary macronutrients are carbohydrates, lipids, and proteins, which are mostly ingested in complex forms not easily absorbed without extensive modification. This process starts in the mouth, where the starches (amylose and amylopectin) and saccharides (mono- and di-) are cleaved by salivary amylase into smaller saccharide units. The stomach's strong acidity quenches this enzymatic activity and provides an environment for starch hydrolysis. Once the starches and other carbohydrates reach the small intestine, α-amylase takes over. This enzyme, a pancreatic juice secreted in response to the hormones secretin and cholecystokinin-pancreozymin, breaks

TABLE 1-7 Sites of Absorption for Vitamins, Minerals, and Nutrients

Stomach	Duodenum	Jejunum	Ileum	Colon
Alcohol	Chloride	Glucose	Pyridoxine	Sodium
	Sulfate	Galactose	Folic Acid	Potassium
	Iron	Fructose	Amino acids	Vitamin K
	Calcium	Vitamin C	Di and tripeptides	Water
	Magnesium	Thiamin	Vitamins A, D, K	
	Zinc	Riboflavin	Vitamin E	
			Fat	
			Cholesterol	
			Bile salts	
			Vitamin B_{12}	

down the somewhat smaller oligosaccharides into their respective disaccharide components and glucose. These products, as well as lactose, sucrose, and other simple sugars, are then absorbed by mucosal cells lining the small intestine.

In the microvilli of these mucosal cells, enzymes degrade the disaccharides into their respective monosaccharide constituents (e.g., maltase breaks maltose down into two glucose molecules). Some monosaccharides (e.g., glucose and galactose) are then actively absorbed, whereas others (e.g., fructose) undergo facilitated diffusion into the bloodstream. Glucose and galactose are more rapidly absorbed than fructose, mannose, xylose, and arabinose. Table 1-7 lists the sites of absorption for glucose and galactose as well as for many other nutrients.

Pancreatic or salivary amylase, enzymes in the gastrointestinal tract, are unable to break down or digest cellulose (a polysaccharide), pectins, gums, and other forms of fiber, which account for a considerable amount of dietary carbohydrate. Collectively, their main utility is as intestinal bulking agents.

Once the monosaccharides have been absorbed and transported to the liver via the portal vein, body tissues can use them for energy or store them as glycogen. The monosaccharides are not the only energy source in the body, as fatty acids also serve in this capacity. The brain relies exclusively on glucose for energy. Glucose becomes phosphorylated when it enters a cell and is no longer able to pass back out. Other than being stored as glycogen or being converted to fat, glucose-6-phosphate is involved in many capacities, including providing energy to cells and providing pentose sugars for nucleic acid and nucleotide biosynthesis.

The glycogen found in the liver is a storage form of glucose. The liver is responsible for releasing sufficient glucose into the bloodstream to maintain a level of 90 to 100 mg of glucose per 100 mL of blood. Glucose-6-phosphatase must cleave the phosphate off this newly formed glucose before it can pass into the bloodstream. Because the liver and muscles have a limited capacity for storing glycogen, excess carbohydrates consumed are stored as fat.

The culprit in glycogen storage disease is typically a glucose-6-phosphatase deficiency in the liver (considered an inborn error of metabolism). In people with this condition, the liver is unable to deliver glucose to the bloodstream since the phosphate cannot be cleaved off the glucose. As a result, the liver becomes engorged with glycogen and hypoglycemia occurs.

When intestinal cells are compromised by disease, deficiency, or genetic abnormalities, intolerance to certain dietary sugars results (e.g., lactose intolerance). Lactose is hydrolyzed to its components, glucose and galactose, by lactase. Approximately 15% of Americans and 90% of African and Asian Americans are lactase deficient, which can lead to such symptoms as bloating, cramping, and osmotic diarrhea. To avoid these problems people can reduce their consumption of lactose-containing foods, pretreat foods with bacterial-derived lactase, or eat lactase-treated dairy products (e.g., Lactaid or Dairy Ease). Calcium supplementation is recommended for people who avoid all products containing lactose.

Lipids

Although gastric lipase is present in the stomach, it only hydrolyzes part of the short chain triglycerides into the corresponding fatty acids and glycerol. Most lipid digestion occurs in the intestine. When fat-containing chyme (partly digested food) passes from the stomach to the small intestine, two distinct events occur. First, enterogastrone is secreted to slow gastric motility and secretion. Second, the hormones secretin and cholecystokinin-pancreozymin are secreted to prompt the secretion of pancreatic and biliary juices, including enzymes and fluids rich in bicarbonate.

Bile, produced by the gall bladder, breaks larger fatty particles into smaller molecules that lipase, a pancreatic enzyme, can hydrolyze. The triacyglycerols (also called triglycerides) are hydrolyzed into fatty acids, monoglycerides, and diglycerides. The products of these reactions—the bile salts, fatty acids, and monoglycerides—then interact with additional fatty molecules to help emulsify them. Once emulsified the lipids are absorbed by microvilli in the small intestine's mucous membrane, whereas the bile salts continue to the ileum to be reabsorbed. Smaller fatty particles (micelles) are absorbed directly into intestinal mucosal cells, where fatty acids are hydrolyzed and new triacylglycerols are formed. Now a β-lipoprotein coat surrounds these triglycerides, along with cholesterol and some phospholipids, creating chylomicrons, which are transported by the lymphatic vessels to the thoracic duct and ultimately into the blood.

Lipids derived from intestinal absorption are removed from the blood via the liver, where triglycerides are hydrolyzed by cellular lipases to fatty acids and glycerol. Glycerol undergoes carbohydrate metabolism, whereas fatty acids return to the bloodstream as part of lipoproteins, which transport water-insoluble fatty acids. When the body requires energy these fatty acids are oxidized via acetyl coenzyme A, initiating the Kreb's cycle (also known as the tricarboxylic or TCA cycle).When the body doesn't need energy, the fatty acids may be eliminated or may be stored as fat for later use. After cholesterol esters are hydrolyzed by pancreatic cholesterol esterase, the process for cholesterol absorption follows a similar sequence of steps.

An alternate route for fatty acids in the liver is to undergo β-oxidation to produce acetoacetic acid, which can then be routed in several directions. Acetoacetic acid can combine with oxaloacetate to become a source of energy, and it can be incorporated in the biosynthesis of fatty acids. When combined with oxaloacetate, it can also undergo degradation to produce acetone, be reduced to β-hydroxybutyric acid, or be hydrolyzed to acetoacetic acid. These three products of fatty acid metabolism are termed ketones (also known as ketone bodies). In diabetes, which involves overproduction of acetoacetate, excessive amounts of acetoacetic acid can lead to ketosis which, if not corrected, can result in acidosis and ketonuria.

As indicated above, lipids (primarily triglycerides) undergo complex digestive and absorptive processes. If a hitch occurs in the sequence, a person can consume more fat than his or her body can manage, resulting in steatorrhea (excessive fat in the feces). Fat malabsorption can cause weight loss, muscle wasting, infertility, dysmenorrhea, diseases associated with vitamin A, D, K, and E deficiencies and, in infants, failure to thrive and growth retardation.[146]

If bile salts are not absorbed, as happens when a person has significant disease of the ileum, they are lost in the stool. These salts form a chelate with calcium, preventing the calcium salt of dietary oxalic acid to form. Oxalic acid then forms a soluble sodium salt, which is available for absorption in the colon and which eventually results in renal oxalate stones. Patients with bile salt malabsorption should avoid foods high in oxalates including spinach, rhubarb, cocoa, chocolate, green beans, peanut butter, collards, and beer.[146]

Protein

Unlike carbohydrates, proteins do not start being digested in the mouth. Once food enters the stomach, hydrochloric acid and the proteolytic enzyme pepsin (the active form of pepsinogen) are released. Pepsin cleaves proteins at specific peptide linkages, specifically those that surround the aromatic amino acids, to produce proteoses, peptones, and large polypeptides.

When the acidic contents of the stomach find their way to the small intestine, secretin and cholecystokinin-pancreozymin are secreted. These two hormones stimulate the pancreas to produce juices that contain enzymes and are high in bicarbonate, which neutralizes the acid. The foods become slightly alkaline, providing the environment for the intestinal enzymes trypsin (active form of trypsinogen), chymotrypsin, carboxypeptidases, and dipeptidases to be most efficient. These enzymes, like pepsin, cleave at specific peptide bonds and further degrade the proteins into much smaller peptides and amino acids. The peptides are absorbed by the microvilli of the intestinal mucosal cells and are hydrolyzed by peptide hydrolases to their constituent amino acids.

The simple amino acids can then either diffuse or undergo active transport from the intestine to the liver via the blood in the portal vein. Amino acids have four primary active transport systems: one for those that are neutral, one for those that are acidic, one for those that are basic, and one for proline and hydroxyproline. From the liver the amino acids can travel to tissues and cells for biosynthesis of proteins and other nitrogenous tissue components. Amino acid catabolism typically involves the loss of the amino group to produce keto acids that can enter the Kreb's cycle and produce energy. Amino acids are not stored in the body and when consumed in excess are degraded and immediately excreted.

Protein is not the sole source of nitrogen for the body. Nonprotein sources are creatine, creatinine, ammonia, uric acid, and urea. Nitrogen balance occurs when the body's use of nitrogen equals what is consumed. If a person's nitrogen balance is negative, it means that utilization of nitrogen is exceeding intake. A negative nitrogen balance can result from a diet deficient in even one of the essential amino acids: histidine, isoleucine, leucine, lysine, methionine, phenylalanine, threonine, tryptophan, and valine.

Vitamins and Minerals

Most vitamins are passively absorbed, going unchanged from the intestine into the bloodstream. (See Table 1-7 for absorption sites.) The presence or absence of other nutrients can influence the degree to which a given vitamin is absorbed. Mineral absorption is much more complicated and typically occurs in three steps.[147] The first, or intraluminal stage, occurs in the stomach and intestine and involves all the chemical reactions and interactions that cations and anions undergo. Both the pH environment and the composition of the diet influence reactions that can occur with cations, but neither affect reactions associated with anions. Soluble in the stomach's acidic milieu, cations become insoluble hydroxide salts in the intestine. To remain available for absorption, minerals must be chelated with dietary substances including amino acids and sugars.

Next, the translocation stage involves the active or passive transport of the minerals or mineral complexes into intestinal mucosal cells. Some anions are small enough to passively diffuse into these cells, but the cation complexes require facilitated diffusion or active transport.

Last, the mobilization stage involves movement of these minerals into the bloodstream or sequestering within the cell. Some of the minerals remain part of a protein complex in the cell, while others are released from the protein to become part of the intracellular pool. Once in the intracellular pool, the minerals are transported by specific proteins (e.g., transferrin for iron transport), by albumin, which can bind to several different minerals, or by amino acid or peptide complexes.[147]

ENERGY

Energy is required for physical activity, for growth/repair of tissues, and for normal metabolic processes and is released continuously via carbohydrate, protein, fat, and alcohol metabolism. One gram of protein and carbohydrate

Calculating Energy Expenditure

Total energy expenditure (TEE) is a combination of energy expended during physical activity, the thermic effect of food, and energy minimally required to maintain vital organ function while the body is in a resting and fasting state. The amount of energy a person expends per day should be correlated with the number of calories he or she takes in.

To calculate TEE you need to know the person's ideal body weight, his or her physical activity level (PAL), his or her resting energy expenditure (REE), and the thermic effect of food (TEF). Factors for PAL are shown in Table 1-8.

Following is the TEE calculation for a 45-year-old woman who is 168 cm tall, weighs 80 kg, works sitting down, and engages in little strenuous activity during leisure hours.

PAL = 1.7 (see Table 1-8)
Ideal body weight = 59 kg (found in several standard reference tables)
REE = 1322 kcal (determined using the Harris-Benedict equations on page 40)
Multiply REE by PAL (1.7) = 1322 × 1.7 = 2248 kcal. Add 10% of 2248 for
   TEF = 225 + 2248 = 2473 kcal (total energy expenditure per day)

TABLE 1-8   Factors for Calculating Physical Activity Levels (PAL)

Lifestyle and Level of Activity	PAL Factor
Bed or chair bound lifestyle	1.2
Seated work: no movement; little to no strenuous work during leisure time	1.4–1.5
Seated work: some requirement to move; little to no strenuous work during leisure time	1.6–1.7
Standing work	1.8–1.9
High level of participation in sports or strenuous work during leisure time (30–60 minutes 4–5 times/week)	+0.3 increment
Strenuous work or very active leisure activities	2.0–2.4

Source: Reference 148.

produces 4 kcal of energy, whereas fat produces 9 kcal and alcohol produces 7 kcal. Evaluating the amount of energy a person expends on a daily basis (total energy expenditure [TEE]) guides dietary plan development to ensure that an appropriate and not excessive number of calories (energy) is consumed.

Everyone expends a certain amount of energy daily based on physical activity, food intake, and other factors (see sidebar above). TEE is a combination of energy expended during physical activity (EEPA), the thermic effect of food (TEF), and resting energy expenditure (REE)—the energy minimally required to maintain vital organ function while the body is in a resting and fasting state. Basal energy expenditure (BEE)—the energy a person uses over 24 hours when mentally and physically at rest in a thermoneutral environment—must be measured at least 12 hours after the last meal.[148]

Energy-Related Terminology

Basal energy expenditure (BEE): A portion of the daily energy expenditure, which represents the minimum amount of energy necessary to sustain life. It is correlated to the basal metabolic rate (BMR) and can be calculated for a specific period of time (BMR × time interval = BEE).

Body mass index (BMI): A gauge of total body fat that is useful for assessing nutritional status and health risk. BMI is derived from the formula: weight(kg)/height(m²). General values for BMI are shown in Table 1-9. You can also find many BMI calculators on the Web, including this one from the Centers for Disease Control and Prevention: www.cdc.gov/nccdphp/dnpa/bmi/calc-bmi.htm

Energy expended during physical activity (EEPA): See Table 1-10 for values.

Fat-free mass (FFM): The amount of metabolically active tissue present. It is measured using reference body composition methods including underwater weighing and measuring total body water using stable isotopes of deuterium or 18-oxygen.

Resting energy expenditure (REE): Expressed as kcal expended in 1 day. REE is calculated using the Harris-Benedict Equations on page 40.

Resting metabolic rate (RMR): Now largely replaced by REE, this is the rate of energy used for metabolism under resting conditions. It is expressed as kcal/kg/hour.

Total energy expenditure (TEE): The amount of energy a person expends on a daily basis, which guides dietary plan development to ensure that an appropriate number of calories is consumed. TEE = REE × PAL factor + TEF.

Thermic effect of food (TEF): Calculated as 10% of (REE × PAL factor).

TABLE 1-9 Body Mass Index

Body Mass Index	Classification
Less than 20	Underweight
20-25	Normal
25-30	Overweight
Greater than 30	Obese

Source: Reference 148.

Recently the total energy expenditure for children was adjusted based on lower EEPA levels than originally proposed. Now the TEE for children is 1.3 to 1.4 times the REE, whereas before it was 1.7 to 2.0 times the REE.[149,150]

Measuring REE accurately is important. Although many equations try to correlate a person's physical characteristics with REE, the Harris-Benedict equations on page 40 are used most commonly.[151] Unfortunately they overestimate REE by 7% to 24%.[152] The REE value can vary due to body size (larger people typically have a higher metabolic rate) and composition (the

Harris-Benedict Equations for Calculating Resting Energy Expenditure (REE)

Men: 66 + [13.7 × weight in kg] + [5.0 × height in cm] –
        [6.8 × age in years] = kcal

Women: 665 + [9.6 × weight in kg] + [1.8 × height in cm] –
        [4.7 × age in years] = kcal

TABLE 1-10   Approximate Energy Expenditure in Physical Activity (EEPA)

Type of Activity	Energy Related to REE	Rate of Energy Expenditure kcal/min
Resting	REE × 1.0	1–1.2
Very light Seated and standing activities, driving, typing, cooking, ironing	REE × 1.5	Up to 2.5
Light Walking 2.5–3 mph, garage work, carpentry, house cleaning, golf, child care	REE × 2.5	2.5–4.9
Moderate Walking 3.5–4 mph, weeding, cycling, skiing, tennis, dancing	REE × 5.0	5.0–7.4
Heavy Walking with load uphill, manual digging, basketball, football, soccer	REE × 7.0	7.5–12

Source: Reference 148.

more fat-free mass [FFM], the more metabolically active tissue present). The REE can also vary with sex, age, and hormonal status. Older people typically have lower REE values due to a gradual loss of FFM, and women's metabolic rate is typically 5% to 10% lower than men's. In addition, thyroid hormone, insulin, cortisol, growth hormone, and hormones associated with the menstrual cycle all influence metabolic rate.

TEF, the energy required for food consumption, makes up 10% of a person's TEE and varies with diet. More energy is needed when carbohydrates and proteins are consumed than when fat is ingested.[153]

A person's activity level, degree of fitness, and body size have a tremendous impact on the percent of TEE represented by EEPA. Using multiples of REE, activities are ranked by the level of energy typically expended (see Table 1-10). Housework, for example, considered a "light" activity, is associated with an energy expenditure of REE × 2.5, or 2.5 to 4.9 kcal/min, whereas heavy manual digging and football are considered "heavy" activities equivalent to REE × 7.0, or 7.5 to 12 kcal/min. Sleeping and reclining, considered "resting," is equivalent to REE × 1.0 or 1 to 1.2 kcal/min.[149] EEPA includes not only all the voluntary physical activity a person engages in but also involuntary energy, such as that expended to maintain posture.[150] Because older people lose fat-free mass, they expend decreased amounts of energy during physical activity and during rest. The rate at which energy is expended is also influenced by the spice content of food. Spicy foods tend to elevate metabolic rate significantly for several hours as compared to unspiced foods.[153]

People accumulate body fat when they consume more calories than they use. A common measure of body fat is the body mass index (BMI), which is calculated as shown on page 39. It is recommended that people limit their caloric intake to maintain a BMI of less than 25.[154] Anyone with a BMI over 25 is considered overweight, and anyone with a BMI equal to or greater than 30 is obese. Anything above 27 is associated with an increased risk of developing health-related problems.

Higher BMI values and/or waist-to-hip ratios have been linked to an increased risk of hypertension and cardiovascular disease.[155,156] Glucose intolerance and insulin resistance frequently develop in obese patients, often leading to type 2 diabetes. An increase in the prevalence of cancers of the breast, cervix, endometrium, ovary, gallbladder and prostate has been linked to excessive caloric consumption in general, but not to fat consumption in particular.[157]

NUTRITION THROUGHOUT THE LIFECYCLE

Pregnancy

When a human egg is fertilized with a sperm, nearly every anatomical, biochemical, and physiological system within the woman's body changes to prepare her for carrying a child to term. The body must be able to provide the essential nutrients for fetal growth and development. It also must gear up for labor and delivery and for feeding the new infant.

Major physiological alterations during the prenatal period include increases in plasma volume, red blood cell volume, cardiac output (increased pulse rate), body water, renal glomerular filtration rate, and respiratory tidal volume, as well as decreases in gastrointestinal and genitourinary motility.[158] The increase in plasma volume results in decreased blood glucose values, serum albumin levels, and concentrations of water-soluble vitamins. The decrease in GI motility allows more nutrients to be absorbed but also causes constipation. Blood pressure tends to fall during the first two trimesters and returns to normal during the third.

Maternal malnutrition can cause fetal growth failure, which results in low birth weight. Fetal growth failure can manifest itself in several ways including reduced number and size of placenta cells, decreased number of brain cells, small head and organs, and altered cell components. The timing, duration, and extent of malnutrition influences its impact on the growing fetus.

Effects on cell size are generally reversible, but can be permanent if the deficiency is long term and many cells are affected. Evaluating a woman's nutrition before she conceives can help identify dietary practices that pose nutritional risk. It's also important to evaluate BMI to determine guidelines for weight gain.

Monitoring nutrition during pregnancy is important because the mother must ingest sufficient nutrients for both herself and the growing fetus. (Table 1-11 lists recommended diet changes during pregnancy.) Total energy needs increase by approximately 15%, especially in the second and third trimesters. A woman's basal metabolic rate (BMR) and level of physical activity largely dictate her total energy requirement. The BMR increases by the fourth month of gestation and remains at 15% to 20% above normal until term. This translates roughly to an increase in the RDA for energy of 200 to 300 kcal/day in the second and third trimesters. Protein should account for some of this increase, adding 19 to 24 g/day for a total of 60 g/day.[159] The BMR returns to normal 4 to 5 days postpartum.

Because the body must provide a continuous supply of fuel at the end of pregnancy, when fetal needs are the greatest (the fetus requires approximately 43 kcal per day per kilogram of fetal weight), the way the body produces energy changes substantially. During pregnancy, 50% to 70% of the mother's fuel comes from glucose, 20% from amino acids, and the remainder from fat. The reason that maternal metabolism shifts—using some fat for fuel—is to allow the fetus to use the glucose. The mother stores fat during the second trimester to prepare for this increased lipolysis. Blood volume and composition also change, so that by the end of the pregnancy the mother's blood volume is 50% higher than at conception.

Several vitamins and minerals should be supplemented during pregnancy. Although vitamin A is potentially toxic and teratogenic in mega doses, the RDA of 4000 IU of vitamin A (800 mcg retinol) should be consumed during pregnancy. Women should carefully evaluate the vitamin A content of their multivitamin to ensure that it does not contain more than 100% of the RDA. Supplementation with vitamin D is likely to be unnecessary during pregnancy. Although vitamin D is instrumental in maintaining calcium homeostasis, the vitamin's concentration in fetal blood is identical to that in maternal blood. Elevated levels of vitamin D can lead to fetal hypercalcemia.

Vitamin B_6, an essential cofactor in amino acid and protein biosynthesis, should be supplemented to 1.9 mg/day from the nonpregnant RDA of 1.3 mg/day. Vitamin B_6 is also necessary for biosynthesis of niacin from tryptophan. Because the placenta concentrates this vitamin, fetal cord blood contains higher amounts than are found in the maternal circulation.

During pregnancy, folic acid requirements increase to support fetal growth and development and increased maternal erythropoiesis. Folic acid deficiency has been linked to congenital birth defects, low birth weight, and preterm labor. Maintaining folic acid at appropriate levels can largely prevent neural tube defects such as spina bifida and anencephaly. Because the neural tube closes so early in fetal development—around 4 weeks after conception—women of childbearing age must increase their consumption of foods containing folic acid or take vitamin supplements that contain the proper amount of folic acid even if they are not planning on becoming pregnant.

The RDAs for the antioxidant vitamins C and E increase during pregnancy: an additional 10 mg/day for vitamin C and an additional 2 IU per day for vitamin E. These increases are easy to accommodate in the typical diet simply by changing the foods eaten, but supplements can be used when necessary. Vitamin E deficiency has been correlated with an increased risk of spontaneous abortion. Low levels of vitamin C are associated with preeclampsia and premature membrane rupture.[160]

Increased iron intake is necessary to form the hemoglobin found in both maternal and fetal red blood cells. Although the fetus accumulates iron largely in the last trimester, reaching a level of about 250 to 300 mg, the mother needs supplementation early in pregnancy to allow for the necessary increase in erythrocyte volume. Infants are rarely anemic at birth because the fetus draws on the mother's iron stores to maintain its own erythropoiesis. The mother should accumulate 700 to 800 mg over the course of the pregnancy, which translates to approximately 15 mg/day on top of the RDA of 18 mg/day. Failure to meet this increase can lead to maternal anemia. Unfortunately, taking iron supplements between meals, necessary for maximal absorption of elemental iron, causes constipation in many women.

Maternal calcium requirements also go up during pregnancy. The fetus, which accumulates nearly 25 g of calcium during gestation, requires most of its calcium in the third trimester (at a rate of 300 mg/day), when skeletal growth is at a maximum. Hormones—especially human chorionic somatomammotropin from the placenta—enhance bone turnover greatly during pregnancy. Estrogen, on the other hand, inhibits bone resorption, which increases secretion of the hormone—parathyroid—that maintains high serum calcium concentrations. To prevent leaching of calcium from the maternal skeleton to support fetal growth and development, calcium intake should increase 300 mg/day to 1300 mg/day during pregnancy.

Increasing the RDAs for zinc, magnesium, and iodide is also recommended during pregnancy. Zinc supplementation has been shown to improve birth weight of babies born to women with low prepregnancy weights and low plasma serum concentrations of zinc.[161] Magnesium supplementation has been correlated with decreased incidence of preeclampsia and premature birth, and with less growth retardation.[162]

To limit constipation women should drink 8 to 10 glasses of fluids per day (64 to 80 oz or 1900 to 2370 mL). Pregnant women's caffeine consumption should not exceed the equivalent of two cups of coffee per day (a total of 16 oz or 474 mL).[163]

The Dietary Guidelines for Americans recommended by the U.S. Department of Agriculture and related Food Guide Pyramid (see Figure 1-1 on page 9) must be altered during pregnancy and lactation to meet the increased demand for nutrients by the developing fetus and to prepare the mother for labor and delivery. Table 1-11 compares the minimum number of daily servings recommended in each food group for pregnant and nonpregnant

TABLE 1-11 Recommended Changes in Diet During Pregnancy

Food Group	Pregnant Woman (servings per day)	Nonpregnant Woman (servings per day)
Breads, cereals, rices, grains	7	6
Fruits and vegetables	5	5
Milk, yogurt, cheeses	3	2
Protein sources	7	5
Fats, oils	3	3

Source: Adapted from *Nutrition During Pregnancy and the Postpartum Period: A Manual for Healthcare Professionals.* California Department of Health Services, Maternal Child Health Branch, 1990.

women. In the last 30 weeks of pregnancy, women's weight should increase 14 oz (0.3 kg) per week.

The lactation process uses approximately 85 kcal per 100 mL of milk produced. Not surprisingly, the RDA for energy—the number of kcal that should be consumed depending on age and gender—increases by 500 kcal/day from the nonpregnancy value. This additional energy need not come entirely from the diet, because maternal fat stores can supply 100 to 150 kcal/day for several months after the birth.

The iron requirement during lactation is lower than it is during pregnancy, but some populations, such as adolescents, may develop an iron deficiency due to a poor diet. On the other hand, breastfeeding mothers' zinc requirement increases postpartum.[164] Although women are advised to continue taking prenatal vitamins after giving birth to ensure adequate intake of calcium, magnesium, zinc, vitamin B_6, and folate, it is generally preferred that these critical vitamins and minerals come from an appropriate diet.[165] Lactating women should also consume 2 to 3 quarts (1900 to 2845 mL) of liquid daily to prevent dehydration.

Infancy

During their first year of life, babies triple their weight and increase their length by approximately 50%. This weight gain depends entirely on their genetic makeup, their environment, and the nutrition supplied by their mother, whereas birth weight is largely dictated by the mother's prepregnancy weight and how much she gains during pregnancy. Immediately after birth babies typically lose about 6% of their body weight due to fluid loss and tissue catabolism. Usually they gain it all back by their 10th day.

A newborn's daily energy expenditure is three to four times greater than an adult's (roughly 90 to 120 kcal/kg vs. 30 to 40 kcal/kg). This amount of energy is necessary because a newborn's REE is relatively high, as are the needs associated with growth and development. A baby is able to use carbohydrates and fats equally as energy sources, but must consume both—not just one or the other—to avoid ketosis or hypoglycemia. Infants' lipid consumption should not be restricted and linoleic acid should make up 3% of the total kcal ingested per day. Carbohydrates, in the form of lactose or other simple sugars, should make up 30% to 60% of the infant's diet.

The newborn's protein requirements per unit of body weight are typically greater than for adults. To ensure a positive nitrogen balance infants must consume the essential amino acids and histidine, which is considered an essential amino acid for infants but not for adults. The amount of protein in breast milk is sufficient for babies up through 6 months of age.

Iron deficiency in newborns is rare because of their prenatal stores, and their food sources contain limited amounts of iron. Children breastfed for only 4 to 6 months, however, are at risk for a negative iron balance and may develop a deficiency after 6 to 8 months.[166] To prevent this, iron supplements or iron-fortified formulas should be introduced (6 mg/day for the first 6 months and then 10 mg/day until age 3).[167] Newborns have no stores of zinc and therefore must receive it in breast milk or infant formula for the first year of life.

Breastfed babies retain nearly two-thirds of the calcium they ingest as compared to the 25% to 30% retention of calcium in babies who drink cow's milk.[167]

Infants who are breastfed usually receive sufficient amounts of all the vitamins they need to meet the RDA, except for vitamin D. To prevent a vitamin D deficiency breastfed infants should receive a supplement or be exposed to sunlight regularly. Breast milk is also low on vitamin K, an essential component of the clotting cascade. In several states, newborns—who do not yet have the necessary intestinal flora to produce vitamin K—are given a prophylactic intramuscular vitamin K injection at birth to prevent hemorrhage.[168]

Babies need plenty of fluids to replace those lost in the feces and urine, as well as through evaporation, but either breast milk or infant formula usually supplies more than enough.

Childhood and Adolescence

Body composition changes during childhood and adolescence, and growth rate and nutrition requirements change, as well. Children should be offered at least three meals and a snack or two per day. Adolescents, too, would benefit from this schedule, but it's difficult to enforce given teens' notoriously bad eating habits and their propensity to miss meals.

The energy RDAs for younger children are currently the subject of some controversy. It has been suggested that the RDA values for children under age 11 (see Table 1-12) may be as much as 25% too high.[169] Although they may very well be elevated, it is still important for a child's diet to be apportioned so that roughly 50% to 60% is in the form of carbohydrates, 25% to 35% is fat and 10% to 15% is protein. As children approach adolescence their energy requirement should be calculated based on calories per unit of height rather than relying on the published RDAs. Likewise, the appropriate protein requirement for teenagers should be calculated based on units of height.

The American Academy of Pediatrics recommends that children and adolescents get their nutrients from a well-balanced diet and does not condone

TABLE 1-12   Energy RDAs for Various Groups

	Age	Weight (Pounds)	Height (Inches)	Energy (kcal)
Males	11–14	99	62	2500
	15–18	145	69	3000
	19–24	160	70	2900
	25–50	174	70	2900
	51+	170	68	2300
Females	11–14	101	62	2200
	15–18	120	64	2200
	19–24	128	65	2200
	25–50	138	64	2200
	51+	143	63	1900
Pregnant				+300
Lactating				+500

Source: Reference 148.

using as a replacement multivitamin supplements that contain minerals and iron.[170] (The one exception is using fluoride supplements to prevent dental caries in areas where water is not fluoridated.) It's essential that the diets of children and teens include sufficient vitamins, calcium, iron, and zinc.[171]

Approximately 45% of the body's skeletal mass is formed during adolescence, but many teens do not consume adequate calcium and vitamin D because they choose foods that do not contain milk (e.g., carbonated beverages).[171] Younger children, in contrast, usually consume milk and milk-containing products regularly, and their calcium retention can approach approximately 100 mg/day.

As children enter adolescence their iron requirement increases proportionately to their increase in blood volume, hemoglobin, and myoglobin synthesis.[172] Boys' increase in muscle mass is correlated with increased blood volume, and girls lose iron every month once they begin menstruating. Iron deficiency is relatively common in young children because they grow fast and expend large amounts of energy without increasing their iron intake accordingly. Foods containing non-heme iron (which is not absorbed as easily as the heme form of iron) are more appealing to children than meats, but they do not consume enough to fulfill the body's needs. As children's taste for meat increases their iron deficiency problems largely disappear, but in the meantime, it's important to find ways to bring iron into their diet or use supplements.

Some children need zinc supplementation, as well. Preschool- and school-aged children typically have a low intake of zinc-containing foods such as meats and seafood. When they enter adolescence, zinc status plays a significant role in the development of secondary sex characteristics.

The adolescent growth spurt is accompanied by significant tissue formation, an increase in energy use, and a corresponding increase in the requirement for the vitamin cofactors (B vitamins) and the antioxidant vitamins E and C, which help keep cells healthy as growth accelerates. Adolescents—especially those who smoke—can become deficient in these protective vitamins if high-fat, low-fiber foods make up a significant component of their diet. A well-balanced diet should not be replaced by multivitamins or vitamin supplements, but using supplements is better than nothing in adolescents with poor eating habits.

The best approach is to foster healthy eating habits among adolescents and try to keep them from becoming overtly preoccupied with their diet, which can lead to eating disorders—a growing problem among adolescent girls.[172]

Older Adults: Over 65

As adults age and enter retirement, their activities and socioeconomic status may change dramatically. Injury, disease, or lack of motivation can cause a person to become less active and prone to obesity, ultimately decreasing the amount of lean body mass, the energy requirement, and the basal metabolic rate. Avoiding obesity and related problems means modifying diet and exercise in accordance with changes in metabolism and energy requirements. The RDA for energy in this population is approximately 2300 kcal/day for men and 1900 kcal/day for women.

Although requirements have not been established for carbohydrate intake per kilogram in older adults, the general guideline that 50% to 60% of the diet should come from carbohydrates applies. These calories should include primarily complex carbohydrates and dietary fibers and only a limited amount of simple sugars. Impaired glucose tolerance, a growing problem for the elderly, can be due to either decreased insulin production or decreased insulin action at receptors on target tissues. When glucose metabolism becomes unpredictable patients are at risk for hypoglycemia or hyperglycemia, which can eventually lead to type 2 diabetes. Consuming complex carbohydrates instead of simple sugars helps control imbalances in glucose metabolism. Lactose intolerance, another sugar-related problem that tends to develop in older people, results from impaired lactase enzyme function.[173] As a result, lactose-containing foods wind up in the intestine, where they cause abdominal cramping, flatulence, and diarrhea.

No requirements have been established for lipid or fat intake in older adults, but keeping fat intake to 30% of total calories consumed is appropriate for this age group. The fats consumed should primarily be monounsaturated and polyunsaturated. Despite the recommendations of some health practitioners, there is little evidence to suggest that severely limiting fat intake in this population makes much of a difference in overall health and well being.[174]

As the aging process reduces skeletal tissue mass, normal stores of protein decrease as well. This means that older adults must maintain the proper amount of protein in their diet for a positive nitrogen balance: 1.0 to 1.25 g/kg/day, an increase from 0.9 g/kg/day of protein for younger adults.[175] Most at risk for reduced protein consumption and malnutrition are elderly

TABLE 1-13 Drug-Nutrient Interactions

Drug Class	Interactions Possible
Psychotherapeutic agents	Altered appetite, decreased ability to remember mealtimes
Diuretics	Depletes Na, K, Mg, Ca, and Zn
H_2 antagonists	Decrease absorption of Ca, Fe, Zn, and vitamins B_{12}, C, and D
Laxatives	Mineral oil use: traps fat-soluble vitamins
	In general: causes potassium depletion
Phenytoin	Tube-fed patients: constituents of "food" adsorbs drug
Antibiotics	Interfere with production of vitamin K
Barbiturates	Interferes with metabolism of vitamin D and folate
Dilantin or phenobarbitol	Interferes with metabolism of vitamins D, K, B_6, and folate
Bile acid resins	Interferes with metabolism of vitamins A, B_{12}, E, and K.
Methotrexate	Folate and Ca

people on a restricted income or who have severe dental problems without the means to pay for dentures.

Adequate fluid consumption, especially water, is critical in the elderly population. Use of laxatives or diuretics, as well as vigorous physical activity that causes perspiration, require replacement of fluids and electrolytes to prevent dehydration. The recommended daily fluid intake in people over age 65 is 30 to 35 mL/kg, with a minimum of 1500 mL/day.[176]

The older population is at risk for a number of drug-nutrient interactions. Medications that alter the absorption, metabolism, distribution, and elimination of dietary nutrients can lead to vitamin or mineral deficiencies. Those that alter the way food tastes can affect appetite and dietary intake. Table 1-13 lists several drug-nutrient interactions.[175]

A nonpharmacological method of treating certain diseases is to change the diet (e.g., lowering salt, fat, cholesterol, or protein). If not monitored closely, however, diet changes may also take a toll on the patient's overall nutritional status.

Older adults should consume 400 IU of vitamin D and 1500 mg of calcium per day to help prevent osteoporosis, which can lead to fractures and severe disability. Weight-bearing exercise in those who can tolerate it is also important to reduce bone loss. Maintaining adequate calcium levels is especially difficult in patients with hypochloridia, in which calcium absorption is impaired by the absence of sufficient hydrochloric acid.[93] Two problems associated with vitamin D production in the elderly is the kidney's limited ability to produce active vitamin D and a lack of sun exposure among institutionalized patients. OTC vitamin D supplements may not be sufficient because they require activation by enzymes from both the liver and the kidney.

Iron stores remain reasonably stable during old age. Anemia develops mainly as a result of chronic blood loss due to peptic ulcer disease or from gastric irritation and bleeding caused by nonsteroidal anti-inflammatory agents. Although reducing the amount of meat consumed doesn't usually affect iron stores, it can lead to zinc deficiency.

The antioxidant vitamins E and C are thought to help prevent macular degeneration and cataract formation in the elderly.[176] Vitamin C levels can be affected by extreme stress, smoking, or medications that impair vitamin C absorption such as H_2 antagonists. The average adult diet usually includes 100 to 250 mg/day of vitamin C, which well exceeds the RDA of 60 mg/day.

REFERENCES

1. Lehninger AL, Nelson DL, Cox MM. Carbohydrates. In: *Principles of Biochemistry.* 2nd ed. New York: Worth Publishers; 1993:308-18.
2. Third National Health and Nutrition Examination Survey, Phase 1, 1988-91. Daily dietary fat and total food-energy intakes. *MMWR Morb Mortal Wkly Rep.* 1994;43:116-7,123-5.
3. National Cholesterol Education Program. Second report of the expert panel on detection, evaluation, and treatment of high blood cholesterol in adults (Adult treatment panel II). *Circulation.* 1994;89:1333-445.
4. Lichtenstein AH, Ausman LM, Jalbert SM, et al. Effects of different forms of dietary hydrogenated fats on serum lipoprotein cholesterol levels. *N Engl J Med.* 1999;340:1933-40.
5. Foley M, Ball M, Chisholm A, et al. Should mono- or poly-unsaturated fats replace saturated fat in the diet? *Eur J Clin Nutr.* 1992;46:429-36.
6. Schaefer EJ, Lichtenstein AH, Lamon-Fava S, et al. Lipoproteins, nutrition, aging, and atherosclerosis. *Am J Clin Nutr.* 1995;61(suppl):726S-40S.
7. Shikany JM. Dietary guidelines for chronic disease prevention. *South Med J.* 2000;93:1157-61.
8. Nestel PJ, Connor WE, Reardon MF, et al. Suppression by diets rich in fish oil of very low density lipoprotein production in man. *J Clin Invest.* 1984;74:82-9.
9. Dimmitt SB. Recent insights into dietary fats and cardiovascular disease. *Clin Exp Pharmacol Physiol.* 1995;22:204-8.
10. Shekelle RB, Shryock AM, Paul O, et al. Diet, serum cholesterol, and death from coronary heart disease: The Western Electric Study. *N Engl J Med.* 1981;304:65-70.
11. Saku K, Zhang B, Ohta T, et al. Quantity and function of high-density lipoprotein as an indicator of coronary atherosclerosis. *J Am Coll Cardiol.* 1999;33:436-43.
12. Austin MA, Breslow JL, Hennekens CH, et al. Low-density lipoprotein subclass patterns and risk of myocardial infarction. *JAMA.* 1988;260:1917-21.
13. Bates CJ. Vitamin A. *Lancet.* 1995;345:31-5.
14. Ross AC. Vitamin A and retinoids. In: Shils ME, Olson J, Shike M, et al., eds. *Modern Nutrition in Health and Disease.* 9th ed. Baltimore: Williams & Wilkins; 1999:305-27.
15. Ross AC, Gardner EM. The function of vitamin A in cellular growth and differentiation, and its roles during pregnancy and lactation. *Adv Exp Med Biol.* 1994;352:187-200.
16. Rothman KJ, Moore LL, Singer MR, et al. Teratogenicity of high vitamin A intake. *N Engl J Med.* 1995;333:1369-73.
17. Oakley GP, Erickson JD. Vitamin A and birth defects: continuing caution is needed. *N Engl J Med.* 1995;333:1414-5.
18. Redlich CA, Blaner WS, Van Bennekum AM, et al. Effect of supplementation with beta-carotene and vitamin A on lung nutrient levels. *Cancer Epidemiol Biomarkers Prev.* 1998;7:211-4.
19. Stephens D, Jackson PL, Gutierrez Y. Subclinical vitamin A deficiency: a potentially unrecognized problem in the United States. *Pediatric Nursing.* 1996;22:377-89, 456.
20. Meigel WN. How safe is oral isotretinoin? *Dermatology.* 1997;195:22-8,38-40.
21. Polyakov NE, Leshina TV, Konovalova TA, et al. Carotenoids as scavengers of free radicals in a fenton reaction: antioxidants or pro-oxidants? *Free Radic Biol Med.* 2001;31:398-404.
22. Palozza P. Prooxidant actions of carotenoids in biologic systems. *Nutr Rev.* 1998;56:257-65.
23. Reddy BS. Micronutrients as chemopreventive agents. *Principles of Chemoprevention.* 1996;139:221-35.
24. Institute of Medicine, Food and Nutrition Board. *Dietary Reference Intakes: Vitamin C, Vitamin E, Selenium, and Carotenoids.* Washington, DC: National Academy Press; 2000.
25. Season, latitude and ability of sunlight to promote synthesis of vitamin D_3 in skin. *Nutr Rev.* 1989;47:252.
26. Fraser DR. Vitamin D. *Lancet.* 1995;345:104-7.
27. DeLuca HF, Zierold C. Mechanisms and functions of vitamin D. *Nutr Rev.* 1998;56:S4-10.

28. Holick MF. McCollum Award Lecture, 1994: Vitamin D: new horizons for the 21st century. *Am J Clin Nutr.* 1994;60:619-30.

29. Chapuy MC, Arlot ME, Duboeuf F, et al. Vitamin D$_3$ and calcium to prevent hip fractures in elderly women. *N Engl J Med.* 1992;327:1637-42.

30. Reid IR. The roles of calcium and vitamin D in the prevention of osteoporosis. *Endocrinol Metab Clin North Am.* 1998;27:389-98.

31. Dawson-Hughes B, Harris SS, Krall EA, et al. Rates of bone loss in postmenopausal women randomly assigned to one of two dosages of vitamin D. *Am J Clin Nutr.* 1995;61:1140-5.

32. Omenn GS. Micronutrients (vitamins and minerals) as cancer-preventive agents. *IARC Sci Publ.* 1996;139:33-45.

33. Langman M, Boyle P. Chemoprevention of colorectal cancer. *Gut.* 1998;43:578-85.

34. La Vecchia C, Braga C, Negri E, et al. Intake of selected micronutrients and risk of colorectal cancer. *Int J Cancer.* 1997;73:525-30.

35. Chesney RW. Vitamin D: can an upper limit be defined? *J Nutr.* 1989;119(suppl 12):1825-8.

36. Shearer MJ. Vitamin K. *Lancet.* 1995;345:229-34.

37. Taylor CT, Chester EA, Byrd DC, et al. Vitamin K to reverse excessive anticoagulation: a review of the literature. *Pharmacotherapy.* 1999;19:1415-25.

38. Allen LV Jr. Nutritional products. In: *Handbook of Nonprescription Drugs.* 10th ed. Washington, DC: American Pharmaceutical Association; 1993:283-311.

39. Meydani M. Vitamin E. *Lancet.* 1995;345:170-5.

40. Acuff RV, Thedford SS, Hidiroglou NN, et al. Relative bioavailability of *RRR*- and all-*rac*-alpha-tocopheryl acetate in humans: studies using deuterated compounds. *Am J Clin Nutr.* 1994;60:397-402.

41. Scott G. Antioxidants – the Modern Elixir? *Chemistry in Britain,* 1995;31:879-82.

42. Blumberg JB, Couris RR, Bernardi VW. The rationale for vitamin E supplementation. *US Pharmacist.* 1998;23:111-22.

43. Lonn EM, Yusuf S. Is there a role for antioxidant vitamins in the prevention of cardiovascular diseases: an update on epidemiological and clinical trials data. *Can J Cardiol.* 1997;13:957-65.

44. Jialal I, Fuller CJ. Effect of vitamin E, vitamin C and beta-carotene on LDL oxidation and atherosclerosis. *Can J Cardiol.* 1995;11(suppl G):97G-103G.

45. The Heart Outcomes Prevention Evaluation Study Investigators. Vitamin E supplementation and cardiovascular events in high-risk patients. *N Engl J Med.* 2000;342:154-60.

46. Stephens NG, Patsons A, Schofield PM, et al. Randomized controlled trial of vitamin E in patients with coronary disease: Cambridge Heart Antioxidant Study (CHAOS). *Lancet.* 1996;347:781-6.

47. Weitberg AB, Corvese D. Effect of vitamin E and beta-carotene on DNA strand breakage induced by tobacco-specific nitrosamines and stimulated human phagocytes. *J Exp Clin Cancer Res.* 1997;16:11-4.

48. Chan JM, Stampfer MJ, Giovannucci EL. What causes prostate cancer: a brief summary of the epidemiology. *Semin Cancer Biol.* 1998;8:263-73.

49. Traber MG, Packer L. Vitamin E: beyond antioxidant function. *Am J Clin Nutr.* 1995;62:1501S-9S.

50. Traber MG. Vitamin E. In: Shils ME, Olson JA, Shike M, et al., eds. *Modern Nutrition in Health and Disease.* 10th ed. Baltimore: Williams & Wilkins; 1999:347-62.

51. Meydani SN, Meydani M, Blumberg JB, et al. Assessment of the safety of supplementation with different amounts of vitamin E in healthy older adults. *Am J Clin Nutr.* 1998;68:311-8.

52. Sauberlich HE. Pharmacology of vitamin C. *Annu Rev Nutr.* 1994;14:371-91.

53. Simon JA. Vitamin C and cardiovascular disease: review. *J Am Coll Nutr.* 1992;11:107-25.

54. Gey KF, Stahelin HB, Puska P, et al. Relationship of plasma level of vitamin C to mortality from ischemic heart disease. *Ann N Y Acad Sci.* 1987;498:110-20.

55. Hemila H. Vitamin C intake and susceptibility to the common cold. *Br J Nutr.* 1997;77:59-72.

56. Barber DA, Harris SR. Oxygen free radicals and antioxidants: a review. *Am Pharm.* 1994;NS34:26-35.

57. Paolini M, Pozzetti L, Pedulli GF, et al. The nature of prooxidant activity of vitamin C. *Life Sci.* 1999;64:273-8.

58. Marcus R, Coulston AM. Water soluble vitamins, the vitamin B complex, and ascorbic acid. In: Hardman JG, Limbird LE, eds. *Goodman and Gilman's The Pharmacological Basis of Therapeutics.* 9th ed. New York: McGraw Hill; 1996:1555-72.

59. Gibbons LW, Gonzalez V, Gordon N, et al. The prevalence of side effects with regular and sustained-release nicotinic acid. *Am J Med.* 1995;99:378-85.

60. Leklem JE. Vitamin B$_6$. In: Shils ME, Olson JA, Shike M, et al., eds. *Modern Nutrition in Health and Disease.* 9th ed. Baltimore: Williams and Wilkins; 1999:413-21.

61. Chandra R, Sudhakaran L. Regulation of immune responses by vitamin B$_6$. *Ann NY Acad Sci.* 1990;585:404-23.

62. Rogers KS, Mohan C. Vitamin B$_6$ metabolism and diabetes. *Biochem Med Metab Biol.* 1994;52:10-7.

63. U.S. Department of Agriculture. *USDA Nutrient Database for Standard Reference*. Washington, DC: Agricultural Research Service; 1999. Release 13.

64. Gregory JF. Bioavailability of vitamin B_6. *Eur J Clin Nutr.* 1997;51(suppl 1):S43-8.

65. Weir MR, Keniston RC, Enriquez JI, et al. Depression of vitamin B_6 levels due to theophylline. *Ann Allergy.* 1990;65:59-62.

66. Institute of Medicine, Food and Nutrition Board. *Dietary Reference Intakes: Thiamin, riboflavin, niacin, vitamin B_6, folate, vitamin B_{12}, pantothenic acid, biotin, and choline*. Washington, DC: National Academy Press; 1998.

67. Refsum H, Ueland PM, Nygard O, et al. Homocysteine and cardiovascular disease. *Annu Rev Med.* 1998;49:31-62.

68. Copeland DA, Stoukides CA. Pyridoxine in carpal tunnel syndrome. *Ann Pharmacother.* 1994;28:1042-4.

69. Johnson SR. Premenstrual syndrome therapy. *Clin Obstet Gynecol.* 1998;41:405-21.

70. Ludwig ML, Drennan CL, Matthews RG. The reactivity of B_{12} cofactors: the proteins make a difference. *Structure.* 1996;4:505-12.

71. Banerjee R. The yin-yang of cobalamin biochemistry. *Chem Biol.* 1997;4:175-86.

72. Scott JM. The bioavailability of vitamin B_{12}. *Eur J Clin Nutr.* 1997;51(suppl 1):S49-S53.

73. Markle HV. Cobalamin. *Crit Rev Clin Lab Sci.* 1996;33:247-356.

74. Delva MD. Vitamin B_{12} replacement, to B_{12} or not to B_{12}? *Can Fam Physician.* 1997;43:917-22.

75. Kapadia CR. Vitamin B_{12} in health and disease: part I—inherited disorders of function, absorption, and transport. *Gastroenterologist.* 1995;3:329-44.

76. Markle HV. Cobalamin. *Crit Rev Clin Lab Sci.* 1996;66:750-9.

77. Malinow MR. Plasma homocyst(e)ine and arterial occlusive diseases: a mini-review. *Clin Chem.* 1995;41:173-6.

78. Zittoun J. Anemias due to disorder of folate, vitamin B_{12} and transcobalamin metabolism. *Rev Prat.* 1993;43:1358-63.

79. Crandall BF, Corson VL, Evans MI, et al. American College of Medical Genetics statement on folic acid: fortification and supplementation. *Am J Med Genet.* 1998;78:381.

80. Kelly GS. Folates: supplemental forms and therapeutic applications. *Altern Med Rev.* 1998;3:208-20.

81. Herbert V. Folic Acid. In: Shils M, Olson J, Shike M, et al., eds. *Modern Nutrition in Health and Disease.* 9th ed. Baltimore: Williams & Wilkins; 1999.

82. Shaw GM, Schaffer D, Velie EM, et al. Periconceptional vitamin use, dietary folate, and the occurrence of neural tube defects. *Epidemiology.* 1995;6:219-26.

83. Shaw GM, Lammer EJ, Wasserman CR, et al. Risks of orofacial clefts in children born to women using multivitamins containing folic acid periconceptionally. *Lancet.* 1995;346:393-6.

84. Hoag SW, Ramachandruni H, Shangraw RF. Failure of prescription prenatal vitamin products to meet USP standards for folic acid dissolution. *J Am Pharm Assoc (Wash).* 1997;NS37:397-400.

85. Refsum H, Ueland PM, Nygard O, et al. Homocysteine and cardiovascular disease. *Annu Rev Med.* 1998;49:31-62.

86. Freudenheim JL, Grahm S, Marshall JR, et al. Folate intake and carcinogenesis of the colon and rectum. *Int J Epidemiol.* 1991;20:368-74.

87. Christensen B. Folate deficiency, cancer and congenital abnormalities: is there a connection? *Tidsskr Nor Laegeforen.* 1996;116:250-4.

88. Jennings E. Folic acid as a cancer preventing agent. *Med Hypotheses.* 1995;45:297-303.

89. Shiroky JB. The use of folates concomitantly with low-dose pulse methotrexate. *Rheum Dis Clin North Am.* 1997;23:969-80.

90. Keshava C, Keshava N, Whong WZ, et al. Inhibition of methotrexate-induced chromosomal damage by folinic acid in V79 cells. *Mutat Res.* 1998;397:221-8.

91. Morgan SL, Baggott JE. Folate antagonists in nonneoplastic disease: proposed mechanisms of efficacy and toxicity. In: Bailey LB, ed. *Folate in Health and Disease.* New York: Marcel Dekker; 1995:405-33.

92. Ivey M, Elmer G. Nutritional supplement, mineral and vitamin products. In: *Handbook of Nonprescription Drugs.* 10th ed. Washington, DC: American Pharmaceutical Association; 1993:474-5.

93. Bouillon R, Carmeliet G, Boonen S. Aging and calcium metabolism. *Baillieres Clin Endocrinol Metab.* 1997;11:341-65.

94. American Pharmaceutical Association. *Therapeutic Options for Osteoporosis Special Report*. Washington, DC: American Pharmaceutical Association; 1993.

95. National Institutes of Health (NIH) Consensus Statement. *Optimal calcium intake*. Rockville, MD: National Institutes of Health; 1994;12(4):1-31.

96. Levy S. Calcium supplements for reducing PMS symptoms. *Drug Topics.* September 21, 1998;52.

97. Garland C, Shekelle RB, Barrett-Connor E, et al. Dietary vitamin D and calcium and risk of colorectal cancer: a 19-year prospective study in men. *Lancet.* 1985;1:307-9.

98. Haines ST, Caceres B, Yancey L. Alternatives to estrogen replacement therapy for preventing osteoporosis. *J Am Pharm Assoc (Wash)*. 1996;NS36:707-15.

99. Goebel SR, Willhite SL. Calcium intake in adolescence. *US Pharmacist*. 1998;23:50-6.

100. Miller DR, Hanel HJ. Prevention and treatment of osteoporosis. *US Pharmacist*. 1999;24:81-90.

101. O'Connell MA. Gastrointestinal tolerance of oral calcium supplements. *Clin Pharm*. 1989;8:425-7.

102. Nolan CR. Aluminum and lead absorption from dietary sources in women ingesting calcium citrate. *South Med J*. 1994;87:894-8.

103. Centers for Disease Control and Prevention. Recommendations to prevent and control iron deficiency in the United States. *MMWR Morb Mortal Wkly Rep*. 1998;47(RR-3):1-26.

104. Institute of Medicine Food and Nutrition Board. *Dietary Reference Intakes for Vitamin A, Vitamin K, Arsenic, Boron, Chromium, Copper, Iodine, Iron, Manganese, Molybdenum, Nickel, Silicon, Vanadium, and Zinc*. Washington, DC: National Academy Press; 2001.

105. Uzel C, Conrad ME. Absorption of heme iron. *Semin Hematol*. 1998;35:27-34.

106. Fairweather-Tait S, Fox T, Wharf SG, et al. The bioavailability of iron in different weaning foods and the enhancing effect of a fruit drink containing ascorbic acid. *Pediatr Res*. 1995;62:785-9.

107. DeSimmons EM, Funk BT. Who should take iron supplements? *US Pharmacist*. 1995;20:26-31.

108. Cook JD, Skikne BS, Baynes RD. Iron deficiency: the global perspective. *Adv Exp Med Biol*. 1994;356:219-28.

109. Ekman M, Reizenstein P. Comparative absorption of ferrous and heme-iron with meals in normal and iron deficient subjects. *Zeitschrift fur Ernahrungswissenschaft* 1993;32:67-70.

110. Beutler E, Lichtman MA, Coller BS, et al. Anemias of Chronic Disease. In: Babior B. ed. *Hematology*. 5th ed. New York: McGraw-Hill Inc; 1995:518-24.

111. Burke W, Cogswell ME, McDonnell SM, et al. Public health strategies to prevent the complications of hemochromatosis. In: Khoury MJ, Burke W, Thomson EJ, eds. *Genetics and Public Health in the 21st Century: Using Genetic Information to Improve Health and Prevent Disease*. New York: Oxford University Press; 2000.

112. Mangione RA. What impact does strenuous activity have on magnesium levels? *US Pharmacist*. 1997;22:102-5.

113. Carlstedt BC. Role of magnesium in cardiovascular wellness. *US Pharmacist*. 1997;22:107-16.

114. Cowan JA. Preface. In: Cowan JA, ed. *The Biological Chemistry of Magnesium*. New York: VCH Publishers; 1995:vii-viii.

115. Institute of Medicine Food and Nutrition Board. *Dietary Reference Intakes: Calcium, Phosphorus, Magnesium, Vitamin D and Fluoride*. Washington, DC: National Academy Press; 1999.

116. Woods KL, Fletcher S, Roffe C, et al. Intravenous magnesium sulfate in suspected acute myocardial infarction: results of the second Leicester Magnesium Intervention Trial (LIMIT-2). *Lancet*. 1992;339:1553-8.

117. McSweeney GW. Fluid and electrolyte therapy and acid-base balance. In: Herfindal ET, Gourley DR, Hart LL, eds. *Clinical Pharmacy and Therapeutics*. Baltimore: Williams & Wilkins; 1992:105-21.

118. Shils ME. Magnesium. In: Shils ME, Olson, JA, Shike M, eds. *Modern Nutrition in Health and Disease*. Vol 1. 8th ed. Philadelphia: Lea & Febiger; 1994:164.

119. Clarkson PM, Haymes EM. Exercise and mineral status of athletes: calcium, magnesium, phosphorous and iron. *Med Sci Sports Exerc*. 1995;27:821-43.

120. Kelepouris E, Agus ZS. Hypomagnesemia: renal magnesium handling. *Semin Nephrol*. 1998;18:58-73.

121. Ascherio A, Hennekens C, Willett WC, et al. Prospective study on nutritional factors, blood pressure, and hypertension among U S women. *Hypertension*. 1996;27:1065-72.

122. Sacks FM, Appel LJ, Moore TJ, et al. A dietary approach to prevent hypertension: a review of the Dietary Approaches to Stop Hypertension (DASH) study. *Clin Cardiol*. 1999;22:6-10.

123. Liao F, Folsom A, Brancati F. Is low magnesium concentration a risk factor for coronary heart disease: the Atherosclerosis Risk In Communities (ARIC) study. *Am Heart J*. 1998;136:480-90.

124. Ascherio A, Rimm EB, Hernan MA, et al. Intake of potassium, magnesium, calcium, and fiber and risk of stroke among U S men. *Circulation*. 1998;98:1198-204.

125. University Medical Center. Drug use issues and actions: guidelines for phosphorous supplementation in adults. *Formulary*. 1998;33:263.

126. Corvilain B, Contempre B, Longombe AO, et al. Selenium and the thyroid: how the relationship was established. *Am J Clin Nutr*. 1993;57(suppl 2):244S-8S.

127. Combs GF Jr, Combs SB. Selenium in Human Diets. In: *The Role of Selenium in Nutrition*. Orlando: Academic Press; 1986:98-107.

128. Levander OA, Beck MA. Interacting nutritional and infectious etiologies of Keshan disease: insights from coxsackie virus B-induced myocarditis in mice deficient in selenium or vitamin E. *Biol Trace Elem Res*. 1997;56:5-21.

129. Itokawa Y. Trace elements in long-term total parenteral nutrition. *Nippon Rinsho*. 1996;54:172-8.

130. Knekt P, Marniemi J, Teppo L, et al. Is low selenium status a risk factor for lung cancer? *Am J Epidemiol*. 1998;148:975-82.
131. Young KL, Lee PN. Intervention studies on cancer. *Eur J Cancer Prev*. 1999;8:91-103.
132. Hercberg S, Galan P, Preziosi P, et al. Background and rationale behind the SU.VI.MAX study, a prevention trial using nutritional doses of a combination of antioxidant vitamins and minerals to reduce cardiovascular diseases and cancers: SUpplementation en VItamines et Mineraux Antio-Xydants Study. *Int J Vitam Nutr Res*. 1998;68:3-20.
133. Aseth J, Haugen M, Forre O. Rheumatoid arthritis and metal compounds: perspectives on the role of oxygen radical detoxification. *Analyst*. 1998;123:3-6.
134. Maher TJ. Chromium and other minerals in diabetes mellitus. *US Pharmacist*. 1999;24:66-76.
135. Koller LD, Exon JH. The two faces of selenium-deficiency and toxicity are similar in animals and man. *Can J Vet Res*. 1986;50:297-306.
136. Borsel JS, Anderson RA. Chromium. In: Frieden, E, ed. *Biochemistry of the Essential Ultratrace Minerals*. New York: Plenum; 1984:175-99.
137. Anderson RA. Chromium, glucose intolerance and diabetes. *J Am Coll Nutr*. 1998;17:548-55.
138. Anderson RA, Cheng N, Bryden NA, et al. Beneficial effects of chromium for people with diabetes. *Diabetes*. 1997;46:1786-91.
139. Ravina A, Slezak L, Rubal A, et al. Clinical use of the trace element chromium (III) in the treatment of diabetes mellitus. *J Trace Elem Exper Med*. 1995;8:183-90.
140. Wise A. Phytate and zinc bioavailability. *Int J Food Sci Nutr*. 1995;46:53-63.
141. Garland ML, Hagmeyer KO. The role of zinc lozenges in treatment of the common cold. *Ann Pharmacother*. 1998;32:63-9.
142. Gibson RS. Content and bioavailability of trace elements in vegetarian diets. *Am J Clin Nutr*. 1994;59:1223S-32S.
143. Prasad AS. Zinc deficiency in women, infants and children. *J Am Coll Nutr*. 1996;15:113-20.
144. Yarze JC, Martin P, Munoz SJ, et al. Wilson's disease: current status. *Am J Med*. 1992;92:643-54.
145. Fosmire GJ. Zinc toxicity. *Am J Clin Nutr*. 1990;51:225-7.
146. Lichtenstein GR, Burke F. Gastrointestinal disease. In: Morrison G, Hark L, eds. *Medical Nutrition and Disease*. Cambridge: Blackwell Science; 1996:204-18.
147. Beyer PL. Digestion, absorption, transport and excretion of nutrients. In: Mahan LK, Escott-Stum S, eds. *Krause's Food, Nutrition & Diet Therapy*. 10th ed. Philadelphia: WB Saunders Company; 2000:12-5.
148. Johnson RK. Energy. In: Mahan LK, Escott-Stum S, eds. *Krause's Food, Nutrition & Diet Therapy*. 10th ed. Philadelphia: WB Saunders Company; 2000:19-30.
149. Food and Nutrition Board, National Research Council, National Academy of Sciences. *Recommended Dietary Allowances*. 10th ed. Washington, DC: National Academy Press; 1989:27.
150. Goran MI, Sun M. Total energy expenditure and physical activity in prepubertal children: recent advances based on the application of the doubly labeled water method. *Am J Clin Nutr*. 1998;68:944S-9S.
151. Harris JA, Benedict FG. *A Biometric Study of Basal Metabolism in Man*. Washington, DC: Carnegie Institute of Washington; 1919: Pub No. 279.
152. Daly JM, Heymsfield SB, Head CA, et al. Human energy requirements: overestimation by widely used prediction equation. *Am J Clin Nutr*. 1985;42:1170-4.
153. McCrory P, Strauss B, Wahlquist ML. Energy balance, food intake, and obesity. In: Hills AP, Wahlquist ML, eds. *Exercise and Obesity*. London: Smith-Gordon and Co Ltd; 1994.
154. Expert Panel on the Identification, Evaluation, and Treatment of Overweight in Adults. Clinical guidelines on the identification, evaluation, and treatment of overweight and obesity in adults: executive summary. *Am J Clin Nutr*. 1998;68:899-917.
155. Shikany JM. Dietary guidelines for chronic disease prevention. *South Med J*. 2000;93:1157-61.
156. Kroke A, Bergmann M, Klipstein-Grobusch K, et al. Obesity, body fat distribution and body build: their relation to blood pressure and prevalence of hypertension. *Int J Obes Relat Metab Disord*. 1998;22:1062-70.
157. Albanes D. Caloric intake, body weight, and cancer: a review. *Nutr Cancer*. 1987;9:199-217.
158. Fagan C. Nutrition during pregnancy and lactation. In: Mahan LK, Escott-Stum S, eds. *Krause's Food, Nutrition & Diet Therapy*. 10th ed. Philadelphia: WB Saunders Company; 2000:167-95.
159. Food and Nutrition Board, National Research Council, National Academy of Sciences; *Recommended Dietary Allowances*. 10th ed. Washington, DC: National Academy Press: 1989:27.
160. Casanueva E, Polo E, Tejero E, et al. Premature rupture of amniotic membranes as functional assessment of vitamin C status during pregnancy. *Ann N Y Acad Sci*. 1993;678:369-70.
161. Tamura T, Goldenberg RL, Johnston KE, et al. Maternal plasma zinc concentrations and pregnancy outcome. *Am J Clin Nutr*. 2000;71:109-13.
162. Lenders CM, Ahlstrom Henderson S. Nutrition in pregnancy and lactation. In: Morrison G, Hark L, eds. *Medical Nutrition and Disease*. Cambridge: Blackwell Science; 1996:69-101.

163. Nehlig A, Debry G. Potential teratogenic and developmental consequences of coffee and caffeine exposure: a review on human and animal data. *Neurotoxicol Teratol.* 1994;16:531-43.

164. Krebs NF. Zinc supplementation during lactation. *Am J Clin Nutr.* 1998;68(suppl 2):509S.

165. Wothington-Roberts BS, Williams SR. *Nutrition in Pregnancy and Lactation.* 5th ed. St. Louis: Mosby; 1993.

166. Kim SK, Cheong WS, Jun YH, et al. Red blood cell indices and iron status according to feeding practices in infants and young children. *Acta Paediatr.* 1996;85:139-44.

167. Trahms CM. Nutrition in infancy. In: Mahan LK, Escott-Stum S, eds. *Krause's Food, Nutrition & Diet Therapy.* 10th ed. Philadelphia: W B Saunders Company; 2000:196-213.

168. Greer FR. Vitamin K deficiency and hemorrhage in infancy. *Clin Perinatol.* 1995;22:759.

169. Cryan J, Johnson RK. Should the current recommendations for energy intake in infants and young children be lowered? *Nutrition Today.* 1997;32:69.

170. Lucas, B. Nutrition in childhood. In: Mahan LK, Escott-Stum S, eds. *Krause's Food, Nutrition & Diet Therapy.* 10th ed. Philadelphia: WB Saunders Company; 2000:239-56.

171. Yates AA, Schlicker SA, Suitor, CW. Dietary reference intakes: the new basis for recommendations for calcium and related nutrients, B vitamins and choline. *J Am Diet Assoc.* 1998;98:699-706.

172. Striegel-Moore RH. Risk factors for eating disorders. *Ann NY Acad Sci.*1997:98-109.

173. Lee MF, Krasinski SD. Human adult-onset lactase decline: an update. *Nutr Rev.* 1998;56:1-8.

174. Harris NG. Nutrition in aging. In: Mahan LK, Escott-Stum S, eds. *Krause's Food, Nutrition & Diet Therapy.* 10th ed. Philadelphia: WB Saunders Company; 2000:287-305.

175. Siegler E, Hark L. Older adults. In: Morrison G, Hark L, eds. *Medical Nutrition and Disease.* Cambridge: Blackwell Science; 1996:142-71.

176. Chernoff R. Thirst and fluid requirements. *Nutr Rev.* 1994;52:S3-5.

177. Seddon JM, Ajani UA, Sperduto RD, et al. Dietary carotenoids, vitamins A, C, and E, and advanced age-related macular degeneration. Eye Disease Case-Control Study Group. *JAMA.* 1994;272:1413-20.

CHAPTER 2

THE PHARMACIST'S ROLE IN DIETARY COUNSELING

Grace M. Kuo, Victoria DeVore, and Lynn Simpson

The public's burgeoning interest in herbal products, vitamins, alternative medicine, and wellness is prompting today's pharmacists to expand their knowledge of nutrition. Pharmacists provide a valuable service by communicating dietary needs to the public, helping patients plan a healthy diet, and giving advice about the confusing array of nutritional aids on the market. Monitoring patients for safe use of dietary supplements and preventing adverse interactions between herbal supplements, medications, and foods are also key roles for pharmacists.

People need proper nutrition to achieve developmental growth, maintain good health, support an active lifestyle, and reduce the risk of heart disease, diabetes, stroke, cancer, and other health problems. Although everyone should eat a well-balanced diet, groups that especially need good nutrition—and therefore stand to benefit the most from pharmacists' assistance—are infants, pregnant and lactating women, people with chronic or acute medical conditions, and the geriatric population.

Nutrients can be derived from foods, from herbs, and from nutritional supplements. Although nutritional supplements can enhance health, some have been found to interfere with prescribed medications, fueling a growing concern in the United States[1-4] that herbal products could have detrimental effects for some people. An estimated one-third of the 1539 to 2055 randomly selected adults in a national survey conducted between 1990 and 1997 used herbal remedies,[4,5] and roughly 15 million patients are at risk of potential drug–herbal supplement interactions.[6]

Of greater concern is that 70% of people who use herbal remedies do not discuss them with their physicians or pharmacists.[7] This lack of communication makes it very difficult for health care professionals to monitor adverse interactions between drugs and herbs or nutritional supplements. Also, many people are unaware of the symptoms they should report to health care professionals when they experience adverse effects from interactions.

PHARMACISTS' NUTRITIONAL SERVICES

In the United States, herbs, vitamins, and nutritional supplements are considered dietary supplements rather than drugs. Consequently, information about dosage and indications, as well as warnings and precautions, do not appear on the product label. For this reason, pharmacists provide a crucial service when they counsel patients about the proper use of nutritional products and discuss possible interactions with medications.

Because pharmacists are more accessible to the public than other health care professionals, you may be patients' only immediate contact for health care information—especially in today's managed care environment, which allows limited time for patient–physician interaction. Among the topics that pharmacists are well qualified to address, for both patients and health care professionals:

- Drugs that deplete the body of nutrients.
- Interactions between prescribed medications.
- Interactions between prescribed medications and food or over-the-counter drugs.
- Interactions between drugs and nutritional or herbal supplements.
- Enteral and parenteral nutrition.
- Pharmaceutical care that includes designing, implementing, and monitoring pharmacotherapeutic plans to produce desirable clinical outcomes for the patient.

Pharmacists are drug experts who are well trained to evaluate adverse events and drug-related interactions, including those associated with herbal medicinals and nutritional supplements. Many adverse events and medication errors occur in the inpatient setting.[8,9] Pharmacists have helped to reduce these adverse events through medication review and pharmaceutical care services.[10,11] Many types of medication errors also occur in outpatient pharmaceutical therapy,[12-14] and pharmacists play an important role in addressing them.[15] Medication errors could come from failure to maintain an accurate list of current medications, drug–drug interactions, failure to inquire about over-the-counter medication and herbal supplement use, unanticipated adverse reactions, failure to take the medication as prescribed, and failure to order appropriate laboratory tests to monitor drug therapy. Because medication error is a growing problem, it is more important than ever that pharmacists get involved in helping patients avoid unnecessary adverse effects from drugs and supplements.

Pharmacists also play a key role in networks of health care professionals who manage patients' nutritional support and drug therapy.[16] Pharmacists on a multidisciplinary team of physicians, nurses, and dietitians can use their expertise in drug therapy management by reviewing medication histories, evaluating the effectiveness of drug therapy, ensuring safe use of medication dosages, preventing undesirable drug-related interactions, and providing education on proper administration of medications.

Pharmacists' Dietary Role

Pharmacists' goals in assisting patients and health care professionals with dietary needs are to:

❑ Assess the parenteral or enteral nutritional needs of patients or their need for nutritional, dietary, or herbal supplements while considering all their medical conditions.

❑ Advise patients on nutritional products and supplements and check for appropriate dose, concentration, formulation, route of administration, planned duration of use, and expiration.

❑ Ensure safe use of nutritional and dietary supplements by monitoring laboratory tests (e.g., serum electrolytes, liver function tests, kidney function tests) and physical examinations (e.g., skin reactions).

❑ Prevent adverse interactions between nutritional and dietary supplements and medications.

❑ Prevent delays in initiating appropriate drug therapy (e.g., chemotherapy or treatments for terminal disease) so patients can seek timely medical care.

❑ Promote public health by encouraging the safe use of nutritional and dietary supplements and by reporting adverse reactions.

Reviews and studies conducted to determine how often pharmacists help maintain the nutritional needs of patients suggest that pharmacists' involvement is increasing. The clinical role of pharmacists in developing interventions in nutritional support that promote optimal pharmaceutical care has been validated.[17] For example, the 1989 National Survey of Hospital-based Pharmacy Services indicated that 28% of pharmacists participate in parenteral–enteral nutritional support teams, 26% counsel patients directly about their medications, and 25% participate in managing drug therapy protocols.[18] In 1995, the National Clinical Pharmacy Services Study showed that pharmacists' participation in these areas had increased, respectively, by 6%, 13%, and 15%.[19]

For years pharmacists have helped provide nutritional support services in the inpatient setting by:

- Assessing the energy needs of patients.[20,21]
- Evaluating drug-related problems in clinical nutrition patients.[22]
- Educating patients and health-care professionals about drug–nutrient interactions.[23]
- Preventing medication errors related to nutrition support.[24]

In a study in which pharmacists provided nutritional support consultation to physicians, the parenteral nutrition therapy that physicians prescribed was more therapeutically effective and allowed patients to make the transition from parenteral to enteral nutrition sooner.[25] Patients could use their gut function more quickly instead of relying on injections to receive nutrition, and could avoid injection site infection. Furthermore, the pharmacist consultation provided better, more cost-effective therapies for patients and health care organizations.

Pharmacists have also provided nutritional support services in the home care setting.[26,27] Many infusion pharmacies mix total parenteral nutrition (TPN) and peripheral parenteral nutrition (PPN) preparations to be delivered to patients' residences or nursing homes. Pharmacists working in this setting offer their expertise in compounding and preparing intravenous admixtures to ensure that nutritional therapies are produced accurately. They also evaluate the patient's medication history to avoid potential drug–food interactions.

Pharmacists play a crucial role in optimizing infant nutrition by counseling pregnant and lactating women.[28] Many medications cross the placenta from the pregnant woman to her baby and may have significant adverse effects during the different trimesters. Similarly, some medications are excreted in breast milk and can have undesirable effects on the nursing baby. Pharmacists are instrumental in giving pregnant women and nursing mothers timely information about nutritional needs and potential drug-related interactions.

In ambulatory care and community pharmacy settings, pharmacists give patients information about the safe use of nutritional supplements and herbal medicinals. They provide counseling services as well as educational materials (e.g., brochures, monograph handouts, video programs, and interactive computer aids) promoting the safe use of herbs, neutraceuticals, and vitamins.

PATIENT HISTORY

As with all medications, whether prescription or over the counter (OTC), it is vital to obtain a detailed patient history before discussing a particular herbal, vitamin, or nutritional remedy. This overview of the patient's health enables you to pinpoint his or her specific problem—which may be different from the one he or she seeks to treat—and to make the most appropriate recommendation, be it an herbal remedy, an OTC medication, referral to another health care provider for a prescription medication, or no drug at all. Generally, the patient history should include the following:

- Age and gender.
- Pregnancy or breastfeeding status.
- Allergies.
- Concurrent medical problems, especially those that could alter or aggravate the effects of the chosen herbal remedy.
- Drug history, including current prescription medications, OTC medications, herbal remedies, nutraceuticals (foods or naturally occurring supplements thought to have beneficial health effects), and social drugs (i.e., caffeine, nicotine, alcohol, and illicit drugs).

A sample form for obtaining a patient history appears in Figure 2-1.

Patient Name: _____

| Last | First | Middle |

Address: _____

| Street | | Apt # |

_____

| City | State | Zip Code |

Telephone: _____ **SS#:** _____ **Gender:** M   F

Date of Birth: _____   **Child Resistant Packaging:** Yes No

Generic Medications if Possible: Yes   No

Prescription Insurance: _____   **ID#:** _____

Cardholder's Name: _____   **Relationship to Cardholder:** _____

MEDICAL INFORMATION

Known Allergies and Drug Reactions   **Current Health Conditions**

Known Allergies and Drug Reactions	Current Health Conditions	
☐ NO KNOWN ALLERGIES/DRUG REACTIONS	☐ ANGINA	☐ KIDNEY DISEASE
☐ ASPIRIN	☐ ANEMIA	☐ LIVER DISEASE
☐ CEPHALOSPORINS	☐ ARTHRITIS	☐ LUNG DISEASE
☐ CODEINE	☐ ASTHMA	☐ PARKINSONS
☐ ERYTHROMYCIN	☐ BLOOD CLOTS	☐ PREGNANCY
☐ PENICILLINS	☐ BREASTFEEDING	☐ ULCER
☐ SULFA DRUGS	☐ CANCER	☐ OTHERS
☐ TETRACYCLINES	☐ DIABETES	☐ _____
☐ XANTHINES (EX. THEOPHYLLINE)	☐ HEART CONDITION	☐ _____
☐ OTHERS:	☐ HIGH BLOOD PRESSURE	

SOCIAL DRUG USE: ☐ Alcohol   ☐ Caffeine   ☐ Tobacco   ☐ Illicit substances

CURRENT PRESCRIPTION MEDICATION REGIMEN:

NAME/DOSE/STRENGTH	FREQUENCY OF USE	INDICATION	PRESCRIBER

CURRENT NONPRESCRIPTION MEDICATION REGIMEN: OTC, HERBAL, NUTRITIONAL

NAME/DOSE/STRENGTH	FREQUENCY OF USE	INDICATION	PRESCRIBER

PHARMACIST'S NOTES: _____

PHARMACIST'S NOTES:

FIGURE 2-1   Patient Profile Form

ACCOMMODATING DIVERSITY

Because pharmacists are at the front line of health care, they deal with patients from all walks of life and all backgrounds. The United States is a culturally diverse nation with many residents who do not speak English as their primary language and who may have different medical traditions and culturally based health beliefs.[29]

As a pharmacist, you must deal not only with cultural barriers but also with such communication obstacles as impaired hearing or vision, dementia, illiteracy, and heightened emotional states (e.g., feelings of anger, embarrassment, or sadness). Some patients may withhold information for personal reasons; others may engage in emotional outbursts that disrupt the counseling process. You must know how to tailor your counseling for each patient.

Health beliefs and religious practices can especially affect the nutritional aspects of medical care. For instance, medication schedules may need to be adjusted for Muslim patients during Ramadan, a month-long period of daily fasting from dawn to sunset. (The dates of Ramadan differ every year because they are based on the Muslim calendar.) This fasting during daylight hours can considerably lower the blood sugar levels of patients who take insulin or oral hypoglycemics and could potentially lead to coma or death.[29]

Many Jewish people follow strict dietary laws that determine whether a food product is kosher and acceptable to be eaten. If you need to recommend a nutritional supplement to a Jewish patient, you may need to determine whether it is considered to be kosher—information that may be available from manufacturers, the Internet, or local rabbis. A helpful Web site on kosher products is http://www.ou.org. Followers of religions that practice vegetarianism as part of their traditional belief, such as Buddhism, may have nutritional deficiencies and require supplementation (e.g., vitamin B_{12}).

Another special group to consider is the elderly, a growing segment of the population. Elderly people typically take many more prescribed medications daily than do younger adults and they consume many OTC drugs and herbal products. In fact, it has been estimated that patients over the age of 65 consume 30% of all prescription drugs and 40% of all OTC products.[31] Because of this high volume of prescribed, OTC, and alternative medicines, the elderly are especially at risk for experiencing side effects or adverse events from drug interactions and can benefit significantly from intervention and counseling by the pharmacist.[32]

COUNSELING TIPS

You can provide a valuable service by counseling patients about dietary supplements, many of which make broad therapeutic claims encompassing everything from the common cold to cancer. In the past, pharmacists simply relayed drug information while counseling patients. It was a passive process, and not terribly effective. Today we understand that good counseling should be interactive. In an interactive counseling session, you use open-ended questions that cannot be answered by a simple "yes" or "no."

Tips on Tailoring Counseling to Your Patient

1. Make scheduled appointments with patients who may require detailed counseling.
2. Consider each patient on an individual basis. Do not simply label someone as visually impaired, hearing impaired, non-English speaking, etc.
3. Keep in mind that the patient is *not* the problem. He or she simply presents a unique situation that requires you to adjust your counseling.
4. Pharmacists should suspect that a language barrier may exist when patients ask no questions, cannot follow simple medication instructions, or always bring someone to the pharmacy with them.
5. Avoid using technical words to describe the patient's medications or medical conditions.
6. Be sure that the counseling area is wheelchair accessible, well lit, and quiet.
7. For patients who are visually impaired, provide directions in large print, use color-coding for different medications, and vary the size of the medication containers.
8. Talk directly to the patient, making good eye contact. Do not focus instead on the caregiver or accompanying family member.

For patients with particularly difficult medication regimens, or patients with low literacy:

9. Use visual aids (e.g., calendar, picture of medications, stick figure warning labels), to enhance understanding.
10. Elicit feedback from patients during the counseling session by having them recite key instructions back to you.

Source: Reference 30.

Open-ended questions are useful for verifying that patients know how to take their medication properly and that they fully understand all pertinent information.

Some key questions you can use are[33]:

- What did your doctor tell you the medication is for?
- How did your doctor tell you to take the medication?
- What did your doctor tell you to expect?

Open-ended questions can also help you determine patients' needs and assess whether their specific ailments are amenable to self-treatment. See the sidebar on page 62 for sample questions to use when patients are selecting herbal remedies and dietary supplements. (For an example of how to use these questions in practice, see the case study on page 64.)

Questions for Patients Seeking Dietary Supplements

- ❏ For what condition are you using this supplement?
- ❏ What current allergies do you have?
- ❏ What plants are you allergic to?
- ❏ What current dietary restrictions do you have?
- ❏ What other medications are you currently taking?
- ❏ What other OTCs, herbs, or supplements are you currently taking?
- ❏ If you have used this product before, how long did you use it? What dosage form of this product did you take? For example, was it a capsule, tea, tablet, tincture, or homeopathic pellet?
- ❏ What other current medical conditions do you have?
- ❏ Is this product going to be used by you or is this remedy for someone else?
- ❏ Which medications you are taking now or have tried in the past have been successful at relieving your symptoms?

TRUST AND EMPATHY

To effectively counsel patients, you must first establish a relationship of trust. That is, patients must feel that you care about their well-being and have their best interests in mind. Establishing trust involves making an effort to become familiarized with the patient, developing a feeling of rapport, maintaining confidentiality, and making patients feel comfortable enough to express themselves and discuss personal matters.

Although the core principle of counseling is to help patients understand how to use their medications properly and manage their disease, you can also help patients understand their symptoms. For example, extensive counseling and nutritional education help patients with diabetes manage the acute and chronic symptoms, such as hyperglycemia, and prevent long-term complications, such as retinopathy, nephropathy, and neuropathy.

Part of building trust is conveying empathy to the patient. Empathy, one of the most essential variables in the communication process, helps patients see that you understand their problems and are sensitive to their needs.[34] Both verbal and nonverbal cues help impart empathy. Verbally, you must exhibit concern and acceptance so that the patient feels encouraged to share anxieties and feelings. Nonverbally, you must use tone of voice, facial expressions, gestures, eye contact, and voice characteristics to reinforce your willingness to help the patient.[30] If you do not seem empathetic, patients will feel that they are not understood and will conclude that the counseling session is not useful or important.

ADVERSE REACTIONS

Warning patients about potential adverse reactions is critical when you are counseling about medications and dietary products. Patients must be

Guidelines for Counseling Patients

❑ Take a thorough patient history, including the patient's age, chief complaints, history of present illness, review of systems, and past family and social history.

❑ Evaluate the patient's current use of medications to identify, and thereby prevent, adverse effects that could arise from interactions between medications, nutritional supplements, and herbal remedies.

❑ Take into consideration the patient's cultural background, medical traditions, and health beliefs.

❑ Establish a relationship of trust with the patient and treat the patient with empathy.

❑ Encourage interactive conversations with patients so that they will have the opportunity to ask nutrition-related questions and to understand the use of their medication(s) or dietary supplement(s).

informed about potentially dangerous side effects or drug interactions to decrease their risk of developing them.

An example of a drug–food interaction that can cause serious harm is the combination of monoamine oxidase (MAO) inhibitors and foods containing tyramine, which can cause an insidious rise in the patient's blood pressure. Some foods that contain tyramine are aged meats and cheeses, beer, red wine, hard liquors, smoked or pickled foods, and yeast-containing products.

Patients also need to be told whether they can drink alcohol while taking their medications or herbal products because alcohol may act synergistically with the supplement, causing potential hepatotoxicity. The recent controversy concerning kava (*Piper methysticum*) provides an excellent example. Kava has long been associated with Polynesia, where it has been used as a ceremonial and ritualistic herb for culminating marriages and welcoming dignitaries and as a medicinal herb for relaxation and urinary tract infections.[35]

In the United States, kava has been used to treat anxiety, stress, and restlessness. Kava's mechanism of action is largely unknown, but the prevailing thought is that the active ingredient of kava is a class of molecules known as kavalactones. These molecules seem to affect the limbic system, the emotional center of the brain, working on the same amino acid sites as the benzodiazepines. While diazepam binds to GABA receptors, however, kava causes more of these receptors to be formed. Because of this relationship to benzodiazepines, pharmacists should caution patients about avoiding alcohol when using kava and also to avoid operating machinery or driving. Reports of arrests while driving under the influence have surfaced in the media when kava is used concurrently with alcohol. There are also concerns about hepatotoxicity when kava is used chronically or with alcohol. Based on anecdotal evidence and case reports concerning the hepatotoxicity of kava, the Food and Drug Administration, American Botanical Council, and other agencies have issued these guidelines[36]:

- Kava should not be used by anyone with liver problems, taking any drug product that has known adverse effects on the liver, or who chronically consumes alcohol.
- Kava should not be taken on a daily basis for longer than 4 weeks without the advice of a health care professional.
- Consumers should discontinue use if symptoms of jaundice (e.g., dark urine, yellowing of the eyes or skin) occur.
- Consumers should consult their physician or pharmacist if they have a history of liver problems or suspect liver problems before using kava or continuing its use.

Case Study

The following case illustrates the importance of using open-ended questions when counseling patients about the use of herbal and nutraceutical remedies.

JS is a 42-year-old woman who visits her community pharmacy (or ambulatory care clinic) because of mild symptoms that she attributes to depression. She explains to you, her pharmacist, that she feels listless, has no energy, has difficulty getting up in the morning, and feels sad many times during the week. She has heard her friends talk about an herbal remedy called St. John's wort that is used to treat depression. Since this herbal remedy is "natural," she feels that it couldn't hurt to try it, and asks you for advice. What important information would you elicit from and relay to JS?

DISCUSSION

A medicinal substance cannot elicit a response unless it first activates a receptor site. This activation requires a coupling reaction, much like a lock and key. Once the key opens the response pathway, both therapeutic and adverse effects can occur. Because there is no way to predict which effect will happen, there are no benign chemical entities, even when they are "all natural," as many patients perceive herbal remedies to be. When counseling JS about St. John's wort, it is very important to ask open-ended questions to assess her level of knowledge, correct misinformation, and add any missing information.[37] The following questions should be asked of any patient who is attempting to self-treat with an herbal remedy.

Have you used this product before? If so, how long did you use it? What dosage form did you take?

Herbal supplements are manufactured in many types of dosage forms. St. John's wort, for example, is dispensed as a capsule, tablet, tea, tincture, liquid, oil, or powder. Without your probing, a patient may not recognize that he or she has used the same chemical ingredient in the past in a different formulation. Your questions can help you ascertain whether the patient had any benefits or problems when using a similar ingredient in the past. The recommended daily dosage of this herb is 900 mg, taken three times daily in 300-mg doses that have been standardized to an extract of 0.3% hypericin. For symptoms of mild to moderate depression, St. John's wort can be taken with food for a maximum of 8 weeks without physician supervision.

Do you have any allergies, especially to any plant material?

Herbal remedies are prepared from any plant part such as the flower, root, bark, fruit, or seed that has medicinal properties. If a patient is allergic to a particular species of plant, he or she may also be allergic to the herbal remedy chosen. For example, people who are hypersensitive to ragweed, asters, chrysanthemums, chamomile, and other members of the Asteraceae compositae (daisy) family might also be allergic to echinacea because it is also a member of this family of plants. Individuals with atopy (a genetic tendency toward allergic conditions) may be more likely to experience an allergic reaction when taking echinacea. Unpublished case reports presented at the American Academy of Allergy, Asthma and Immunology (AAAAI) 2000 annual meeting describe 23 cases of allergic reactions to echinacea consistent with IgE-mediated hypersensitivity.[38]

Echinacea is mostly used for upper respiratory tract infections such as the common cold and influenza because of its reported antiviral and immune system stimulatory effects. Echinacea seems to have indirect antiviral activity, possibly by stimulating interferon-like effects. This herbal increases phagocytosis and increases lymphocyte activity, possibly by promoting release of tumor necrosis factor, interleukin-1, and interferon. Echinacea preparations seem to decrease the severity and duration of symptoms associated with influenza-like upper respiratory infections if started when symptoms are first noticed and used for 7–10 days.[38]

Allergies to St. John's wort, another well known herbal remedy, or to its active ingredients, are rare.[36] The flowering tops of the plant contain its medicinal properties.

What other medical conditions do you have?

By asking this question, you can identify other health care providers that patients are seeing and encourage patients to talk to providers about including herbal remedies in their therapeutic plans. JS, our case-study patient, claimed that she has hypertension, which is currently controlled by medication, diet, and exercise. She should be instructed to let her primary care physician know about the addition of St. John's wort to her medication regimen.

What prescription medications, OTC medications, or herbal remedies are you currently taking?

This question allows you to determine whether adding an herbal to the patient's regimen will cause an interaction between the herbal and a drug, an herbal, or a disease state. St. John's wort has recently been discovered to cause several drug interactions of concern. As a CYP3A4 enzyme inducer, St. John's wort may reduce the efficacy of oral contraceptives, protease inhibitors, and cyclosporin.[39] Potential adverse interactions could also occur with digoxin, theophylline, and selective serotonin reuptake inhibitors (SSRIs). Because St. John's wort most likely exerts its antidepressive actions through the reuptake of serotonin,[40] it is important to warn patients about the use of other serotonergic drugs, such as the triptans for migraines, other SSRIs used for depression, and dextromethorphan for cough suppression.

In JS's case, she takes verapamil for her hypertension. Because St. John's wort may affect the concentrations of some calcium channel blockers by modulating P-glycoprotein,[41] you must tell JS that when she starts taking St. John's wort she needs to monitor her blood pressure closely for any changes.

Is this product going to be used by you or is it for someone else?

An appropriate question to ask about any medication, this is especially important for herbal remedies, which, unlike prescription or OTC medications, are not regulated by the FDA. Herbal remedies should be used with caution in children and in women who are pregnant or lactating. The elderly, too, should be watched carefully when they use herbal remedies because of possible polypharmacy and the detrimental effects that can occur in someone with compromised renal or liver function.

Are any of the medications you are currently taking, or have any remedies you've tried in the past, relieved your symptoms?

This question lets you know about remedies a patient has tried and which ones have worked. It also helps you determine what makes the patient's symptoms worse and what makes them better, as well as whether the symptoms are cyclic or continuous.

In the final part of the counseling session, you tell the patient about side effects associated with the herbal remedy, explain how to take it most effectively, and discuss how long it will take to experience any therapeutic effects. In the case of JS, side effects associated with St. John's wort include photosensitivity, headache, nervousness, itching, gastrointestinal irritation, and restlessness. JS should be counseled about the importance of wearing sunscreen and avoiding sun exposure. Having her space out her doses so she takes them with meals may help minimize gastrointestinal effects. It is important to reiterate the dose to be taken and to tell her not to use other medications without consulting a health care provider.

Although St. John's wort might have some MAO-inhibitory activity, a tyramine-free diet is not currently advocated.[42] Tyramine is contained in a number of foods, such as aged meats and cheeses, beer, red wine, hard liquors, smoked or pickled foods, and yeast-containing products. Without dietary restriction of tyramine, it may be prudent to discuss the symptoms of hypertensive crisis associated with it: increased blood pressure, headache, stiff neck, nausea, vomiting, and clammy skin. If these symptoms develop, she should seek emergency care. JS should also be reminded that she may have to wait several weeks before experiencing the beneficial effects of this remedy.

JS should be encouraged to discuss her problem with her primary care provider to rule out potential physical causes of her symptoms and to have her depression assessed properly. Most importantly, you should maintain an open dialogue with JS so that she considers her pharmacist to be a trusted and accessible partner on her health care team.

REFERENCES

1. Eliason BC, Kruger J, Mark D, et al. Dietary supplement users: demographics, product use, and medical system interaction. *J Am Board Fam Pract*. 1997;10:265-71.
2. Fugh-Berman A. Herbal medicinals: selected clinical considerations, focusing on known or potential drug-herb interactions [letter]. *Arch Intern Med*. 1999;159:1957-8.
3. Fugh-Berman A. Herb-drug interactions. *Lancet*. 2000;355:134-8.
4. Eisenberg DM, Davis RB, Ettner SL, et al. Trends in alternative medicine use in the United States, 1990-1997: results of a follow-up national survey. *JAMA*.1998;280:1569-75.
5. Johnston BA. One-third of nation's adults use herbal remedies. *Herbalgram*. 1997;40:49.
6. Smolinske SC. Dietary supplement-drug interactions. *J Am Med Womens Assoc*. 1999;54:191-2,195.
7. Eisenberg DM, Kessler RC, Foster C, et al. Unconventional medicine in the United States: prevalence, costs, and patterns of use. *N Engl J Med*. 1993;328:246-52.
8. Bond CA, Raehl CL, Franke T. Medication errors in United States hospitals. *Pharmacotherapy*. 2001; 21:1023-36.
9. Webster CS, Merry AF, Larsson L, et al. The frequency and nature of drug administration error during anaesthesia. *Anaesth Intensive Care*. 2001; 29:494-500.
10. Alderman CP, Farmer C. A brief analysis of clinical pharmacy interventions undertaken in an Australian teaching hospital. *J Qual Clin Pract* 2001;21:99-103.
11. Bond CA, Raehl CL, Franke T. Clinical pharmacy services, hospital pharmacy staffing, and medication errors in United States hospitals. *Pharmacotherapy*. 2002;22:134-47.
12. Kaufman DW, Kelly JP, Rosenberg L, et al. Recent patterns of medication use in the ambulatory adult population of the United States: the Slone survey. *JAMA*. 2002;287:337-44.
13. Steven ID, Malpass A, Moller J, et al. Towards safer drug use in general practice. *J Qual Clin Pract*. 1999;19:47-50.
14. Britten N, Brant S, Cairns A, et al. Continued prescribing of inappropriate drugs in general practice. *J Clin Pharm Ther* 1995;20:199-205.
15. Jones JK, Fife D, Curkendall S, et al. Coprescribing and codispensing of cisapride and contraindicated drugs. *JAMA*. 2001;286:1607-9.
16. Pfau PR, Rombeau JL. Nutrition. *Med Clin North Am*. 2000;84:1209-30.
17. McDermott LA, Albrecht JT, Good DH, et al. Documentation of clinical interventions in nutritional support. *Top Hosp Pharm Manage*. 1993;13:32-45.
18. Raehl CL, Bond CA, Pitterle ME. Pharmaceutical services in U.S. hospitals in 1989. *Am J Hosp Pharm*.1992;49:323-46.
19. Raehl CL, Bond CA, Pitterle ME. 1995 National Clinical Pharmacy Services Study. *Pharmacotherapy*. 1998;18:302-26.
20. Brown RO, Dickerson RN, Hak EB, et al. Impact of a pharmacist-based consult service on nutritional rehabilitation of nonambulatory patients with severe developmental disabilities. *Pharmacotherapy*. 1997;17:796-800.
21. Bonal JF. Clinical pharmacy in inpatient care. *Pharmacotherapy*. 2000;20:264S-72S.
22. Cerulli J, Malone M. Assessment of drug-related problems in clinical nutrition patients. *JPEN J Parenter Enteral Nutr*. 1999;23:218-21.
23. Gauthier I, Malone M, Lesar TS, et al. Comparison of programs for preventing drug-nutrient interactions in hospitalized patients. *Am J Health Syst Pharm*. 1997;54:405-11.
24. Lustig A. Medication error prevention by pharmacists: an Israeli solution. *Pharm World Sci*. 2000;22:21-5.
25. McDermott LA, Albrecht JT, Good DH. Nutritional support: pharmacists' influence on the prescribing process. *Top Hosp Pharm Manage*. 1994;14:30-9.
26. Woloschuk DM, Nazeravich DR, Gray LJ, et al. Establishment of a bone marrow transplant satellite pharmacy. *Can J Hosp Pharm*. 1993;46:5-11.

27. The increasing role of the pharmacist in home care. *Caring*.1994;13:42-6.
28. Logsdon BA. Drug use during lactation. *J Am Pharm Assoc (Wash)*. 1997;NS37:407-18.
29. Jacobson J. Inspiring patients to meet their treatment goals. *Am J Health Syst Pharm*. 2000;57:1032, 1035.
30. Rantucci MJ. *Pharmacists Talking with Patients: A Guide to Patient Counseling*. Baltimore: Williams & Wilkins, 1997:172-9.
31. Salom IL, Davis K. Prescribing for older patients: how to avoid toxic drug reactions. *Geriatrics*. 1995:50(10):37-43.
32. Kay B, Crowling GH, Jr, Kershaw VL, et al. Perspectives on pharmacy's role in managed care. *Am J Health Syst Pharm*. 1998;55:1482-8.
33. Tindall WN, Beardsley RS, Kimberlin CL. *Communication Skills in Pharmacy Practice*. Philadelphia: Lea and Febiger; 1989.
34. Northouse LL, Northouse PG. Communication variables in health care. In: *Health Communication: Strategies for Health Professionals*. 3rd ed. Stamford, CT: Appleton & Lange; 1998:23-78.
35. Singh YN, Blumenthal M. Kava: an overview. *HerbalGram*. 1997;39:33-57.
36. Blumenthal M, Klein J, Hall T, et al. *The Complete German Commission E Monographs. Therapeutic Guide to Herbal Medicine*. Austin: The American Botanical Council; 1998.
37. Allen LV Jr, Berardi RR, DeSimone EMI, et al. *Handbook of Nonprescription Drugs*. 12th ed. Washington, DC: American Pharmaceutical Association; 2000.
38. Jellin JM, Gregory PJ, Batz F, et al. *Pharmacist's Letter/Prescriber's Letter Natural Medicines Comprehensive Database*. 4th ed. Stockton, CA: Therapeutic Research Faculty; 2002.
39. Ernst E. Second thoughts about the safety of St. John's wort. *Lancet*. 1999;354:2014-6.
40. Yu PH. Effect of the hypericum perforatum extract on serotonin turnover in the mouse brain. *Pharmacopsychiatry*. 2000;33:60-5.
41. Fisunov A, Lozovaya N, Tsintsadze T, et al. Hyperforin modulates gating of P-type Ca2+ current in cerebellar Purkinje neurons. *Pflugers Arch*. 2000;440:427-34.
42. Miller LG. Herbal medicinals: selected clinical considerations focusing on known or potential drug-herb interactions. *Arch Intern Med*. 1998;158:2200-11.

CHAPTER 3

DRUG–NUTRIENT INTERACTIONS

Grace Earl, Jennifer Malinowski, Debra Skaar

C hapter 3 will provide you with information to identify and manage drug–nutrient interactions (DNIs). The process for managing DNIs differs based on practice setting. For example, in the acute care setting, pharmacists usually participate in a multidisciplinary team that develops protocols for managing DNIs. In the ambulatory care setting, however, pharmacists play a direct role in counseling patients and promoting self-management of DNIs. In this situation, the pharmacist's responsibility includes evaluating the medication profile, medical and surgical history, and dietary practices to reveal factors that predispose patients to DNIs.

This chapter is organized by therapeutic area and each section offers counseling tips to help you develop a practical plan for managing acute and chronic interactions.

DEFINITIONS AND CLINICAL APPLICATIONS

DNIs can significantly impact the pharmacologic action of the target drug—resulting in a therapeutic, inadequate, or toxic response. Many DNIs stem from pharmacokinetic interactions affecting drug absorption and metabolism. For example, drug absorption can be enhanced when the anti-infective drug atovaquone (Mepron) is taken with a high-fat meal. This drug is indicated for *Pneumocystis carinii* pneumonia, and counseling patients to take it with foods high in fat can improve bioavailability and treatment outcome.

DNIs can also arise from pharmacodynamic interactions. For example, when patients consume a diet containing significant quantities of vitamin K, they can lose the anticoagulant effect of warfarin (Coumadin). Vitamin K is a cofactor necessary for activation of clotting factors and reverses the effect of warfarin. As a result, consuming significant quantities of vitamin K places the patient at great risk for treatment failure and can cause a thromboembolic event such as deep vein thrombosis, pulmonary embolism, or stroke.

Interactions can also result in nutrient depletion. For example, potassium and magnesium depletion secondary to diuretic use may precipitate ventricular

---

Drug–Nutrient Interactions (DNIs)

DNIs can significantly impact the pharmacologic action of the target drug—resulting in a therapeutic, inadequate, or toxic response. Many DNIs stem from pharmacokinetic interactions affecting drug absorption and metabolism.

The influence of a meal affects the rate and extent of drug absorption. Accelerating or decreasing the rate of absorption will alter the time (Tmax) to achieve the peak drug plasma concentration (Cmax). Factors that diminish the extent of absorption, or bioavailability (F), of a drug will decrease the area under the concentration–time curve (AUC).

---

arrhythmias. Also, chronic administration of glucocorticoids affects calcium metabolism, causing osteoporosis. You can help patients manage these interactions by prescribing electrolyte and mineral supplements.

INTERACTION MECHANICS

The pharmacokinetic principles and terminology used to describe DNIs are similar to those for drug–drug interactions. As shown in Tables 3-1 and 3-2, the influence of a meal affects the rate and extent of drug absorption. Accelerating or decreasing the rate of absorption will alter the time (Tmax) to achieve the peak drug plasma concentration (Cmax). Factors that diminish the extent of absorption, or bioavailability (F), of a drug will decrease the area under the concentration–time curve (AUC). For example, calcium found in milk products binds to quinolone and tetracycline antibiotics, decreasing bioavailability.[1]

Pharmacists play a major role in identifying significant DNIs by critically evaluating pharmacokinetic studies in the literature. By recognizing changes in Cmax or AUC, you can also predict the potential for adverse effects.

The significance of the side effects will depend on the therapeutic window of the drug. With a large therapeutic window, you will see a therapeutic effect over a wide range of drug plasma concentrations. A DNI causing a small change in AUC or Cmax is unlikely to cause an immediate systemic response. It is important to remember, though, that the likelihood of drug toxicity increases with drugs having a narrow therapeutic range. This scenario was reported with Theo 24, a long-acting theophylline sustained-release dosage form. When taken with a meal, it resulted in immediate and complete release of the drug, causing significant drug toxicity (known as dose-dumping phenomenon).[2]

Drug Clearance

DNIs affect drug clearance by altering drug metabolism. Metabolism via the cytochrome P450 system (CYP) is an important route of elimination for many drugs. The CYP system is composed of oxidative enzymes located in

TABLE 3-1   Drug–Nutrient Interactions:
Increased Absorption with Food

Drug	Instructions
Antibiotics	
Cefuroxime	Take with milk
Clarithromycin	Take with a meal
Nitrofurantoin	Take with a meal
Antifungal	
Griseofulvin	Take with a meal
Antiprotozoal	
Atovaquone	Take with a meal high in fat
Antiviral	
Saquinavir	Take with a meal high in fat
Cholesterol-Lowering	
Lovastatin	Take with an evening meal

TABLE 3-2   Drug–Nutrient Interactions: Decreased
Absorption with Food

Taking these medications with food may decrease the
effectiveness of the drug. Separate from a meal by 1 or 2 hours.

Antibiotics	**Cardiovascular Agents**
Amoxicillin	
Penicillin V	***ACE Inhibitors***
Trimethoprim	Moexipril, Captopril, Quinapril
Ciprofloxacin	
Erythromycin	***Beta Blocker***
	Acebutolol, Nadolol
Antitubercular Agent	
Ethambutol	***Calcium Channel Blocker***
Isoniazid	Nicardipine, Nitrendipine
Rifampin	
	Anti-inflammatory Agents
Antiviral	Tolmetin, Penicillamine
Indinavir	
Zalcitabine	**Parkinson's Disease**
	Carbidopa/Levodopa
Antifungal	
Itraconazole	**Alzheimer's Disease**
	Tacrine
Hyperthyroidism	
Propylthiouracil	

* Note: Some drugs may cause significant abdominal discomfort when taken on an empty stomach. Because this discomfort outweighs the effects on drug absorption, it may be prudent to advise patients to take this medication with food.

the gastrointestinal (GI) tract and the liver. Many drug–drug interactions have been identified that involve the CYP3A4, 2D6, 1A2, and 2C enzymes.[3]

Drugs or nutrients can act to inhibit or induce the activity of the enzyme. An inducer, such as phenytoin, increases the rate of oxidative activity, thus increasing clearance of the drug substrate. Grapefruit juice, on the other hand, inhibits the CYP3A4 enzyme, diminishing the rate of metabolism and increasing the drug plasma concentration. Grapefruit juice affects CYP enzymes in the GI tract that reduce pre-systemic clearance, and does not affect hepatic CYP enzymes.

Food–Drug Interactions

DNIs, or food–drug interactions, may be caused by specific nutrients such as protein, carbohydrate, fat, and amino acids (such as tyramine).[1] Meals high in fat may increase drug absorption. This effect is secondary to stimulation of gastrointestinal enzymes and bile.[4] Meals containing a high percentage of fat are used to develop pharmacokinetic models on food–nutrient interactions. These models, however, may not apply to daily living since the average person eats a variety of foods.

There are other interactions involving the GI tract. Taking a medication with food delays gastric emptying and delays absorption of drugs.[1] The increased viscosity associated with ingestion of polymers such as fibers and suspensions may delay GI transit time and delay absorption.[4]

Water, soda, and fruit juices can affect the dissolution rate of drugs. In most circumstances patients are encouraged to take their medications with a drink. However, if a beverage significantly reduces the gastric pH, it may alter the dissolution and degradation of the drug. Controlled release, delayed release, or enteric coated dosage formulations can also be affected.[4]

The presence of food in the GI tract increases blood flow to the intestines via the capillaries of the splanchnic system.[1] Drugs with first high-pass metabolism—such as beta-blocking agents (e.g., metoprolol and propranolol) and antiarrhythmic agents (e.g., propafenone)—are rapidly delivered to the portal system, bypassing the liver, and increasing the overall bioavailability.

DIETARY, MEDICAL, AND SURGICAL HISTORY

Before dispensing medications with a high risk of DNIs, you should always try to interview the patient to gather specific dietary practices. For example, what percentage of total calories does the patient derive from dietary carbohydrate, fat, and protein? Because timing of medications with food may increase the likelihood of some interactions, you should also determine the size and frequency of meals and snacks.

Serious systemic effects can result from an acute change in blood pressure or heart rate. When nifedipine, a calcium channel-blocking agent, is taken with food an increase in Cmax and AUC may cause an immediate decrease in blood pressure.

Dietary, Medical, and Surgical History

Before dispensing medications with a high risk of DNIs, you should always try to interview the patient to gather specific dietary practices. For example, what percentage of total calories does the patient derive from dietary carbohydrate, fat, and protein? Because timing of medications with food may increase the likelihood of some interactions, you should also determine the size and frequency of meals and snacks.

Pharmacists should also:

❑ Ask specific questions to determine the potential for any known serious DNIs like warfarin with vitamin K, or monoamine oxidase (MAO) inhibitors and tyramine.
❑ Provide major educational interventions or minor counseling (such as take with food, avoid milk).
❑ Promote patient self-management.

Pharmacists can ask specific questions to determine the potential for any known serious DNIs, such as warfarin with vitamin K or monoamine oxidase (MAO) inhibitors and tyramine. You can also provide major educational interventions or minor counseling (such as take with food, avoid milk). In addition, you should always promote patient self-management.

Reviewing the medical and surgical history, and results of the physical examination may provide useful information. For example:

- Any delay or shortening of GI transit time may affect drug absorption.
- Diabetic gastroparesis delays gastric emptying.[4]
- Factors such as achlorhydria in the elderly may affect absorption of drugs that require an acid milieu.
- Surgical removal of a portion of the GI tract (short bowel syndrome, gastrectomy), or inflammatory bowel disease (Crohn's disease) may decrease the absorptive capacity of the GI tract.[4]
- Medications administered via feeding tubes placed below the level of the pylorus (jejunostomy tube) bypass the stomach.
- Ketoconazole absorption requires an acid environment and should not be administered via a jejunostomy tube.
- Patients who are unable to eat may experience prolonged periods without enteral stimulation, causing atrophy of the intestinal mucosa.
- Decreases in splanchnic blood flow associated with heart failure and liver disease may decrease systemic absorption of drugs.
- The presence of anatomic, pathologic, or iatrogenic factors may affect GI tract function and subsequently impair drug absorption.

ACUTE CARE

Enteral Nutrition

The drug–nutrient interaction between enteral nutrition formulas and phenytoin has been a topic of discussion and controversy among health care providers for nearly 20 years. When hospitalized patients cannot eat normally, early enteral nutrition is usually started.

Phenytoin remains a first-line drug for prophylaxis for treatment of generalized tonic-clonic or partial seizures in adult patients. It is manufactured in a variety of convenient dosage forms, including injection, suspension, tablet, and capsule. Phenytoin is absorbed at a slow rate after oral or enteral administration.

Conditions that slow gastrointestinal transit time can decrease bioavailability of phenytoin.[5] In addition, considerable interpatient variability as well as clinically relevant differences in bioavailability exist with various dosage forms.[6] Phenytoin also exhibits concentration-dependent elimination; therefore, small changes in bioavailability can result in disproportionate increases in serum concentration. For these reasons, the interaction between phenytoin and enteral nutrition formulas is clinically important.

Several studies have described the interaction between continuous nasogastric feedings and oral phenytoin absorption. One investigator studied 20 neurosurgery patients who were receiving phenytoin suspension (1000 mg loading dose followed by 300 mg/day).[7] The first 10 study patients received concomitant phenytoin suspension and continuous nasogastric feedings (Isocal). On day 8, the tube feedings were discontinued. Trough phenytoin serum concentrations were measured. The mean serum phenytoin concentration was 2.59 mcg per milliliter in the first phase of the study. After the enteral feedings were stopped for 7 days, the mean phenytoin serum concentration increased to 10.22 mcg per milliliter (p < 0.0001).

The next 10 study patients were started on phenytoin suspension but were not administered enteral formula until day 7. The initial trough phenytoin serum concentration was 9.80 mcg per milliliter. After being crossed over to receive nasogastric feedings for 7 days, the serum concentrations dropped to 2.72 mcg per milliliter (p < 0.0001).

This study demonstrated that enteral formulas interfere with absorption of phenytoin suspension. This interaction is critical when patients are initiated on phenytoin. Administration of phenytoin during initiation or continuation of enteral formulas may result in failure to achieve therapeutic phenytoin serum concentrations (as demonstrated in the first study group). In addition, the DNI may cause declining drug concentrations in patients stabilized on phenytoin (as seen in the second study group).

To minimize the risk of this drug–nutrient interaction, pharmacists should follow the recommendations in the following sidebar.

A number of studies have also been conducted to determine the cause of the drug–nutrient interaction between enteral feedings and phenytoin.[8-9] In one particular study by Hooks,[8] a phenytoin suspension was mixed with an

Minimizing the Risk of DNIs with Nasogastric Feedings and Phenytoin

To minimize the risk of a drug–nutrient interaction between nasogastric feedings and phenytoin, pharmacists should recommend that:

❏ Nasogastric feedings be stopped two hours before the daily dose of phenytoin.
❏ The suspension be administered via the feeding tube and then the tube should be flushed with 60 ml of water.
❏ Two additional hours should elapse before the tube feedings are resumed.
❏ The rate should be recalculated to ensure complete administration of the enteral formula over the remaining 20 hours.
❏ Despite these maneuvers, however, patients typically require large doses of phenytoin (range 800–1600 mg/day) to maintain therapeutic serum concentrations.

Source: Reference 7.

enteral formula (Osmolite). The amount of phenytoin recovered was significantly less than with a control solution. Because some enteral formulas contain intact protein in the form of sodium and calcium caseinates, and because phenytoin binds to serum proteins (albumin 90% in vivo), Hooks hypothesized that a physical interaction between phenytoin and intact protein may decrease the bioavailability of the drug.

Electrolytes may also play a role in this interaction. Antacids containing calcium and magnesium have been shown to decrease the bioavailability of a single dose of phenytoin.[10] Other factors that may decrease bioavailability are direct binding of the drug to the feeding tube.[9] Enteral tube feedings may also affect gastrointestinal pH by lowering the gastrointestinal tract pH below the point of critical solubility where phenytoin, a weak acid, is absorbed.[9]

Pharmacists should closely screen special populations, such as patients with head injury, for altered phenytoin pharmacokinetics. Patients with head injury require doses of phenytoin up to 800 mg every 8 hours. Critical care researchers have suggested that traumatic injury increases hepatic drug metabolism, resulting in lower than expected phenytoin serum concentrations.[11-12] During convalescence, the effect abates and serum phenytoin concentrations can increase.[11] In cases where large doses of phenytoin suspension are not successful in maintaining therapeutic drug concentrations, you may consider intravenous phenytoin or fosphenytoin as alternatives.

Although the mechanism of the phenytoin–enteral nutrition interaction remains controversial, the potential danger of subtherapeutic or toxic phenytoin serum concentrations is real. The narrow therapeutic range, nonlinear pharmacokinetics, and multitude of drug interactions with phenytoin complicate management of this drug–nutrient interaction.

Treating Electrolyte Depletion

When treating electrolyte depletion, a cost-effective principle to follow is this: treat the patient, not the number. For asymptomatic patients, oral administration of electrolytes may be sufficient for repletion. The parenteral route can be used for situations when patients are symptomatic, or when the patient has an existing intravenous (IV) site and is in a monitored setting (vital signs, electrocardiogram).

You should counsel patients receiving medications that cause electrolyte depletion to report symptoms of muscle weakness, cramping, palpitations, or chest pain. Electrolyte deficiencies may be aggravated by conditions such as dehydration following exertion or exercise, and illnesses causing diarrhea and vomiting.

Parenteral Nutrition

Critically ill patients and those patients with malnutrition due to cancer and hypermetabolism may require total parenteral nutrition (TPN) support during their hospitalization. Evidence from animal studies demonstrates that TPN alters oxidative activity of hepatic cytochrome P450 enzymes.[13] Studies performed in humans confirm that TPN interacts with the cytochrome P450 system and accounts for changes in drug clearance. A number of enzymes have been examined including CYP3A2, also known as erythromycin demethylase. Similar effects on drug clearance have also been demonstrated during malnutrition and sepsis, but the extent of these interactions and their clinical significance has not been fully defined.

Electrolyte Depletion During Acute Care

Electrolyte depletion can occur in both the inpatient and outpatient setting. Because critically ill inpatients are more likely to be treated aggressively for their underlying condition, the resulting electrolyte depletion can cause arrhythmias and respiratory failure.[14] To prevent these dangerous side effects, you should review the patient's medication profile to detect drugs causing electrolyte depletion and develop a prospective plan for monitoring and ordering electrolytes. Following guidelines for acute electrolyte replacement and continued maintenance dosing may help keep values within the normal range.

When treating electrolyte depletion, a cost-effective principle to follow is this: treat the patient, not the number. For asymptomatic patients, oral administration of electrolytes may be sufficient for repletion. The parenteral route can be used for situations when patients are symptomatic, or when the patient has an existing intravenous (IV) site and is in a monitored setting (vital signs, electrocardiogram).

You should counsel patients receiving medications that cause electrolyte depletion to report symptoms of muscle weakness, cramping, palpitations, or chest pain. Electrolyte deficiencies may be aggravated by conditions such as dehydration following exertion or exercise, and illnesses causing diarrhea and vomiting.

Potassium Depletion

Potassium and magnesium depletion can cause cardiac arrhythmias such as ventricular tachycardia.[15] Patients with heart failure may be treated with high doses of diuretics or diuretic combinations. As a result, these patients may be at greater risk for developing lethal arrhythmias.

One case exists where a drug–nutrient interaction can actually be used to avoid a cardiovascular side effect. Sympathomimetic drugs can reduce plasma concentrations of potassium by shifting potassium ions across the cell membrane. This interaction can be used to treat patients with elevated potassium levels. Sympathomimetics such as albuterol have been administered via metered-dose inhaler to treat hyperkalemia in outpatient dialysis centers.[16]

In the case of renal failure, administer IV potassium chloride very cautiously. Administering electrolytes with food and adhering to usual dosage ranges will diminish osmotic diarrhea caused by electrolyte supplements.

For more rapid oral repletion, select immediate release formulations. For example, potassium given as a powder mixed with water will increase the blood levels more rapidly as compared to sustained release dosage forms.

Phosphate Depletion

Because phosphate is necessary for respiratory muscle function, low phosphate levels may cause respiratory failure and result in emergent intubation or prolonged weaning from the ventilator. Hypophosphatemia, a complication of diabetic ketoacidosis, refeeding syndrome, and protein-calorie malnutrition in the intensive care unit,[17] can also depress cardiac function and neuromuscular function, resulting in myopathy.[18]

Magnesium Depletion

Severe hypomagnesemia induces muscle spasm and causes tetany and ventricular arrhythmias.[17] Intravenous administration of magnesium can actually promote renal magnesium excretion when high concentrations of magnesium are presented to the renal tubule. As a result, magnesium should be replaced over a number of days. Oral magnesium supplementation may be used for mild, asymptomatic patients, while IV administration is reserved for symptomatic situations such as muscle spasm, tetany, seizures, or ventricular arrhythmias.

Tables 3-3, 3-4, and 3-5 detail drugs causing potassium, magnesium, and phosphorus depletion.

TABLE 3-3 Drugs Causing Potassium Depletion

Thiazide diuretics	hydrochlorothiazide
Loop diuretics	furosemide, bumetanide, torsemide, ethacrynic acid
Mineralocorticoids	fludrocortisone, licorice
Glucocorticoids	methylprednisolone
Antifungal agent	amphotericin B

TABLE 3-4 Drugs Causing Magnesium Depletion

Thiazide diuretics	hydrochlorothiazide
Loop diuretics	furosemide, bumetanide, torsemide, ethacrynic acid
Antibiotics (Aminoglycosides)	gentamicin, tobramycin, amikacin
Antiviral agent	foscarnet
Antiprotozoal agent	pentamidine
Antifungal agent	amphotericin B
Immunosupressant	cyclosporine
Antineoplastic agent	cisplatin

TABLE 3-5 Drugs Causing Phosphate Depletion

Phosphate binders	aluminum and calcium-containing antacids, sevelamer, calcium acetate
Antiulcer agent	sucralfate
Diuretic (Carbonic anhydrase inhibitor)	acetazolamide
Parenteral nutrition solutions without phosphate	

COMMUNITY MANAGEMENT

Cardiology

Warfarin (Coumadin)

Warfarin is an anticoagulant associated with a significant number of drug–food interactions. It acts by inhibiting hepatic reductase, an enzyme responsible for converting the storage form of vitamin K to the active form (vitamin K_1). Dietary intake of vitamin K interferes with the pharmacologic action of warfarin, resulting in the need for higher doses to achieve the same effect.[19]

Fluctuating quantities of vitamin K in the diet may lead to unexplained variability in the international normalized ratio (INR).[20-36] Excessive intake of dietary vitamin K may cause subtherapeutic anticoagulation and subsequent clot formation. Although serious clinical events are rare, two cases of fluctuating vitamin K levels have been identified that were associated with development of acute myocardial infarction and thrombosis of an aortic valve prosthesis, respectively.[29,33] Reduction in vitamin K in the diet may lead to a supra therapeutic INR, which increases the risk of bleeding in patients previously stabilized on a specific dose.[19]

You should counsel patients taking warfarin to consume a well-balanced diet that maintains a *consistent* amount of vitamin K.[19] The current recommended dietary allowance (RDA) of vitamin K is 0.5–1 mcg/kg body weight.[19] You can tell patients that they do not need to eliminate all foods containing vitamin K. As shown in Table 3-6, many of the foods containing vitamin K are nutritious and contain fiber. This is particularly beneficial for patients with, or at risk for, atherosclerotic heart disease, a diagnosis that supports the consumption of fresh vegetables.

To help patients taking warfarin comply with dietary recommendations, you should make sure that they:

- Have a list of foods high in vitamin K such as green leafy vegetables, beans, green tea, chickpeas, and certain types of oils.
- Receive supplemental written material as well as face-to-face counseling.[37]
- Avoid daily variability in the quantity of food intake, especially foods high in vitamin K.[38,39]
- Inform you before taking any nutritional or herbal supplements, as well as prescription and nonprescription drugs.

Endogenous vitamin K may be affected by a number of pharmacologic interventions. Broad-spectrum antibiotics may reduce the endogenous biosynthesis of vitamin K_2 (menaquinone), resulting in a potentially high INR and an exaggerated response to warfarin.[40,41] Broad-spectrum antibiotics destroy intestinal flora responsible for synthesizing vitamin K, possibly increasing the risk of bleeding. In contrast, intravenous fat emulsions are associated with warfarin resistance.[42] These emulsions contain soybean oil alone or in combination with safflower oil. Both of these oils are sources of plant-derived phytosterols, which contain vitamin K. Since vitamin K_1 may be added directly to TPN to prevent deficiency, the risk for warfarin antagonism increases.[43]

If you anticipate exogenous or endogenous vitamin K fluctuations, you should check the INR frequently and monitor patients daily. Scenarios associated with fluctuation include:

- Illness (where intake is reduced),
- Initiation of a weight reduction diet (where intake is likely to be increased), or
- Starting supplemental oral or IV vitamin K_1 (phytonadione).

You should base any dose adjustments or vitamin K_1 administration on the INR. The recommendations of the Sixth American College of Clinical Pharmacy Consensus Conference on Antithrombotic Therapy Guidelines provide clear guidelines for dosing.[19] You should also monitor the patient for signs and symptoms of bleeding or clot formation.

TABLE 3-6   Vitamin K Content in Selected Foods

Foods	Portion Size (Household Measure)	Vitamin K Content
Coffee brewed	80 oz (10 cups)	Low
Cola, regular and diet	3½ oz	Low
Fruit juices, assorted types	3½ oz	Low
Milk	3½ oz	Low
Tea, black, brewed	3½ oz	Low
Bread, assorted types	4 slices	Low
Cereal, assorted types	3½ oz	Low
Flour, assorted types	8 oz (1 cup)	Low
Oatmeal, instant, dry	8 oz	Low
Rice, white	4 oz (½ cup)	Low
Spaghetti, dry	3½ oz	Low
Butter	3 oz (6 tbsp)	Low
Cheddar cheese	3½ oz	Low
Eggs	2 large	Low
Margarine	3½ oz (7 tbsp)	Medium
Mayonnaise	4 oz (8 tbsp)	High
Oils		
Canola, salad, soybean	3½ oz	High
Olive	3½ oz	Medium
Corn, peanut, safflower	3½ oz	Low
Sesame, sunflower	3½ oz	Low
Sour cream	4 oz	Low
Yogurt	3½ oz	Low
Apple	1 medium	Low
Banana	1 medium	Low
Blueberries	5¼ oz (⅔ cup)	Low
Cantaloupe pieces	5¼ oz	Low
Grapes	8 oz (1 cup)	Low
Grapefruit	½ medium	Low
Lemon	2 medium	Low
Orange	1 medium	Low
Peach	1 medium	Low
Abalone	3½ oz	Low
Beef, ground	3½ oz	Low
Chicken	3½ oz	Low
Mackerel	3½ oz	Low
Meatloaf	3½ oz	Low
Pork, meat	3½ oz	Low
Tuna	3½ oz	Low
Turkey, meat	3½ oz	Low

TABLE 3-6   Vitamin K Content in Selected Foods (continued)

Foods	Portion Size (Household Measure)	Vitamin K Content
Asparagus, raw	7 spears	Medium
Avocado, peeled	1 small	Medium
Beans, pod, raw	8 oz (1 cup)	Medium
Broccoli, raw and cooked	4 oz (½ cup)	High
Brussel sprouts	3 sprouts	High
Cabbage, raw, shredded	12 oz (1½ cup)	High
Cabbage, red, shredded	12 oz	Medium
Carrot	5¼ oz (⅔ cup)	Low
Cauliflower	8 oz	Low
Celery	2½ stalks	Low
Coleslaw	6 oz (¾ cup)	Medium
Collard greens	4 oz	High
Cucumber peel, raw	8 oz	High
Cucumber, peel removed	8 oz	Low
Eggplant	10 oz (1¼ cup)	Low
Endive, raw, chopped	16 oz (2 cups)	High
Green scallion, chopped	5¼ oz (⅔ cup)	High
Kale, raw leaf	6 oz (¾ cup)	High
Lettuce, shredded	14 oz (1¾ cups)	High
Mushrooms	12 oz (1½ cup)	Low
Mustard greens, raw	12 oz	High
Onion, white	5¼ oz	Low
Parsley, chopped & cooked	12 oz	High
Peas, green, cooked	5¼ oz	Medium
Pepper, green, raw	8 oz	Low
Potato	1 medium	Low
Pumpkin	4 oz (½ cup)	Low
Spinach, raw leaf	12 oz	High
Tomato	1 medium	Low
Turnip greens, raw	12 oz	High
Watercress, raw	24 oz (3 cups)	High
Honey	2½ oz (5 tbsp)	Low
Jell-O Gelatin	2½ oz (⅓ cup)	Low
Peanut butter	3 oz (6 tbsp)	Low
Pickle, dill	1 medium	Medium
Sauerkraut	8 oz	Medium
Soybean, dry	4 oz	Medium

Reprinted with permission from Lexi-Comp, Inc., Hudson, Ohio.
To convert to metric equivalent: 1 fluid ounce = 30 ml, 1 oz = 30 g.

Helping Patients Comply with Dietary Recommendations

To help patients taking warfarin comply with dietary recommendations, pharmacists should make sure that patients:

❏ Have a list of foods high in vitamin K such as green leafy vegetables, beans, green tea, chickpeas, and certain types of oils.
❏ Receive supplemental written material as well as face-to-face counseling.
❏ Avoid daily variability in the quantity of food intake, especially foods high in vitamin K.
❏ Inform you before taking any nutritional or herbal supplements, as well as prescription and nonprescription drugs.

Inflammatory Conditions

Glucocorticoids

Glucocorticoids are the most common drug-induced cause of osteoporosis.[44] Although glucocorticoids induce osteoporosis by affecting sex hormones and inhibiting bone formation, researchers do not know how these agents impair calcium absorption. Urinary calcium is increased in patients receiving glucocorticoids, which results in a negative calcium balance. However, it does not change parathyroid hormone (PTH) and calcitonin concentrations—two markers of normal calcium homeostasis.

Administering moderate- to high-dose steroids can cause osteoporosis and osteopenia.[38,45-52] During the first 6 months of steroid therapy, bone loss is accelerated and is proportional to the dose and duration of treatment.

The incidence of fractures associated with long-term glucocorticoid use is estimated between 30% and 50%.[53] High cumulative dose exposure over time and prednisone (or equivalent) doses at or above 7.5 mg daily pose an increased risk for bone loss. In addition, alternate-day dose regimens do not appear to lessen bone loss compared to daily regimens.[54,55] Inhaled steroids can also cause bone loss.[56-58]

The American College of Rheumatology Task Force on Osteoporosis endorses diagnostic recommendations for the detection of glucocorticoid-induced osteoporosis.[44] Before beginning a long-term therapy (greater than 6 months), patients should obtain a baseline bone mineral density measurement of both the spine and hip. All patients should receive follow-up measurements of bone density after 6 to 12 months of continuous steroid therapy.

Prevention of steroid-induced osteoporosis should include discontinuation of the drug whenever clinically feasible. While treating patients with steroids, use the lowest effective dose to produce a clinical effect for the shortest amount of time. Although inhaled steroids have been associated

---

Nonpharmacologic Interventions for Preventing Osteoporosis

Pharmacists should counsel patients receiving long-term steroids on non-pharmacologic interventions to improve bone health. Key interventions include:

- ❏ Stopping smoking.
- ❏ Decreasing caffeine intake.
- ❏ Preventing falls.
- ❏ Maintaining a calcium intake of 1500 mg/day.[44]

---

with bone loss, they have less effect compared to systemic therapy and should be used whenever possible.[44]

Pharmacists should counsel patients receiving long-term steroids on non-pharmacologic interventions to improve bone health. Key interventions are listed in the sidebar above.

For patients receiving long-term steroids, pharmacists should also:

- Recommend supplements for patients who have insufficient amounts of calcium in the diet.
- Recommend Vitamin D (either 800 IU/day or 50,000 IU three times per week) or calcitriol (0.5 mcg/day) supplementation.[44]
- Prudently monitor serum and urine calcium levels for the possible development of hypercalcemia with hypercalcuria.
- Educate all postmenopausal women on the benefits of hormone replacement therapy, unless contraindicated.
- Use hydrochlorothiazide to blunt the hypercalcuria associated with glucocorticoids.
- Treat patients who have already developed a fracture with a bis-phosphonate or calcitonin.
- Recommend a bone mineral density assessment at 6–12 months following a fracture to monitor the effectiveness of the therapeutic intervention.[44]

Neurology

Anticonvulsants

The anticonvulsant agents phenytoin and phenobarbital decrease calcium absorption in the intestine.[43,59] These patients have normal calcitriol concentrations and researchers believe that the mechanism does not involve vitamin D metabolism.[60]

Although chronic administration of anticonvulsant agents can lead to rare cases of osteomalacia and rickets, most patients obtain sufficient vitamin D from their diet to counteract this effect. Pharmacists should educate patients receiving these agents chronically to maintain their intake of foods with high vitamin D and calcium content and to take supplements if necessary. You should also recommend the nonpharmacologic interventions outlined in the "Glucocorticoid" section. Pharmacists can also recommend vitamin D$_2$ (ergocalciferol) to prevent and treat osteomalacia and rickets, in combination with a calcium supplement.[43,59] Carbamazepine, which has not been associated with alterations in calcium metabolism, can serve as an alternative to phenytoin and phenobarbital.[43]

Phenytoin can also reduce folic acid concentrations, possibly resulting in folic acid deficiency and development of macrocytic anemia.[43] Compounding this problem, folic acid supplementation is associated with decreased phenytoin concentrations. To avoid this potential interaction, you should initiate a patient on a daily multivitamin containing folic acid, or add 1 mg folic acid daily to the patient's drug regimen at the onset of therapy. This early supplementation will lessen the influence of pharmacokinetic alterations and possibly prevent the onset of folic acid deficiency.[43,61]

Grapefruit Juice

As detailed in Table 3-7, the list of DNIs reported with grapefruit juice continues to grow. Significant pharmacokinetic effects on AUC, Cmax, and half-life have been demonstrated. Grapefruit juice inhibits intestinal CYP3A4 enzymes and increases bioavailability by decreasing presystemic clearance of drugs administered via the oral route. The inhibitory effects last for up to 24 hours.[62] The reaction is most prominent in drugs with poor oral bioavailability and when there is repeated daily use of grapefruit juice.[63] Interactions with cisapride,[64] statins,[65] and cyclosporine[66] are the most notable, due to their potential for side effects.

Grapefruit juice, pulp, and skin contain flavonoid and nonflavonoid components. Flavonoids, such as naringin and naringenin, give citrus fruits their characteristic flavor.[67] A nonflavonoid substance is dihydroxybergamottin, a furanocoumarin, which has been shown to be a potent inhibitor of CYP enzymes in *in vitro* studies. Flavonoids and nonflavonoids are considered to be potential causative agents of this interaction. Whole grapefruit, fresh squeezed juice, and frozen concentrates have all caused DNIs.[68] However, processing alters the composition of the juice, and is a likely reason for variable and inconsistent study results.[4]

Are grapefruit interactions clinically significant? This is still being debated. Clearly, grapefruit–drug interactions mediated via CYP3A4 can result in clinically and statistically significant increases in drug plasma concentrations. One study demonstrated QT prolongation on the electrocardiogram when terfenadine 60 mg was taken with 8 oz (240 ml) of grapefruit juice from frozen concentrate daily for 7 days.[69] This study did not show any clinical evidence of an arrhythmia, but did demonstrate a change in a surrogate marker (QT prolongation). Other drug–drug interactions arising from CYP3A4 inhibition have also resulted in serious adverse events. For example, there are

TABLE 3-7 Drug Interactions with Grapefruit Juice

Medication	Potential Side Effect
Antihypertensives Amlodipine, Felodipine Nicardipine, Nisoldipine, Nitrendipine Nifedipine	decreased blood pressure, dizziness
Subarrachnoid Hemorrhage Nimodipine	decreased blood pressure
Rate Control **(Calcium Channel blocker)** Verapamil	decreased heart rate
Antiarrhythmics Amiodarone Quinidine	prolonged QT Interval, Torsades des Pointes
Immunosuppressants Cyclosporine	increased blood pressure, nephrotoxicity
Sedatives Midazolam, Triazolam, Diazepam	drowsiness, sleepiness
Antianxiety Buspirone	dizziness
Anticonvulsant, Neuropathy Carbamazepine	drowsiness, sleepiness
Statins Lovastatin, Atorvastatin, Simvastatin	rhabdomyolysis, muscle weakness, pain note: fluvastatin & pravastatin not affected
Prokinetic Agent Cisapride, restricted use	prolonged QT Interval, Torsades des Pointes
Antiviral Agent **(Protease inhibitor)** Saquinavir	hyperglycemia, paresthesias

reports of rhabdomyolysis from macrolide–lovastatin interaction.[70,71] Therefore, the possibility of a clinically significant adverse event occurring from a grapefruit juice interaction exists, and you should counsel patients on this interaction.

In general, you should alert patients to the drug interactions with grapefruit juice listed in Table 3-7. Make sure to tell them that drinking grapefruit juice every day may increase the possibility of an interaction, and that the interaction can occur with fresh squeezed juice and processed frozen concentrates sold in grocery stores. Unfortunately, separating the medication by a number of hours after drinking the juice will not diminish the interaction. If patients want to include grapefruit juice in their diet, they should avoid drinking it every day, and limit the amount to one glass (8 oz, 240 mL) or less.

A number of cardiovascular medications are affected by grapefruit juice.[67] For example:

- A three-fold increase in AUC was demonstrated with felodipine. This was the most significant pharmacokinetic effect seen with the calcium channel blocking agents.[68]
- No effect was seen with diltiazem and amlodipine.[72]
- Quinidine, bioavailability of 70%, was minimally affected by grapefruit juice (no affect on AUC),[73] whereas amiodarone had an increase in AUC (F = 50%).[74]
- Warfarin, an anticoagulant, does not interact with grapefruit juice, and concomitant use did not show any changes in INR.[75]

Cyclosporine, an immunosupressant, prevents organ rejection following cardiac, renal, and liver transplant and for autoimmune disorders. The bioavailability of cyclosporine is poor, and a new microemulsion formulation was developed to improve bioavailability. When taken with grapefruit juice, bioavailability of both formulations was improved.[66,76] Kane[76] discourages using these drugs in combination with grapefruit juice because the interaction is variable and risks of hypertension and nephrotoxicity outweigh the benefits of lowering the dose of cyclosporine. This interaction may also extend to tacrolimus, a newer immunosupressant, metabolized by the CYP3A4 pathway.

The new generation of sedatives and antidepressants are generally considered to have less serious side effects than older tricyclic antidepressants. Patients taking these agents should be alerted that grapefruit juice can increase drug levels. Patients with respiratory disease and liver disease are at greatest risk for central nervous system depression and respiratory depression from sedatives and antidepressants. Therefore, these patient groups are at greatest risk for grapefruit juice–drug interactions and should be carefully screened.

Psychiatry

Monoamine Oxidase Inhibitors

Monoamine oxidase inhibitors (MAO inhibitors) were developed in the 1950s to treat a number of psychiatric diagnoses such as depression and bipolar disorder.[77] Currently, these medications are not considered first-line agents. Newer drugs, such as tricyclic antidepressants, serotonin reuptake inhibitors, lithium, and valproic acid, have a more positive risk–benefit profile.

TABLE 3-8   Monoamine Oxidase Inhibitors

Nonselective inhibitors of MAO A and B

Antidepressants
Phenelzine (Nardil, Parke-Davis)
Tranylcypromine (Parnate, SmithKline Beecham)
Isocarboxazid (Marplan, Oxford)

Antibiotics
Linezolid (Zyvox, Pharmacia & Upjohn)
Weak inhibitor

Selective inhibitor of MAO B

Parkinson's Disease
Selegiline (Eldepryl, Somerset)
Selective inhibition seen at doses ≤ 10 mg/day

The agents used to treat depression are nonselective, irreversible inhibitors of MAO-A and B. Selegiline, a drug used for Parkinson's disease, is a selective, irreversible inhibitor of MAO-B.[78] Linezolid (Zyvox), an antibiotic, is a nonselective, reversible, MAO inhibitor.[79] Table 3-8 gives examples of MAO inhibitors.

Monoamine oxidase is ubiquitous in the body. It inactivates endogenous amines in the gastrointestinal tract and in brain tissue. MAO inhibitors are effective for treating depression by increasing the biologic presence of norepinephrine and serotonin. Tyramine, an amine found in a number of foods, is detoxified in the intestine via MAO enzymes.

Monoamine oxidase enzymes are divided into a Class A and B. As shown in Table 3-8, the drugs are either irreversible or reversible. Because the effects of irreversible inhibitors persist for weeks, there are implications for drug–drug interactions and DNIs.

Hypertensive emergencies resulting in stroke and death have been attributed to ingesting tyramine-containing foods while taking MAO inhibitors. Symptoms of hypertensive emergencies include headache and confusion as well as nausea, palpitations, and diaphoresis.[80] Gardener et al.[80] carefully reviewed the published reports and developed criteria for restricting foods containing more than 6 mg of tyramine per serving. Since linezolid is a weak inhibitor of monoamine oxidase, the manufacturer recommends restricting tyramine to less than 100 mg per meal.[79]

Most sources agree that aged cheeses and cured meats should be restricted due to high tyramine content. Fava beans or broad bean pods in Middle Eastern foods such as falafel contain L-dopa, a precursor to dopamine. Broad bean pods should be avoided since they have caused hypertensive crises.[80] Tap beers—alcoholic and nonalcoholic—contain tyramine. Table 3-9 gives direction on intake of tyramine-containing foods with MAO inhibitors.

TABLE 3-9   Direction on Intake of Tyramine-Containing Foods for Patients on MAO Inhibitors

Food	Allowed	Minimize Intake	Not Allowed
Beverages	Milk, decaffeinated coffee, tea, soda	Chocolate beverage, caffeine-containing drinks, clear spirits	Acidophilus milk, beer, ale, wine, malted beverages
Breads/cereals	All except those containing cheese	None	Cheese bread and crackers
Dairy products	Cottage cheese, farmers or pot cheese, cream cheese, ricotta cheese, all milk, eggs, ice cream, pudding (except chocolate)	Yogurt (limit to 4 oz per day)	Aged cheese, American, camembert, cheddar, gouda, gruyere, mozzarella, parmesan, provolone, romano, roquefort, stilton
Meat, fish, and poultry	All fresh or frozen	Aged meats, hot dogs, canned fish and meat	Chicken and beef liver, dried and pickled fish, summer or dry sausage, pepperoni, dried meats, meat extracts, bologna, liverwurst
Starches – potatoes/rice	All	None	Soybean (including paste)
Vegetables	All fresh, frozen, canned, or dried vegetable juices except those not allowed	Chili peppers, Chinese pea pods	Fava beans, sauerkraut, pickles, olives, Italian broad beans
Fruit	Fresh, frozen, or canned fruits and fruit juices	Avocado, banana, raspberries, figs	Banana peel extract
Soups	All soups not listed to limit or avoid	Commercially canned soups	Soups that contain broad beans, fava beans, cheese, beer, wine, any made with flavor cubes or meat extract, miso soup
Fats	All except fermented	Sour cream	Packaged gravy
Sweets	Sugar, hard candy, honey, molasses, syrups	Chocolate candies	None
Desserts	Cakes, cookies, gelatin, pastries, sherbets, sorbets	Chocolate desserts	Cheese-filled desserts

TABLE 3-9 Direction on Intake of Tyramine-Containing Foods for Patients on MAO Inhibitors (continued)

Food	Allowed	Minimize Intake	Not Allowed
Miscellaneous	Salt, nuts, spices, herbs, flavorings, Worcestershire sauce	Soy sauce, peanuts	Brewer's yeast, yeast concentrates, all aged and fermented products, monosodium glutamate, vitamins with Brewer's yeast

Reprinted with permission from Lexi-Comp Inc., Hudson, Ohio.

Enforcing these dietary restrictions may be difficult. Sweet et al.[81] performed a survey of 139 patients treated with MAO inhibitors for a number of psychiatric disorders. The results revealed that 90% of patients reported eating some type of cheese on a weekly basis. These foods are so pervasive in the normal diet that the surveyors recommend counseling patients before initiating therapy with MAO inhibitors.[81]

Gastrointestinal

Proton Pump Inhibitors

Proton pump inhibitors suppress acid, which may prevent the release of cyanocobalamin from dietary protein.[38] This in turn results in the inability to form intrinsic factor, which is needed to absorb vitamin B_{12} in the ileum.[82] Since B_{12} deficiency is rarely reported, no specific recommendations have been identified for preventing it.

Patients receiving vitamin B_{12} supplementation orally have clinically reduced absorption when the vitamin is administered concomitantly with proton pump inhibitors.[83] In this case, you should switch the patient to an alternative acid suppressant such as H_2 receptor antagonists or sucralfate, and counsel the patient to separate the vitamin administration from proton pump inhibitor by 2 hours. In case of symptomatic B_{12} deficiency, you should consider administering vitamin B_{12} intramuscularly or subcutaneously with concomitant use of proton pump inhibitors.[78] Also, make sure that patients who are on long-term proton pump inhibitor therapy are aware of this adverse effect, and counsel them on the symptoms of vitamin B_{12} deficiency (such as fatigue and tingling in the hands and feet).

Infectious Disease

Fluoroquinolones

Divalent cations such as calcium, iron, magnesium, and zinc interact with several oral fluoroquinolones, resulting in decreased absorption of the antibiotic. These cations chelate antibiotics in the gut lumen, resulting in decreased antimicrobial effectiveness.[84-89]

You should counsel patients to separate administration of these agents from the antibiotic. In general, most fluoroquinolones should be given 2 hours before or 4–6 hours after supplementation.[78] One exception to this interaction (with calcium) is gatafloxacin. Results from a single dose pharmacokinetic study with 400 mg gatafloxacin administered at the same time as 1000 mg calcium carbonate showed no effect on the absorption of the antibiotic.[90] However, separating these agents from the antibiotic may not be reliable for every patient. Therefore, pharmacists should counsel patients on how to monitor for decreased antibiotic effectiveness daily (such as increased temperature or worsening symptoms), and consider switching the antibiotic to the intravenous route, or temporarily discontinuing the supplement.

Tetracyclines

Similarly, the tetracycline antibiotics also chelate the divalent cations, resulting in decreased absorption of the antibiotic.[78] Dietary sources of divalent cations also contribute to reduced antibiotic effectiveness. The interaction is more common with tetracycline, compared to doxycycline.[91] Nevertheless, a potential interaction exists, even with the intravenous formulation of doxycycline.[92]

As with the fluoroquinolones, you should instruct patients to separate calcium, zinc, iron, and magnesium from the antibiotic by at least 2 hours before or 4–6 hours after intake. Patients should also separate dairy products and antibiotics using the same guidelines. Certain iron products that are associated with a reduced likelihood of this interaction include tablets (versus capsules), enteric coated (versus regular) tablets, sustained release formulations, and gluconate and fumarate salts (versus the sulfate salt).[78,93,94] In spite of this, patients should still separate all dosage forms of iron from the tetracyclines as much as possible. As with the fluoroquinolones, you should also monitor patients for decreased antimicrobial effectiveness, such as increased temperature or increased infectious symptoms.

Isoniazid

Isoniazid is an antituberculosis agent that competitively inhibits formation of pyridoxine, vitamin B_6.[78] This interaction ultimately results in secondary vitamin B_6 deficiency, which manifests as peripheral neuropathy. Approximately one quarter of all patients receiving 6 mg/kg/day or greater of isoniazid will experience this effect.[37,95,96] All patients taking prescription isoniazid should receive 25–50 mg vitamin B_6 orally each day. Lower doses are insufficient in preventing peripheral neuropathy associated with vitamin B_6 deficiency.[97] You should also educate patients on the signs and symptoms of peripheral neuropathy, such as numbness or tingling in the hands and feet, and tell them to contact their doctor immediately if any of these symptoms present. Alcoholic, diabetic, and malnourished patients are at greatest risk for peripheral neuropathy.[98]

Weight Reducing Agents

Orlistat

Orlistat is a potent inhibitor of GI lipases and is used to treat obesity. Lipase is necessary for digestion of fat. In addition to the desired effects of weight reduction, fat-soluble vitamin absorption may be impaired. Although limited data exist, beta carotene and vitamin E absorption are reduced 30% and 60% respectively when given at the same time as orlistat.[99] Pharmacists should encourage patients taking orlistat to take a multivitamin supplement daily and to separate administration from orlistat by at least 2 hours.

IMPLEMENTING POLICIES AND PRACTICES IN HEALTH CARE ORGANIZATIONS

In a health care system, the responsibility to provide patient education on drug–nutrient interactions is mandated by the Joint Commission on Accreditation of Healthcare Organizations (JCAHO).[100] Pharmacy administrators should support the multidisciplinary process for developing policies on managing DNIs and educating the hospital staff.[101,102]

The task force or committee addressing these issues should include a physician, nutritionist, nurse, and pharmacist. The committee should conduct a continuous quality improvement process to review available literature, identify and maintain the listings of DNIs, and educate providers on significant interactions.

Computer software programs should make the process of identifying DNIs easier. You can program clinical information systems to alert you to DNIs. Instructions printed at the point-of-care either as part of the medication order or as a label should provide specific instructions for managing the interaction. When combined with in-service training, this method has been shown to improve nurse awareness of DNIs.[103]

Patient education tools can include medication lists highlighting drugs that they must separate from food or take with a meal. You can also develop pamphlets that provide detailed information on diets for complicated interactions that occur with target drugs such as warfarin and MAO inhibitors.

SUMMARY AND CONCLUSION

Pharmacists play a key role in evaluating the medication profile and screening for DNIs. This chapter has discussed major DNIs that can have a significant impact on drug therapy and the interventions necessary to manage these interactions, such as advising the patient to take medications with or without food. Patients taking warfarin and MAO inhibitors, however, may require more formal education on dietary restrictions. The pharmacist may have to consult with the prescriber to suggest a therapeutic drug monitoring plan and additional electrolyte, vitamin, and mineral supplements.

The pharmacist should play an active role in educating patients and other health care professionals about DNIs. First, organize and collect drug information resources on the topic. Then, as new drugs are approved for use, you can screen for interactions, and anticipate the impact on disease management programs.

The pharmacist also has a keen understanding of drug pharmacokinetics and can critically evaluate data presented in the literature to determine the significance of the interactions. Using sophisticated software programs in medication profiling systems pharmacists can more easily screen for these interactions.

Patients have direct access to pharmacists, who are highly visible and easily accessible health care professionals. By advising patients on the potential risks and benefits associated with the DNI, you play a vital role in improving patient treatment outcomes.

REFERENCES

1. Fleischer D, Li C, Zhou Y. Drug, meal and formulation interactions influencing drug absorption after oral administration. *Clin Pharmacokinet.* 1999;36:233-54.
2. Hendeles L, Weinberger M, Milavetz G, et al. Food-induced "dose dumping" from a once-a-day theophylline product as a cause of theophylline toxicity. *Chest.* 1985;87:758-65.
3. Michalets EL. Update: clinically signficant cytochrome P-450 drug interactions. *Pharmacotherapy.* 1998;18:84-112.
4. Singh BN. Effects of food on clinical pharmacokinetics. *Clin Pharmacokinet.* 1999;37:213-55.
5. Krueger KA, Garnett WR, Comstock TJ, et al. Effect of two administration schedules of an enteral nutrient formula on phenytoin bioavailability. *Epilepsia.* 1987;6:706-12.
6. Manson JI, Beal SM, Magarey LJ. Bioavailability of phenytoin from various pharmaceutical preparations in children. *Med J Aust.* 1975;2:590-2.
7. Bauer LA. Interference of oral phenytoin absorption by continuous nasogastric feedings. *Neurology.* 1982;32:570-2.
8. Hooks MA, Longe RL, Taylor AT, et al. Recovery of phenytoin from an enteral nutrient formula. *Am J Hosp Pharm.* 1986;43:685-8.
9. Cacek AT, DeVito JM, Koonce JR. In vitro evaluation of nasogastric administration methods for phenytoin. *Am J Hosp Pharm.* 1986;43:689-92.
10. Carter BL, Garnett WR, Pellock JM, et al. Effect of antacids on phenytoin bioavailability. *Ther Drug Monit.* 1981;3:333-40.
11. Markowsky SM, Skaar DJ, Christie JM, et al. Phenytoin protein binding and dosage requirements during acute and convalescent phases following brain injury. *Ann Pharmacother.* 1996;30:443-8.
12. Boucher BA, Kuhl DA, Fabian TC, et al. Effect of neurotrauma on hepatic drug clearance. *Clin Pharmacol Ther.* 1991;50:487-97.
13. Earl-Salotti GL, Charland SL. The effect of parenteral nutrition on hepatic cytochrome P-450. *JPEN J Parenter Enteral Nutr.* 1994;18:458-65.
14. Aubier M, Murciano D, Lecocguic Y, et al. Effect of hypophosphatemia on diaphragmatic contractility in patients with acute respiratory failure. *N Engl J Med.* 1985;313:420-4.
15. Cohn JN, Kowey PR, Whelton PK, et al. New guidelines for potassium replacement in clinical practice: a contemporary review by the national council on potassium in clinical practice. *Arch Intern Med.* 2000;160:2429-36.
16. Gennari FJ. Current concepts: hypokalemia. *N Engl J Med.* 1998;339:451-8.
17. Weisinger JR, Bellorin-Font E. Magnesium and phosphorus. *Lancet.* 1998;352:391-6.
18. Brown GR, Greenwood JK. Drug- and nutrition-induced hypophosphatemia: mechanism and relevance in the critically ill. *Ann Pharmacother.* 1994;28:626-32.
19. Hirsch J, Dalen JE, Anderson D, et al. Oral anticoagulants: mechanism of action, clinical effectiveness, and optimal therapeutic range. *Chest.* 2001;119(suppl 1): 8S-21S.
20. O'Reilly RA, Rytand DA. "Resistance" to warfarin due to unrecognized vitamin K supplementation. *N Engl J Med.* 1980;303:160-1.

21. Lader E, Yang L, Clarke A. Warfarin dosage and vitamin K in osmolite. *Ann Intern Med.* 1980;93:373-4.
22. Griffith LD, Olvey SE, Triplett WC. Increasing prothrombin times in a warfarin-treated patient upon withdrawal of Ensure Plus. *Crit Care Med.* 1982;10:799-800.
23. Westfall LK. An unrecognized cause of warfarin resistance. *Drug Intell Clin Pharm.* 1981;15:131.
24. Lee M, Schwartz RN, Sharifi R. Warfarin resistance and vitamin K. *Ann Intern Med.* 1981;94:140-1.
25. Zallman JA, Lee DP, Jeffrey PL. Liquid nutrition as a cause of warfarin resistance. *Am J Hosp Pharm.* 1981;38:1174.
26. Parr MD, Record KE, Griffith GL, et al. Effect of enteral nutrition on warfarin therapy. *Clin Pharm.* 1982;1:274-6.
27. Kempin SJ. Warfarin resistance caused by broccoli. *N Engl J Med.* 1983;308(20):1229-30.
28. Watson AJ, Pegg M, Green JR. Enteral feeds may antagonise warfarin. *Br Med J.* 1984;288:557.
29. Walker FB 4th. Myocardial infarction after diet-induced warfarin resistance. *Arch Intern Med.* 1984;144:2089-90.
30. Howard PA, Hannanman KM. Warfarin resistance linked to enteral nutrition products. *J Am Diet Assoc.* 1985;85:713-5.
31. Karlson B, Leijd B, Hellstrom K. On the influence of vitamin K-rich vegetables and wine on the effectiveness of warfarin treatment. *Acta Med Scand.* 1986;220:347-50.
32. Martin JE, Lutomski DM. Warfarin resistance and enteral feedings. *JPEN J Parenter Enteral Nutr.* 1989;13:206-8.
33. Chow WH, Chow TC, Tse TM, et al. Anticoagulation instability with life-threatening complication after dietary modification. *Postgrad Med J.* 1990;66:855-7.
34. Pedersen FM, Hamberg O, Hess K, et al. The effect of dietary vitamin K on warfarin-induced anticoagulation. *J Intern Med.* 1991;229:517-20.
35. Taylor JR, Wilt VM. Probable antagonism by green tea. *Ann Pharmacother.* 1999;33:426-8.
36. Qureshi GD, Reinders TP, Swint JJ, et al. Acquired warfarin resistance and weight-reducing diet. *Arch Intern Med.* 1981;141:507-9.
37. Booth SL, Sadowski JA, Weihrauch JL, et al. Vitamin K_1 (phyloquinone) content of foods: a provisional table. *J Food Comp Anal.* 1993;6:109-20.
38. Kirk J. Significant drug nutrient interactions. *Am Fam Physician.* 1995; 51:1175-82.
39. Coumadin (warfarin sodium) [package insert]. Wilmington, DE: DuPont Pharma; January 2001.
40. Trovato A, Nuhlicek DN, Midtling JE. Drug nutrient interactions. *Am Fam Physician.* 1991; 44:1651-8.
41. Ansell J, Hirsch J, Dalen J, et al. Managing oral anticoagulant therapy. *Chest.* 2001;119(suppl 1):22S-38S.
42. Lutomski DM, Palascak JE, Bower RH. Warfarin resistance associated with intravenous lipid administration. *JPEN J Parenter Enteral Nutr.* 1987;11:316-8.
43. Brown R, Dickerson R. Drug–nutrient interactions. *Am J Managed Care.* 1999;5:345-55.
44. American College of Rheumatology Task Force on Osteoporosis Guidelines. Recommendations for the prevention and treatment of glucocorticoid-induced osteoporosis. *Arthritis Rheum.* 1996;39:1791-801.
45. Adinoff AD, Hollister JR. Steroid-induced fractures and bone loss in patients with asthma. *N Engl J Med.* 1983;309:265-8.
46. Verstraeten A, Dequeker J. Vertebral and peripheral bone mineral content and fracture evidence in postmenopausal patients with rheumatoid arthritis: effect of low dose corticosteroids. *Ann Rheum Dis.* 1986;45:852-7.
47. Dykman TR, Gluck OS, Murphy WA, et al. Evaluation of factors associated with glucocorticoid-induced osteopenia in patients with rheumatic diseases. *Arthritis Rheum.* 1985;28:361-8.
48. Michel BA, Bloch DA, Fries JF. Predictors of fractures in early rheumatoid arthritis. *J Rheumatol.* 1991;18:804-8.
49. Michel BA, Bloch PA, Wolfe F, et al. Fractures in rheumatoid arthritis: an evaluation of associated risk factors. *J Rheumatol.* 1993;20:1666-9.
50. Cooper C, Coupland C, Mitchell M. Rheumatoid arthritis, corticosteroid therapy and hip fracture. *Ann Rheum Dis.* 1994;54:49-52.
51. Saag KG, Koehnke R, Caldwell JR, et al. Low dose long-term corticosteroid therapy in rheumatoid arthritis: an analysis of serious adverse events. *Am J Med.* 1994;96:115-23.
52. Marystone JF, Barrett-Connor EL, Morton DJ. Inhaled and oral corticosteroids: their effect on bone mineral density in older adults. *Am J Public Health.* 1995;85:1693-5.
53. Adachi JD, Bensen WG, Hodsman AB. Corticosteroid-induced osteoporosis. *Semin Arthritis Rheum.* 1993;22:375-84.
54. Gluck OS, Murphy WA, Hahn TJ, et al. Bone loss in adults receiving alternate day glucocorticoid therapy: a comparison with daily therapy. *Arthritis Rheum.* 1981;24:892-8.

55. Ruegsegger P, Medici TC, Anliker M. Corticosteroid-induced bone loss: a longitudinal study of alternate day therapy in patients with bronchial asthma using quantitative computed tomography. *Eur J Clin Pharmacol.* 1983;25:615-20.

56. Ward MJ. Inhaled corticosteroids: effect on bone? *Respir Med.* 1993;87(suppl A):33-6.

57. Boyd G. Effect of inhaled corticosteroids on bone. *Respir Med.* 1994;88(suppl A):45-52.

58. Hanania NA, Chapman KR, Sturtridge WC, et al. Dose-related decrease in bone density among asthmatic patients treated with inhaled corticosteroids. *J Allergy Clin Immunol.* 1995;96(5 Pt 1):571-9.

59. Tjellesen L. Metabolism and action of vitamin D in epileptic patients on anticonvulsive treatment and healthy adults. *Dan Med Bull.* 1994;41:139-50.

60. Gilman AG, Rall TW, Nies AS, et al., eds. *Goodman and Gilman's The Pharmacological Basis of Therapeutics.* 8th ed. New York: Pergamon Press; 1990.

61. Lewis DP, VanDyke DC, Wilhite LA, et al. Phenytoin-folic acid interaction. *Ann Pharmacother.* 1995;29:726-35.

62. Lilja JJ, Kivisto KT, Neuvonen PJ. Duration of effect of grapefruit juice on the pharmacokinetics of the CYP3A4 substrate simvastatin. *Clin Pharmacol Ther.* 2000;68:384-90.

63. Lilja JJ, Kivisto KT, Backman JT, et al. Effect of grapefruit juice dose on grapefuit juice–triazolam interaction: repeated consumption prolongs triazolam half-life. *Eur J Clin Pharmacol.* 2000;56:411-5.

64. Kivisto KT, Lilja JJ, Backman JT, et al. Repeated consumption of grapefruit juice considerably increases plasma concentrations of cisapride. *Clin Pharmacol Ther.* 1999;66:448-53.

65. Kantola T, Kivisto KT, Neuvonen PJ. Grapefruit juice greatly increases serum concentrations of lovastatin and lovastatin acid. *Clin Pharmacol Ther.* 1998;63:397-402.

66. Ku YM, Min DI, Flanigan M. Effect of grapefruit juice on the pharmacokinetics of microemulsion cyclosporine and its metabolite in healthy volunteers: does the formulation difference matter? *J Clin Pharmacol.* 1998;38:959-65.

67. Ameer B, Weintraub RA. Drug interactions with grapefruit juice. *Clin Pharmacokinet.* 1997;33:103-21.

68. Bailey DG, Dresser GK, Kreeft JH, et al. Grapefruit–felodipine interaction: effect of unprocessed fruit and probable active ingredients. *Clin Pharmacol Ther.* 2000;68:468-77.

69. Benton RE, Honig PK, Zamani K, et al. Grapefruit juice alters terfenedine pharmacokinetics, resulting in prolongation of repolarization on the electrocardiogram. *Clin Pharmacol Ther.* 1996;59:383-8.

70. Spach DH, Bauwens YE, Clark CD, et al. Rhabdomyolysis associated with lovastatin and erythromycin use. *West J Med.* 1991;154:213-5.

71. Grunden JW, Fisher KA. Lovastatin-induced rhabdomyolysis possibly associated with clarithromycin and azithromycin. *Ann Pharmacother.* 1997;31:859-63.

72. Vincent J, Harris SI, Foulds G, et al. Lack of effect of grapefruit juice on the pharmacokinetics and pharmacodynamics of amlodipine. *Br J Clin Pharmcol.* 2000;50:455-63.

73. Damkier P, Hansen LL, Brosen K. Effect of diclofenac, disulfiram, itraconazole, grapefruit juice and erythromycin on the pharmacokinetics of quinidine. *Br J Clin Pharmacol.* 1999;48:829-38.

74. Libersa CC, Brique SA, Motte KB, et al. Dramatic inhibition of amiodarone metabolism induced by grapefruit juice. *Br J Clin Pharmacol.* 2000,49:373-8.

75. Sullivan DM, Ford MA, Boyden TW. Grapefruit juice and the response to warfarin. *Am J Health Syst Pharm.* 1998;55:1581-3.

76. Kane G, Lipsky JJ. Drug–grapefruit juice interactions. *Mayo Clin Proc.* 2000;75:933-42.

77. Livingston MG, Livingston HM. Monoamine oxidase inhibitors: an update on drug interactions. *Drug Saf.* 1996;14:219-27.

78. *Drug Facts and Comparisons.* 55th ed. St. Louis, MO: Facts and Comparisons, Inc; 2001.

79. Zyvox (linezolid) [package insert]. Kalamazoo, MI: Pharmacia & Upjohn Company; 2000.

80. Gardner DM, Shulman KI, Walker SE, et al. The making of a user friendly MAOI diet. *J Clin Psychiatry.* 1996;57:99-104.

81. Sweet RA, Brown EJ, Heimberg RG, et al. Monoamine oxidase inhibitor dietary restrictions: what are we asking patients to give up? *J Clin Psychiatry.* 1995;56:196-201.

82. Termanini B, Gibril F, Sutliff VE, et al. Effect of long-term gastric acid suppressive therapy on serum vitamin B_{12} levels in patients with Zollinger–Ellison syndrome. *Am J Med.* 1998;104:422-30.

83. Marcuard S, Albernaz L, Khazanie PG. Omeprazole therapy causes malabsorption of cyanocobalamin (vitamin B_{12}). *Ann Intern Med.* 1994;120:211-5.

84. Polk RE, Healy DP, Shai J, et al. Effect of ferrous sulfate and multivitamins with zinc on absorption of ciprofloxacin in normal volunteers. *Antimicrob Agents Chemother.* 1989;33:1841-4.

85. Polk RE. Drug–drug interactions with ciprofloxacin and other fluoroquinolones. *Am J Med.* 1989;87:76S-81S.

86. Lomaestro BM, Bailie GR. Quinolone-cation interactions: a review. *Drug Intell Clin Pharm.* 1991;25:1249-58.

87. Lehto P, Kivisto KT. Different effects of products containing metal ions on the absorption of lomefloxacin. *Clin Pharmacol Ther.* 1994;56:477-82.

88. Kara M, Hasinoff BB, McKay DW, et al. Clinical and chemical interactions between iron preparations and ciprofloxacin. *Br J Clin Pharmacol.* 1991;31:257-61.

89. LePennec MP, Kitzis MD, Terdjman M, et al. Possible interaction of ciprofloxacin with ferrous sulphate. *J Antimicrob Chemother.* 1990;25:184-5

90. Tequin (Gatafloxacin) [package insert]. Princeton, NJ: Bristol-Myers Squibb Company; 1999.

91. Rosenblatt JE, Barrett JE, Brodie JL, et al. Comparison of in vitro activity and clinical pharmacology of doxycycline with other tetracyclines. *Antimicrobial Agents Chemother.* 1966;6:134-41.

92. Venho VM, Salonen RO, Mattila MJ. Modification of the pharmacokinetics of doxycycline in man by ferrous sulfate or charcoal. *Eur J Clin Pharmacol.* 1978;14:277-80.

93. Neuvonen PJ. Interactions with absorption of tetracyclines. *Drugs.* 1976;11:45-54.

94. D'Arcy PF. Nutrient–drug interactions. *Adverse Drug React Toxicol Rev.* 1995;14:233-54.

95. Biehl JP, Vilter RW. Effect of isoniazid on vitamin B_6 metabolism: its possible significance in producing isoniazid and neuritis. *Proc Soc Exp Biol Med.* 1954;85:389-92.

96. Bender DA, Russell-Jones R. Isoniazid-induced pellagra despite vitamin B_6 supplementation. *Lancet.* 1979;2:1125-6.

97. Chan TYK. Pyridoxine ineffective in isoniazid-induced psychosis [letter]. *Ann Pharmacother.* 1999;33:1123-4.

98. Ward E. Tuberculosis. In: Young LY, Koda-Kimble MA, eds. *Applied Therapeutics: The Clinical Use of Drugs.* 6th ed. Vancouver, WA: Applied Therapeutics Inc; 1995:1-15.

99. Xenical (orlistat) [package insert]. Nutley, NJ: Roche Laboratories Inc; 1999.

100. Joint Commission. *Comprehensive Accreditation Manual for Hospitals.* Oakbrook Terrace, IL: Joint Commission on Accreditation of Healthcare Organizations; 2001: PF.1.5.

101. Nowlin DB, Blanche W. Refining a food–drug interaction program. *Am J Health Syst Pharm.* 1998;55:114,122-3.

102. Teresi ME, Morgan DE. Attitudes of healthcare professionals toward patient counseling on drug–nutrient interactions. *Ann Pharmacother.* 1994;23:576-80.

103. Gauthier I, Malone M, Lesar TS, et al. Comparison of programs for preventing drug–nutrient interactions in hospitalized patients. *Am J Health Syst Pharm.* 1997;54:405-11.

Thanks to Barbara Nansteil, MS, AHIP, Wilkes University, for assistance with research for Chapter 3.

CHAPTER 4

ERGOGENIC AIDS

Robert E. C. Wildman and Louis J. Ciliberti, Jr.

F or centuries, people have searched for ways to maximize physical performance. Ergogenic dietary aids—those that help the body increase its ability to work—were used by the ancients to improve athletic competitiveness and achieve military prowess.

Foods considered performance-enhancing changed with the times. The Greek physician Galen recorded that many of the Olympic athletes in the seventh century BC ate a vegetarian-style diet that included cheese, figs, and breads.[1-3] During the fifth century BC, Stymphalos, who was a champion Olympic long-distance runner, endorsed meats.[4] The selected meats, cheeses, figs, and breads were equivalent to today's power bars.

Organs of animals noted for strength and ferocity were also highly prized as performance enhancers.[1] Consuming the heart or testicles of a bull, for example, could transfer desirable attributes of those animals.

We can look all the way back to the ancient Egyptians for records of the first sport drinks, which were concocted from the hooves of asses boiled in oil, with rose petals and rose hips added for flavor.[1] Legend has it that Persian physicians provided iron supplements to weary soldiers who hemorrhaged from wounds. And medieval knights allegedly used various stimulants and "magic potions" to enhance ferocity and performance during prolonged battles.

Today the sport food and supplement industry boasts sales of roughly a billion dollars in the United States alone.[1,2] This chapter will provide an overview of many of the most popular substances touted to have ergogenic properties. Some are supplements and others are components of sport drinks and bars.

ARGININE, ORNITHINE, AND LYSINE (GROWTH HORMONE SECRETAGOGUES)

The infusion of the essential amino acid lysine and two nonessential amino acids, arginine and ornithine, is a growth hormone (GH) secretagogue. This infusion may have clinical benefit for patients who have sustained

---

What Are Ergogenic Aids?

The term "ergogenic" is of Greek origin, from *ergon* meaning "work" and *gennan* "to produce." Ergogenic substances or methods attempt to increase performance by promoting or supporting the development of greater physical power, strength, and endurance. They also provide neurological stimulation, and may help people develop fit and athletic bodies.

---

burns.[1,2,5-7] Donati and colleagues[5] reported that infusing severely burned patients (i.e., burned over 20% to 60% of body surface area) with 20 g of ornithine α-ketoglutarate (OKG) secured positive nitrogen balance by the 5th day of supplementation (9th day post-trauma). Cumulative N-balance, or the sum of daily N-balance measures, was achieved by the 21st day. The supplemented patients also presented higher plasma protein levels, lower mean losses of body weight, and better subjective scores of tissue repair when compared to unsupplemented patients. In a similar investigation by De Bant and colleagues,[6] they observed reduced urinary 3-methyl histidine (3-MH) and hydroxyproline levels in burn patients who were supplemented with OKG (30 g/d). People who weight train are particularly interested in the anti-catabolic properties of GH secretagogues. This is because muscle protein balance is the algebraic sum of protein synthesis and catabolism. Therefore, reducing muscle protein catabolism could lead to greater muscle mass development.

Whether or not oral supplementation of these amino acids can have similar GH secretagogue effects is still unclear. There are practical considerations that must be taken into account. Certainly, oral supplementation of these amino acids at the infusion dosages noted above might be difficult to tolerate in the intestinal tract due to their potential osmotic influence. In addition, competitive amino acid absorption needs to be considered as ornithine, arginine, and lysine all compete with each other as well as with cystine for the same transporter.[2] Furthermore, potential toxicity might be a concern and has not been explored.

Lower supplemental doses have been tested, but the results are inconclusive and even positive reports are incomplete.[7] Isidori and colleagues[8] reported that the combined supplementation of arginine and lysine (1.2 g each) resulted in an increase in GH, while neither did so independently. Suminski and colleagues[9] also noted that a mixed supplement of arginine and lysine (1.5 g each) raised GH during resting conditions. However, supplementation prior to a bout of resistance training failed to further augment the training-induced elevation in GH. The results of this investigation suggest that supplementation may be most effective several hours after a workout.

Corpas and colleagues[10] reported that the elderly may not respond to oral arginine as young people do. Older men (69 ± 5 years) were compared to young men (26 ± 4 years) after both were supplemented with arginine and lysine (3 g each) for 14 days. Blood samples were obtained at intervals between 8:00 pm and 8:00 am on the day before and after supplementation. The results showed that GH was not elevated in the older men in response to supplementation, and that GH levels were positively related to serum arginine.

In related studies Marcell and colleagues[11] observed that arginine (5 g) failed to increase GH levels in both older men and younger men. Here the basal GH was more than two-fold greater in the young men (i.e., 543.6 +/- 84.0 vs. 211.5 +/- 63.0 ng/mL). They also reported that arginine did not increase GH levels above unsupplemented levels after a bout of resistance training in the older men, and actually hindered the elevation of GH in the young men.

Fogelholm and colleagues[12] provided 2 g of arginine, ornithine, and lysine to competitive weightlifters. Here again GH levels were not increased above those in a placebo trial, nor were insulin levels. In support, Lambert and colleagues[13] reported that neither a supplement of arginine and lysine (2.4 g) or ornithine and tyrosine (1.85 g) increased GH levels in the blood of male bodybuilders. Their experimental design also included a GH releasing test, with 0.5 mcg GH-releasing hormone/kg body weight infused to assess GH secretory response, which was the same with supplementation and with placebo.

In an endurance trial, Eto and colleagues[14] provided supplemental glutamate-arginine to highly trained cyclists. Their GH levels as well as insulin and cortisol levels during rest did not differ from those of a group using placebo. However, in comparison to the control group, amino acid supplementation diminished the exercise-induced elevations in GH and cortisol. Thus the hindering influence of GH secretagogues upon exercise-induced GH elevation in younger people has been noted in two studies.[11-14]

Although the results of the studies above tell us a little about how supplements affect hormonal levels, less is known about how they influence athletic performance. In one of few studies in this area, Ceremuzynski and colleagues[15] reported that arginine supplementation (6 g/day for 3 days) improved the exercise (i.e., treadmill) capacity of patients with stable angina pectoris. These findings were supported in a follow-up study involving patients with stable coronary artery disease.[16] Some scientists have speculated that arginine has the potential, at least in theory, to improve endurance by serving as a precursor of nitric oxide, which seems to be a potent local vasodilator. A study involving arginine supplementation in rats supports these findings.[17]

Colombani and colleagues[18] set out to assess the impact of arginine/aspartate supplementation (15 g/day) on trained runners treated for 2 weeks prior to a marathon, evaluating blood indices of energy metabolism, enzymes, and metabolic hormones. Plasma levels of carbohydrate (e.g., glucose, lactate, pyruvate) and fat metabolites (e.g., fatty acids, glycerol, beta-hydroxybutyrate), cortisol, insulin, ammonia, lactate dehydrogenase, and creatine kinase as well as the respiratory exchange ratio (RER) were unaffected by the supplementation. However, the levels of somatotropic hormone, glucagon, urea, and arginine were raised, while the level of most of the remaining plasma amino acids, as well as their sum, were lowered.

Terms Associated with Ergogenic Aids

❑ **Aminate** means to combine with ammonia.
❑ **Aromatization** refers to the catalytic activity of aromatase in the conversion of testosterone to estrogen.
❑ **Catabolism** is the breaking down in the body of complex chemical compounds into simpler ones.
❑ **Concomitant** refers to simultaneous or concurrent.
❑ **Ergolytic** refers to having the ability to reduce physical performance.
❑ **Secretagogues** are agents that promote secretion, the movement of a physiologically active substance out of the cell or organ in which it is formed.
❑ **Somatotropic** agents stimulate body growth.
❑ **Vasodilators** cause dilation of the blood vessels.

Conflicting information regarding the efficacy of these GH secretagogues might be attributed to different dosage levels. Also, it is important to identify a mechanism for the GH effect if it occurs. The possibility that these amino acids interact directly with receptors in anterior pituitary gland tissue is a starting point. The findings of Villalobas,[19] working with rat tissue, support this theory. The study reported that roughly 40% of anterior pituitary gland cells had receptors for these amino acids. In addition, the metabolic influence and potential blunting of exercise-induced GH release by these amino acids require much greater investigation.

ASPARTIC ACID

Blood ammonia concentrations are known to increase during high-intensity exercise of longer duration, which in turn is associated with fatigue.[1] As aspartic acid is involved in the formation of urea and thus in the metabolism of ammonia, it is possible that supplementation increases urea formation and reduces the potential for ammonia-related premature fatigue. In addition, aspartic acid has been suggested to slow glycogen depletion in muscles during endurance activity by slowing glycogen breakdown. Here the carbon skeleton of aspartic acid would serve as a source of oxaloacetate (OAA), which would combine with fatty acid-derived acetyl coenzyme A (CoA) to limit the need for glucose-derived OAA (via pyruvate carboxylase). This could also postpone fatigue associated with glycogen depletion. Only a handful of research studies have been conducted to test the efficacy of aspartate supplementation, but the data are increasing.

Hagan and colleagues[20] provided 7.2 g of potassium and magnesium aspartate to seven males during a 24-hour period prior to their walking on a treadmill for 90 minutes at 62% VO_2max. In this general experimental design the supplementation influenced cardiorespiratory (i.e., VO_2, CO_2, BP, HR, RER(RQ)), hematological (i.e., % change in plasma volume) and metabolic

Abbreviations Associated with Ergogenic Aids

- ❏ **BP** refers to blood pressure.
- ❏ **CO$_2$** is carbon dioxide.
- ❏ **HR** is heart rate.
- ❏ **RER** refers to respiratory exchange ratio and is used interchangeably with RQ.
- ❏ **RQ** is respiratory quotient.
- ❏ **VO$_2$max (or VO$_2$peak)** refers to the maximal amount of oxygen consumption in a minute (ml/min).

parameters (i.e., serum creatine kinase, lactate, lactate dehydrogenase), and body temperature in comparison to control trials.

Soon after, Maughan and Sadler[21] provided 6 g of potassium-magnesium aspartate over a 24-hour period to young males who then cycled at 75% VO$_2$max until they were exhausted. Time before exhaustion with the aspartic acid supplement (82.7 minutes) varied little from the times posted by the unsupplemented control group (85.4 minutes). In addition, aspartic acid supplementation did not influence plasma ammonia concentrations as well as other markers of energy metabolism (i.e., glucose, lactate, or free fatty acids [FFA]).

deHaan and colleagues[22] also reported that aspartic acid supplementation (i.e., K$^+$ and Mg^{2+}/aspartic acid salts) failed to improve metabolic parameters (i.e., adenosine triphosphate (ATP), creatine phosphate, lactate) or force generation in the electrically stimulated quadriceps of rats, nor were there changes in submaximal endurance time in humans. Elsewhere, aspartic acid supplementation did not allow rats to swim longer till exhaustion, nor did it influence liver and muscle glycogen content at 60 minutes of swimming in comparison to controls.[23] Interestingly, the rats supplemented with aspartic acid presented a lower plasma FFA at exhaustion.

Meanwhile, Tuttle and colleagues[24] reported that 24-hour supplementation of aspartic acid prior to high-intensity resistance training also failed to lower ammonia concentrations during and after the exercise. Colombani and colleagues[18] provided an arginine/aspartate supplement (15 g) to runners for 14 days prior to running a marathon and measured gas exchange during and blood samples before, during, and after a marathon. While the level of the supplemented amino acids (and GH) was increased, the level of other amino acids decreased and glucose, lactate, FFA, and ammonia were unchanged. They concluded that aspartate/alanine supplementation failed to provide a metabolic benefit during the run.

But there is some suggestion of positive benefits associated with aspartic acid supplementation at a higher dosage. Lancha and colleagues[25] reported that supplementation of aspartic acid, asparagine, and carnitine extended time to exhaustion by 40% during an endurance trial in rats. As mentioned, aspartic acid and asparagine are precursors for OAA, which combines with acetyl CoA derived from either fatty acids, glucose or leucine to form the preliminary tricarboxylic (TCA) cycle substrate acid (see discussion of branched chain amino acids below). It should be noted that this research laboratory also reported myocyte ultrastructural aberrations associated with this supplementation in rats.[26]

BORON

Supplemental boron may increase testosterone levels.[1] This notion derived from an earlier study in which postmenopausal women took boron supplements (3 mg/day) after following a low boron diet.[27] During the period of supplementation their serum estrogen and testosterone increased. However, when Green and Ferrando[28,29] provided boron supplements (2.5 mg/day) to male bodybuilders for 7 weeks, increases in their testosterone levels, lean body mass, and strength were comparable to those from training alone. Other investigators also reported that supplemental boron failed to alter circulating hormone levels.[30,31]

However, researchers for another study[32] involving boron supplementation reported a significant increase in plasma 17-β estradiol (E2) concentration and a nonsignificant trend for plasma testosterone (T) levels to be increased. The ratio of E2/T was increased significantly, which raises questions about supplementation in males. In a related report,[33] boron supplementation increased plasma estrogen levels, while rats showed an increase in plasma testosterone and vitamin D and a decrease in high-density lipoprotein (HDL) cholesterol levels.

Clearly more investigation is needed in the area of boron supplementation, with studies using a broader range of individuals and physiological conditions as well as different doses and concomitant substances. Since elevations in plasma estrogen seem to be more common than elevations in testosterone, it is important to understand why this occurs. For instance, if the increased estrogen level results from aromatization of testosterone, then boron supplementation would theoretically need a concomitant aromatization-inhibiting factor. Furthermore, information regarding boron toxicity is needed. One mg daily will probably be adequate to help meet boron requirements and 10 mg may be safe in light of high urinary excretion.[33]

BRANCHED CHAIN AMINO ACIDS (BCAA)

The BCAA (leucine, isoleucine, and valine) have been touted to be ergogenic because they reduce fatigue associated with high-intensity activity sustained for a long period of time.[1] However, some scientists speculate that BCAA supplementation, more specifically leucine supplementation, may actually be ergolytic by potentially decreasing the content of a TCA cycle intermediate. Little scientific research is available on BCAA as a supplement for athletes based on measured metabolic and performance parameters. More recently a newer ergogenic role for leucine has been offered, in that it can directly stimulate muscle protein synthesis.[1]

Skeletal muscle has the ability to break down and oxidize seven amino acids, namely the BCAA and glutamate, aspartate, asparagine, and alanine.[1] Alanine can be deaminated and its carbon skeleton derivative (i.e., pyruvate) oxidized in muscle tissue. However, during endurance exercise, there would be a net alanine formation and positive alanine balance in muscle tissue and in circulation.

The key (i.e., rate determining reaction) to utilizing the BCAA is the enzyme system branched chain α-ketoacid dehydrogenase (BCKADH).[1] At rest only about 4% of this enzyme complex is active in human skeletal muscle, but its activity increases several times over during exercise following an overnight fast.[34,35] This allows for an increased BCAA oxidation during exercise. However, the activity of BCKADH is influenced by metabolic state and is inversely activated by glycogen levels.[34,36-39] If glycogen stores are higher, such as after glycogen loading, the degree of activation of BCKADH would be lower. Also, the ingestion of carbohydrate (e.g., sport drink) during endurance activity may also limit BCKADH activity.

The available research indicates that BCAA supplementation before and during activity may not increase energy. Furthermore, leucine catabolism may steal an intermediate of the TCA cycle (namely α-ketoglutarate) in the process. While three acetyl CoA molecules are produced from the carbon skeleton of leucine, the removal of α-ketoglutarate is potentially problematic as acetyl CoA requires OAA to enter the TCA cycle. OAA is α-ketoglutarate-derived and substitutive OAA will need to come via pyruvate carboxylase, which itself is regulated by the metabolic state of the muscle cell and requires ATP. As described by Lancha and colleagues[40] the activity of pyruvate carboxylase increases during exercise for both sedentary and trained rats. Yet this may not be a concern as the carbon skeletons of asparagine and aspartic acid both serve as precursors for OAA.[1,41]

During sustained high-intensity exercise, working skeletal muscle will increase its uptake of circulating BCAA, which then can become a fuel source. This will result in a reduction in the level of BCAA in the plasma, and some scientists think this could be a significant cause of central fatigue. The mechanism here would be indirect, as BCAA (and other amino acids) compete with tryptophan for the same transporter to cross the blood brain barrier.[1,42]

When the ratio of BCAA:tryptophan decreases, the transport of tryptophan will increase and this amino acid will serve as a precursor for serotonin. This suggests that the rate-limiting step in the production of serotonin is indeed tryptophan transport.[1,42-44] Furthermore, tryptophan circulates to some degree bound to albumin, which begins to bind more and more fatty acids liberated from adipocytes. This further decreases the BCAA:tryptophan ratio and in turn increases tryptophan transport. Serotonin is associated with sedation, so increased serotonin production via increased tryptophan availability may cause central fatigue.

While the theory that central fatigue is caused by a lower BCAA:tryptophan ratio seems plausible, researchers have not been able to demonstrate that it is true, or that BCAA supplementation just prior to or during exercise extends performance.[42] In fact, they have studied the issue by trying BCAA supplements to extend performance and tryptophan supplements to bring on fatigue.[1,42]

Van Hall and colleagues[45] tested endurance trained males with a sucrose solution (6%) with or without amino acids during a cycling bout of 70%–75% maximal power output until exhaustion. Tryptophan was provided at 3 g/L while the BCAA were provided at either 6 or 18 g/L of carbohydrate solution. The researchers reported that BCAA supplementation increased plasma levels and reduced brain tryptophan uptake by 8%–12% while tryptophan supplementation resulted in a 7- to 20-fold increase in tryptophan uptake. Yet despite these significant manipulations of tryptophan, time to exhaustion during the exercise trial was not affected by the difference in treatments. The results of this study suggest that manipulation of tryptophan supply to the brain either has no additional effect upon serotoninergic activity during exercise to exhaustion, or that manipulation of serotoninergic activity does not contribute functionally to mechanisms of fatigue.

Similarly, BCAA supplementation did not influence time until exhaustion of endurance-trained males cycling at 75% VO_2max.[46] Here the cyclists began the bout with reduced muscle glycogen stores and were provided either flavored water or a 6% carbohydrate solution with or without BCAA (7 g/L). While the carbohydrate solution definitely extended performance, the addition of the BCAA did not make a further difference. Other researchers have also reported that BCAA supplementation may not push back central fatigue during higher intensity endurance activity[47] or improve completion time for an endurance bout (100 km cycling trial).[48]

On the other hand, two publications[49,50] suggest that BCAA supplementation may improve endurance performance, but the way these studies were designed makes practical application of the data a concern. For instance, carbohydrate intake was not controlled in one study[49] and not provided in the second study.[50] Incontrovertibly, the foundation of ergogenicity during endurance activity is carbohydrate status and its provision in addition to hydration. Furthermore, the studies above strongly suggest that there was no advantage to BCAA supplementation with carbohydrates over using carbohydrates alone.

Although BCAA supplementation may not prolong higher intensity endurance activity, newer rationales for supplementation have emerged. BCAA supplementation may limit glutamine reductions following an exhaustive exercise bout (e.g., marathon, triathlon). This might then thwart reductions in immunocompetence and increased incidence of infection following the exercise. Bassit and coinvestigators[51] reported that BCAA supplementation can limit plasma glutamine reductions following an endurance bout (Olympic distance triathlon) as well as inhibit the reduction of interleukin-1 (IL-1) production which occurred in a nonsupplemented group. This could be directly related to decreased symptoms of infections as well as an increased potential for lymphocyte proliferation in supplemented athletes.

In addition, Coombes and colleagues[52] reported reductions in the level of plasma markers for muscle tissue damage in the days that followed a bout of endurance exercise. Here BCAA were provided at 12 g/day for 2 weeks

---

How Much Caffeine?

Are all soft drinks created equal? Not as far as caffeine content is concerned. Most cola drinks like Coca Cola and Pepsi have about 35 mg caffeine per 12 oz serving. Diet Coke has significantly more (45 mg) as does Pepsi One, a low calorie version of Pepsi (55 mg). But another diet cola, Canada Dry Diet Cola, has under 10 mg.

Benign-sounding A & W Crème Soda, at 29 mg, rivals the popular colas in "buzz" power. Dr. Pepper, a cola hybrid, and Sunkist orange both contain 41 mg caffeine. Iced tea drinks vary widely in caffeine content—Nestea Iced Tea contains 16.5 mg, and Snapple Raspberry Tea almost twice as much, 31 mg.

Mountain Dew delivers a super jolt (55 mg), but can't rival the real Jolt drink, which tops the charts at a whopping 72 mg caffeine. That's the maximum amount allowed by the Food and Drug Administration (FDA) per 12 oz serving—great if your goal is to pull an all-nighter. But if you're having trouble sleeping, stick to Sprite, 7-Up, or Fresca. Their caffeine content? Zero.

---

prior to a 2-hour cycling bout at 70% VO_2max and creatine kinase and lactate dehydrogenase were used as plasma markers of muscle tissue damage.

Lastly and independently, leucine supplementation may directly induce protein synthesis in skeletal muscle. Anthony and colleagues[53] recently described how leucine probably upregulates protein synthesis in skeletal muscle by enhancing both the activity and synthesis of proteins involved in mRNA translation. Furthermore, the potentially positive influence of leucine upon protein synthesis can be maximized when it is associated with insulin. Will leucine become the next "big" bodybuilding supplement? If so, it would seem likely that leucine supplementation would be recommended in conjunction with carbohydrate.

CAFFEINE

Caffeine is a methylxanthine compound that occurs naturally in plant sources such as coffee bean, tea leaf, kola nut, and cacao seed.[1] The average 8-oz (237 mL) cup of coffee contains 50–150 mg of caffeine, while tea has about 50 mg/cup and caffeinated cola drinks about 35 mg/12 oz (356 mL). Chocolate contains some caffeine; most of its methylxanthine is derived from theobromine. The term "caffeine" is used in a general sense to include other methylxanthines (e.g., theobromine, theophylline).

Once caffeine is absorbed, most tissue will take it up from circulation. But brain tissue appears to be particularly sensitive to caffeine, and this causes wakefulness or sleep latency in some people. At least some of the stimulatory effects of caffeine are attributable to its inhibition of phosphodiesterase. Phosphodiesterase hydrolyzes the second messenger molecule cyclic adenosine monophosphate (cAMP). Thus, caffeine could prolong the influence of hormones utilizing cAMP as a second messenger, such as glucagon and epinephrine. However, caffeine-related neural stimulation probably occurs before caffeine reaches its potency threshold for this enzyme. Caffeine probably inhibits the activity of chloride channels in neural membranes, resulting in stimulation of physical activity.

Adenosine seems to inhibit neural activity, both direct action at postsynaptic sites as well as presynaptic neurotransmitter release.[1] Because caffeine and adenosine are similar in molecular design, they will compete for the same binding sites. Thus caffeine is an adenosine antagonist. To counter this antagonism, more adenosine receptors are produced in brain tissue and more caffeine must be consumed to effectively compete with them.

Also, once caffeine ingestion ceases, adenosine interacts unchallenged for adenosine receptors, whose numbers have been augmented by chronic caffeine consumption. This probably accounts for many of the symptoms associated with caffeine withdrawal, such as tiredness, which may affect both normal activity and athletic performance. Additionally, some of the effects of caffeine may be indirect, as caffeine ingestion is typically associated with increased plasma epinephrine levels, which may have a central stimulatory influence.

Caffeine is a potential ergogenic aid for several reasons.[1] First, caffeine and related substances stimulate the central nervous system (CNS). Secondly, caffeine may have direct effect upon muscle fiber calcium transport and glycogen breakdown, which may increase performance. Thirdly, caffeine may stimulate the mobilization of FFA from adipose tissue.

Early reports of caffeine enhancing endurance exercise showed that ingesting 330 mg of caffeine 1 hour prior to cycling at 80% VO_2max by trained individuals extended the time till exhaustion from 76 to 90 minutes.[54] A subsequent study[55] presented data that 250 mg of caffeine one hour prior to exercise and then every 15 minutes in the first 1½ hour of an endurance bout could increase both work output and VO_2 by roughly 7%. Both of these studies suggested that fat utilization was augmented by approximately 30% as a result of caffeine ingestion. While some questioned the methodology of earlier studies, these studies evoked tremendous interest in caffeine as an ergogenic aid.[56] Conlee[57] summarized the factors that need to be controlled, and they include the nature of the exercise (i.e., modality), level of tested power output, and dose of caffeine used.

During the decade that followed, there were many studies involving caffeine and performance and the results were somewhat equivocal. Now it seems that caffeine may have an ergogenic effect, but the right conditions must exist for it to be effective. [57,58] Results from several studies using caffeine doses between 3 and 13 mg/kg in elite and recreationally trained athletes running or cycling at 80% to 90% VO_2max showed they improved their performance between 20% and 50%.[58-61] Doses between 3 and 6 mg/kg did not result in urinary caffeine levels above the International Olympic Committee (IOC) acceptable limit, and side effects were uncommon. But at doses of 9 mg/kg and higher, several of the athletes did present urinary caffeine levels above the limits accepted by the IOC. Furthermore, side effects such as dizziness, insomnia, headache, and gastrointestinal distress were noted in several of the athletes.

Caffeine ingestion was associated with an increase in plasma epinephrine and FFA at rest and during the first 15 minutes of exercise. FFA and epinephrine were not significantly affected by a 3 mg/kg dose of caffeine, but performance was improved. Furthermore, caffeine ingestion did seem to "spare" muscle glycogen utilization, but this effect was limited to the first 15 minutes of the exercise.

Some athletes may find caffeine beneficial for shorter and higher intensity workouts.[62,63] For instance, 250 mg of caffeine was reported by Collomp and colleagues[63] to prolong cycling time till exhaustion at 100% VO_2max from 5:20 to 5:49. Also, 150–200 mg of caffeine (i.e., coffee) improved treadmill performance by 4.2 seconds (i.e., 1500 m) in well-trained runners.[64] In this study, the athletes ran 1.1 km and then were instructed to run 400 m as fast as they could. Caffeine allowed all athletes to run faster during the 400 m all-out run, and the average VO_2 was also higher following coffee ingestion. Thus, caffeine consumption does seem to have an ergogenic effect in efforts of this nature.

However, the research on sprinting is less clear and requires further assessment. For instance, two studies reported that caffeine consumption failed to improve maximal power output, muscular endurance, or total work in shorter tests.[65] However, 250 mg of caffeine was reported to improve performance in repeated bouts of freestyle sprinting by swimmers.[66–68]

How well caffeine supplementation works may be influenced by regular caffeine consumption and other dietary factors. For instance, lower doses of caffeine (i.e., < 9 mg/kg) may dampen the effect of caffeine on the CNS and fat metabolism.[69] Some researchers have speculated that caffeine should be withdrawn from the diet of habitual caffeine consumers for at least 4 days to accurately assess the ergogenic effect of caffeine.

More recent studies have challenged this idea. For instance, Van Soeren and colleagues[70] reported that the ergogenic effects of caffeine on a cycling bout in chronic caffeine consumers were no different before or after a 4-day withdrawal period. Also, carbohydrate consumption just before or during exercise may dampen the ergogenic potential of caffeine. For instance, Weir and colleagues[71] reported that a high-carbohydrate diet and carbohydrate ingested just before a race negated some of the effect of caffeine upon FFA mobilization from adipose tissue. But a review by Spriet[72] cited several studies that showed neither a high-carbohydrate diet nor carbohydrate consumed before exercise negated the ergogenic effects of caffeine.

CARNITINE

Carnitine (β-hydroxy-γ-trimethylammonium butyrate) is found in a variety of human tissue, though it is very concentrated in muscle. Two amino acids, lysine and methionine, are used to make carnitine, and synthesis occurs in the liver and kidneys. Carnitine transport mechanisms are necessary to

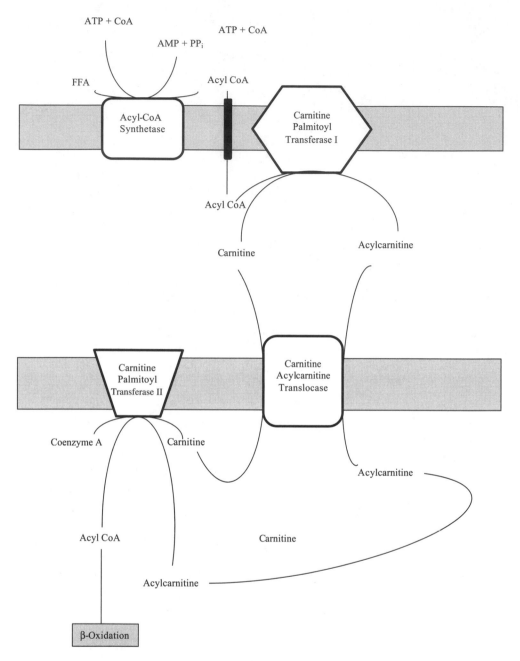

FIGURE 4-1   Movement of Longer Chain Fatty Acids into the Mitochondria
                 Matrix Requires Carnitine

move long chain fatty acids (LCFA) into the mitochondrial matrix, which is
the predominant site of fatty acid oxidation (see Figure 4-1). Short chain fatty
acids are able to diffuse into the mitochondrial matrix without assistance.[2]

The first step in the movement of "activated" LCFA from the cytosol to
the mitochondrial matrix is the conversion of long chain acyl CoAs to acylcarnitine. Performing this task is carnitine palmitoyl transferase I (CPTI),

which is present in the outer mitochondrial membrane. The combination of the fatty acid and carnitine (i.e., acylcarnitine) is then able to permeate the inner mitochondrial membrane by moving through the carnitine acylcarnitine translocase antiport system. It seems that one acylcarnitine molecule enters the matrix in exchange for one free carnitine molecule moving from the matrix to the mitochondrial intermembrane space. Once inside the matrix, acyl-CoA molecules are reformed by another carnitine dependent enzyme complex called carnitine palmitoyl transferase II (CPT II). Acyl-CoA molecules are then available for oxidation, while the free carnitine is available for the exchange.[2]

Once the role of carnitine was established, researchers hoped that it could be an ergogenic aid or even increase normal fat utilization for weight loss in nonexercising individuals. However, decades of studies have failed to demonstrate that carnitine supplementation is useful in either of these tasks.[1] In a recent review, the literature evaluated suggests that carnitine supplementation does not enhance fatty acid utilization or spare glycogen, nor does it postpone the onset of fatigue.[73] Furthermore, it was stated that carnitine supplementation does not help people lose fat or weight, nor will it improve exercising VO_2max. And carnitine does not appear to shorten or aid recovery from exercising to exhaustion.[74]

Although numerous studies failed to show enhanced ergogenic or metabolic effects from routine supplementation with carnitine, one study[75] did report that carnitine has some ergogenic merit. In this study, moderately trained young men ingested 2 g of carnitine just before a maximal exercise bout on a cycle ergometer. The researchers reported an increase in the subjects' maximal oxygen uptake and power output.

In general, it seems that carnitine may not have an independent ergogenic effect. However, as a substance crucial for the oxidation of LCFAs, which are the majority of fatty acids oxidized, carnitine may support the actions of other supplements or pharmaceuticals. You would be hard-pressed to find a "fat burner" supplement that did not include carnitine. For instance, both Ripped Fuel and Metabolife contain carnitine. Certainly, research investigating the supportive effect of carnitine is warranted.

Carnitine supplementation may be beneficial to people with special clinical considerations.[76–79] For instance, in patients with end-stage renal disease, endogenous carnitine stasis is negatively impacted by decreased synthesis compounded by carnitine lost during dialysis. People requiring dialysis tend to demonstrate a reduction in skeletal muscle carnitine levels relative to length of time on dialysis. The decreased tissue level is associated with decreased exercise performance, and it seems that carnitine supplementation is effective in increasing total muscle carnitine levels and increasing VO_2max. Meanwhile, propionyl-L-carnitine (PLC) has been reported to be more effective in improving muscle metabolism in individuals with peripheral arterial disease.

Because urinary excretion of carnitine increases relative to intake levels, the supplement has generally been viewed as safe. However, Lancha[80] reported that supplementation of carnitine at 90 mg/kg body weight, along with asparagine and aspartate, led to utrastructural anomalies in the soleus muscle of swimming-trained rats. The anomalies included small regions of myofibril degeneration, Z-line streaming and disruption, as well as mitochondrial disorganization and disruption. Such findings warrant further investigation.

CHOLINE AND LECITHIN (PHOSPHOTIDYLCHOLINE)

Choline, a component of a number of important metabolites, functions in ways that might benefit performance. It provides acetylation to the neurotransmitter acetylcholine; irreversible oxidation to betaine, a methyl group donor, which participates in homocysteine metabolism; and phosphorylation to phosphocholine, which is the first step in generating the membrane phospholipid lecithin.

Scientists have reported that plasma choline levels decrease following a bout of endurance exercise.[81] Supplementation seems to ameliorate this effect, but it does not improve endurance performance.[82] Other research efforts[83,84] have suggested that choline supplementation by itself does not positively influence endurance performance. However, in one study[85] choline supplementation combined with carnitine and caffeine improved VO_2max and increased fatty acid utilization. Choline may not be ergogenic by itself and short term, but further investigation is needed regarding choline's potential as a synergistic factor.

CHROMIUM

Supplementation with the essential mineral chromium is touted to aid in weight reduction, increase lean body mass, and maximize the actions of insulin. Chromium is marketed mostly in the form of chromium picolinate, but other forms such as chromium nicotinate and chromium chloride supplements are also available. The picolinate (i.e., tryptophan derivative) form makes chromium absorption more efficient, probably by decreasing the interaction or chelation of chromium (Cr^{3+}) to negatively charged entities (e.g. phytates) in the digestive tract that would reduce absorption.[2]

Chromium is the biologically active component of glucose tolerance factor (GTF).[2,86] This compound appears to maximize the effects of insulin and aid in normal insulin function.[87,88] Athletes with insufficient chromium intake find supplementation promotes optimal insulin effectiveness and also optimizes carbohydrate and lipid metabolism.[89-91] However, allowance would need to be made for the person to first achieve "normal" chromium status. Before a supplement study involving chromium (or any other essential nutrient) begins, participants need to have good base levels of the nutrient.

Numerous recent studies have shown chromium supplementation to be ineffective for weight loss, increasing lean body mass, or improving muscular strength.[92–101] In a double-blind investigation by Lukaski and colleagues,[92] subjects given chromium supplements for 8 weeks (3.3–3.5 μmoles/day) while participating in a resistance training program showed no greater changes in body composition or gains in strength in comparison to a placebo group. It was reported that supplementation did increase both serum chromium concentrations and urinary chromium excretions.

Another double-blind study conducted by Clancy and colleagues[94] at the University of Massachusetts yielded similar results. Here football players utilized chromium picolinate (200 mcg/day) for 9 weeks during a strength training program. Chromium supplementation again failed to significantly influence skin fold measurements, percentage of body fat, or lean body mass and strength measurements.

Hallmark and colleagues[95] also conducted a study involving chromium supplementation. Sixteen untrained individuals were supplemented with 200 mcg/day of chromium for 12 weeks during a resistance-training program. Researchers reported no significant changes in body composition, percent body fat, strength, or lean body mass (LBM). Likewise, Hasten and co-workers[96] performed a double-blind study of 37 men and 22 women, all of whom were untrained and college age. Here once again, no significant differences in strength gains were found after 12-week supplementation of 200 mcg/day of chromium picolinate. However, the females receiving chromium supplement gained 2.5 kg of body weight.

Campbell and colleagues[101] conducted a study of older men (age 56–69) provided with 924 mcg of chromium daily (chromium picolinate) who participated in a high-intensity resistance training program for 12 weeks. The exercise increased fat-free mass, whole body muscle mass, and vastus lateralis type II fiber area, but chromium supplementation provided no additional benefit.

Collectively, research suggests that chromium is probably not effective in increasing lean body mass, favorably altering body composition, or improving strength in either trained or untrained individuals, regardless of age. There appears to be a limit to how much chromium can be absorbed by tissue, as measured by the amount excreted in urine. Yet what has not been investigated is the potential concomitant effect of chromium supplementation in combination with other nutritional factors. Like carnitine, chromium is often added to "fat burner" supplements such as Ripped Fuel and Metabolift, which are both marketed by TwinLabs.

Information pertaining to the safety of chromium is limited, but a recent case study reveals that exogenous chromium picolinate may become toxic when ingested at 6–12 times the recommended dosage over the course of many months.[102] Such ingestion caused renal impairment in test subjects, who required dialysis to restore renal function. At this time, exogenous chromium is considered safe when consumed in recommended quantities. However, in vitro studies performed by Stearns and colleagues[103,104] have suggested that chromium can accumulate in cultured cells and cause chromosomal damage.

COENZYME Q$_{10}$ (UBIQUINONE)

Coenzyme Q$_{10}$ is also commonly referred to as CoQ$_{10}$ and ubiquinone, yet the terms are not entirely synonymous from a biochemical perspective. Ubiquinone is an aromatic ring system with isoprenoid units attached, which seems to vary between organisms. In mammals, ubiquinone has 10 isoprenoid units, hence Q_{10}. Ubiquinone is found in mitochondria as a component of the electron transport chain, and also as a mobile component within the matrix.[2]

The ubiquinone content in skeletal muscle will allow for two roles, namely respiratory chain activity and antioxidation.[2] Both of these areas have raised interest as to the ergogenic potential (i.e., aerobic performance and oxidative stress reduction) of ubiquinone supplementation.[2,105] Ubiquinone therapy is being studied in cases of heart failure, as well.

Braun and colleagues[106] provided 100 mg of ubiquinone/day for 8 weeks to male cyclists, who then failed to significantly improve their cycling performance, VO_2max, submaximal physiological parameters, or lipid peroxidation. In another investigation,[107] ubiquinone (100 mg) was formulated into a coenzyme athletic performance system (CAPS) which triathletes ingested three times daily for 4 weeks. CAPS also contained cytochrome c (500 mg), inosine (100 mg), and vitamin E (200 IU). Again, no significant improvement in endurance was observed, nor were there changes in blood glucose, lactate, or FFA at exhaustion.

In other studies[108–112] ubiquinone supplementation failed to improve aerobic performance or favorably alter plasma metabolic indices. In contrast, Ylikoski and colleagues[113] reported that ubiquinone supplementation (90 mg/day) improved indices of physical performance, including VO_2max in Finnish top-level cross-country skiers.

In general, ubiquinone has not enhanced athletic performance, but supplementation (either alone or in combination) may improve exercise-related events that may have an impact on tissue and general health. For instance, Vasankari and colleagues[114] provided 60 mg of ubiquinone in combination with 294 mg vitamin E and 1 g of vitamin C and found improvements in serum and low-density lipoprotein antioxidant potential in endurance athletes. In another investigation[115] ubiquinone supplementation (10 mg/kg/day for 4 weeks) was reported to markedly suppress exercise-induced lipid peroxidation in organs such as liver, heart, and gastrocnemius tissue in rats. However, postexercise rise in creatine kinase, an indicator of muscle tissue damage, was not affected by supplementation.

Ubiquinone is generating attention for its effects in certain clinical situations, especially in cases of heart failure.[116-119] Clinical investigations have not always demonstrated benefits from ubiquinone supplementation, as either a primary or adjunctive treatment of chronic congestive heart failure. However, a growing body of evidence suggests that there may be at least a minimal benefit to supplementing with 100 mg daily.[116-120] In a meta-analysis[119] of several controlled clinical trials of congestive heart failure patients, Soja and Mortensen reported that several cardiac parameters were improved by ubiquinone treatment. These parameters included ejection fraction, stroke volume, cardiac output, cardiac index, and end diastolic volume index. Further investigative efforts are needed to better understand the potential application of ubiquinone, used independently and as adjunctive therapy, for the treatment of chronic cardiac failure.

CREATINE

Creatine is derived from arginine, glycine and methionine and requires two organs (liver and kidneys) for production.[1] As creatine circulates it is taken up by skeletal and cardiac muscle, and by other tissue—including the brain—via a creatine transport protein (CREAT).[1,120] Intracellular creatine is then phosphorylated by creatine kinase to form creatine phosphate (CP), which then serves as a small high energy phosphate reserve and a mechanism for rapidly regenerating ATP anaerobically. As skeletal muscle ATP can become exhausted in one second during supramaximal bouts of exercise, the phosphate group from CP is transferred to ADP (adenosine diphosphate) to regenerate ATP via creatine kinase. Creatine phosphate regenerating of ATP, along with adenylate cyclase, allows for ATP concentrations to remain at operational level for a longer period of time during very high intensity exercise.

Roughly 1.6% of cellular creatine will undergo spontaneous and nonenzymatic cyclization, forming creatinine which is then excreted in the urine.[1] The skeletal muscle of a typical adult male may contain about 3–5 g of creatine/kg of tissue. As Benzi[121] points out, a 70 kg male might have a creatine pool of roughly 120 g or a little more than a ¼ lb. Meanwhile, a typical American diet might provide about 1–2 g of creatine daily, with meat eaters consuming more than vegetarians. Several more exhaustive reviews[122-125] of creatine metabolism are available.

Creatine has been one of the most popular ergogenic supplements, and is usually marketed in the form of creatine monohydrate. Although dosage protocols can vary, manufacturers often recommend that creatine be ingested with carbohydrate for maximal tissue retention.[126-127] Carbohydrate consumption may increase creatine transport into tissue because greater quantities of insulin are produced, but this is speculative.[1] Creatine is marketed as powder, pills, or concentrated liquids which are dropped beneath the tongue or drunk.

Recommendations for creatine supplementation will vary. Initially creatine "loading" (approximately 20–25 g/day for 5–7 days) followed by a "maintenance" intake (roughly 2–5 g/day.)[1] was recommended. These recommended levels may be based on the results published by Hultman and colleagues.[128] In their study they provided 20 g (loading) of creatine daily for 6 days and observed a 20% rise in creatine levels. Furthermore, the rise in muscle creatine levels was maintained for 30 days by ingesting only 2 g/day (maintenance). They determined that ingesting 3 g a day would increase muscle creatine levels by the same amount, but it takes longer (measured at 28 days).

Lower doses of creatine daily prove more economical, and this regimen is a popular alternative to loading. In addition, newer practices for creatine supplementation are based on body weight. For instance, 0.25 g of creatine monohydrate/kg body weight was used in a recent study.[129] This is probably appropriate when investigating a specific population (e.g., rowers, wrestlers, soccer players) due to the highly similar physical characteristics among subjects.[1]

Supplements are often broken up over the course of the day if a loading dose is used (e.g., 5 g, four times/day). For alternative dosing, creatine users may pay more attention to anecdotal information they hear in the gym or read in magazines and on Web sites than they do to physician's recommendations. Greenwood and colleagues[130] noted different levels of consumption of creatine among collegiate Division I athletes. Some young men interviewed by an author of this chapter knew of serious weight trainers who supplemented at levels ≥ 40 g/day.

Creatine consumption to increase muscle fiber CP levels is generally effective, according to various studies.[1] As mentioned, Hultman and colleagues[128] determined that total muscle creatine concentration in men was increased by 20% after 6 days of supplementing 20 grams of creatine monohydrate. Meanwhile Volek and colleagues[131] reported an increase of creatine in muscle by 22%. Green and colleagues[127] also reported increases in muscle tissue creatine levels after supplementation.

As discussed by Greenhaff,[132] muscle creatine levels probably do not increase substantially for everyone. In their study, five of eight participants had significant augmentations of muscle creatine (i.e., 15%–32%), yet the remaining three participants demonstrated only modest augmentations of roughly 5%–7%. The degree of augmentation of muscle creatine levels would dictate the development of higher levels of creatine phosphate during recovery periods, and strongly influence whether improvements in performance are realized.[132]

Individual differences in creatine accumulation during supplementation may be affected by basal dietary creatine and endogenous synthesis of creatine and CREAT, as influenced by training. This may explain why creatine supplementation has failed to produce an ergogenic response in some highly trained and elite athletes,[133-135] but has in others.[129,136,137] Also from an ergogenic perspective, it is important to consider that an increase in muscle creatine (and associated water) should lead to increases in muscle and total body mass. Thus, improvements in energy properties must exceed any potential detriments associated with greater workload associated with moving a greater mass. Whether or not this is a detriment for those participating in ballistic sports, such as sprinting and volleyball, requires further attention.

Research shows creatine supplementation (especially a loading dosage of 5 g four times/day) increases strength and power.[1] For instance, one study[137] revealed that creatine supplementation extended all-out treadmill running by 13% in sprinters. Meanwhile, Birch[138] observed that creatine supplementation increased measures of power output during repeated bouts of maximal isokinetic cycling. Another study[139] revealed that creatine supplementation resulted in a greater knee extension torque production as measured on a Cybex II isokinetic dyanamometerm.

Meanwhile, Earnest[140] observed that creatine supplementation led to a 6% increase in the subjects' 1-RM (1-repetition maximum) free weight bench press. Yet another study[141] demonstrated that creatine supplemented men were able to complete 10 bouts of 6-second high-intensity exercise on a friction-loaded cycle ergometer, while a placebo-treated group was not able to complete the regimen. Becque and colleagues[142] reported a greater improvement in 1-RM effort with creatine supplementation versus a placebo. Increases in strength were also reported by Stone and coinvestigators,[143] whose American football player subjects improved their 1-RM bench press, combined 1-RM squat and bench press, and static vertical jump (SVJ) power output and peak rate of force development for SVJ. Kreider[144] also reported improvements in measures of strength in NCAA Division I football players.

And several studies[1,143-145] have reported increases in body mass and LBM and decrease in fat mass in response to creatine supplementation. At this time, the nature of these gains is not well understood. Clearly, augmented muscle creatine levels will increase both LBM and total mass. Furthermore, increased intracellular (and extracellular) creatine will have an osmotic effect. In muscle this would swell the myocytes. In fact, some researchers believe that "creatine swelling" of skeletal myocytes leads to increased protein synthesis. It is then possible that this anabolic influence may be cumulative, with increased overload stimulus associated with greater work from supplementation. Therefore, increased LBM is likely to be a combination of increased muscle, total body protein, and water.

For shorter duration studies (e.g., 1 week) expanding these body composition compartments is likely to contribute nearly all the increased mass. However, adaptive enhancements in other tissue (e.g., bone) may contribute a small yet significant amount of mass during chronic supplementation. Reductions in fat mass may be due to diluting as LBM expands, and also to increased fat oxidation associated with hypertrophic activities. The metabolic aspects associated with creatine supplementation await further study.

At this time most of the evidence supporting creatine as a credible ergogenic aid has involved people engaging in high-intensity activities. Whether creatine supplementation is effective in training for more endurance-based activities remains to be seen. Preliminary investigations[146,147] have failed to demonstrate an ergogenic effect on endurance performance. But if, for instance, a long-distance runner sprints periodically during an endurance run, creatine supplementation may improve performance during that phase of the run.[148]

An endurance athlete thinking of taking creatine supplements needs to consider several issues. First, will the extra weight become a performance detriment, especially if the terrain is varied (e.g., mountain climbs) and will changes in altitude affect oxygen supply? And second, will the endurance bout include intermittent periods of sprinting? This could be the case in the "final kick" of distance runs and breakaways and sprint finishes in distance cycling.[1]

As creatine becomes more popular among athletes and noncompetitive weight trainers, concerns about its potential toxicity (e.g., creatine or contaminants) and impact on disease risk factors have been raised.[149-151] Clearly, more research is needed in this area. Shorter duration studies lasting just a few weeks do not show harmful effects. For instance, Mihic and coinvestigators[145] reported that creatine supplementation does not increase blood pressure and that creatine kinase levels in the plasma do not influence renal performance. In a related effort, Poortmans and Francaux[149] reported that long-term creatine supplementation does not impair renal function. Schilling and colleagues[151] performed a retrospective study of long-term creatine users and reported that markers of concern were not different for non-users. Meanwhile, in preliminary echocardiographic assessment, Wildman and coinvestigators[152] reported that creatine loading does not alter heart size or function versus control subjects. But more investigation into creatine's influence on the cardiovascular system is warranted, as well as research on how it affects cerebral tissue and cognition.[1]

DHEA (PRASTERONE) AND ANDROSTENEDIONE

Dehydroepiandrosterone (DHEA) is a steroid hormone that is produced by and released from the adrenal glands.[153-155] DHEA can be sulfated (i.e., DHEAS) and both of these hormone forms circulate to tissue where they are converted into androgens and/or estrogens (see Figure 4-2). For most people the level of plasma DHEA and DHEAS peaks during their 20s and 30s and then declines steadily as they age.[156-158] However, there appear to be individual variations within age groups as well as variations depending on gender, race, and health status. Investigators have reported an inverse relationship between circulating DHEA levels and incidences of heart disease, various cancers, and several other age-related diseases.[159-161]

DHEA is made via cholesterol that first undergoes conversion to pregnenolone, which can then be converted to 17-hydroxypregnenolone that can then be converted to dehydroepiandrosterone.[162,163] Most of the DHEA formed in the adrenal glands is quickly modified by the addition of sulfate to form DHEAS. DHEA can also be sulfated in the liver. While DHEAS is relatively inactive, removal of the sulfate group by tissue will reactivate the steroid structure. DHEA circulates both independently and loosely bound to albumin and sex hormone-binding globulin while DHEAS circulates strongly bound to albumin.[164-166] With the exception of their precursor cholesterol, DHEA and DHEAS are the steroids found in the highest quantity in the blood.[153-155]

Humans produce high levels of DHEA—it is possible that more than 50% of the total androgens in adult male tissue are derived from DHEA. For women, the conversion of DHEA to estrogens may represent as much as 75% of total estrogen in tissue before menopause and 100% after menopause.[167-169] Deriving such a significant proportion of their peripheral active sex steroids from DHEA allows for local control of sex steroid levels as dictated by the needs of specific tissue. The ability of target tissue to convert DHEA and DHEAS into androgens and/or estrogens relies on the presence of steroidogenic and metabolizing enzyme systems such as 3β-hydroxysteroid dehydrogenase/Δ^5-Δ^4-isomerase (3β-HSD).[163]

Only a few human trials have been published that test whether DHEA supplementation can increase testosterone levels and adaptations to resistance training in healthy people. Dehennin and colleagues[170] reported that a single dose of DHEA (50 mg) was readily absorbed, as 50% to 75% was

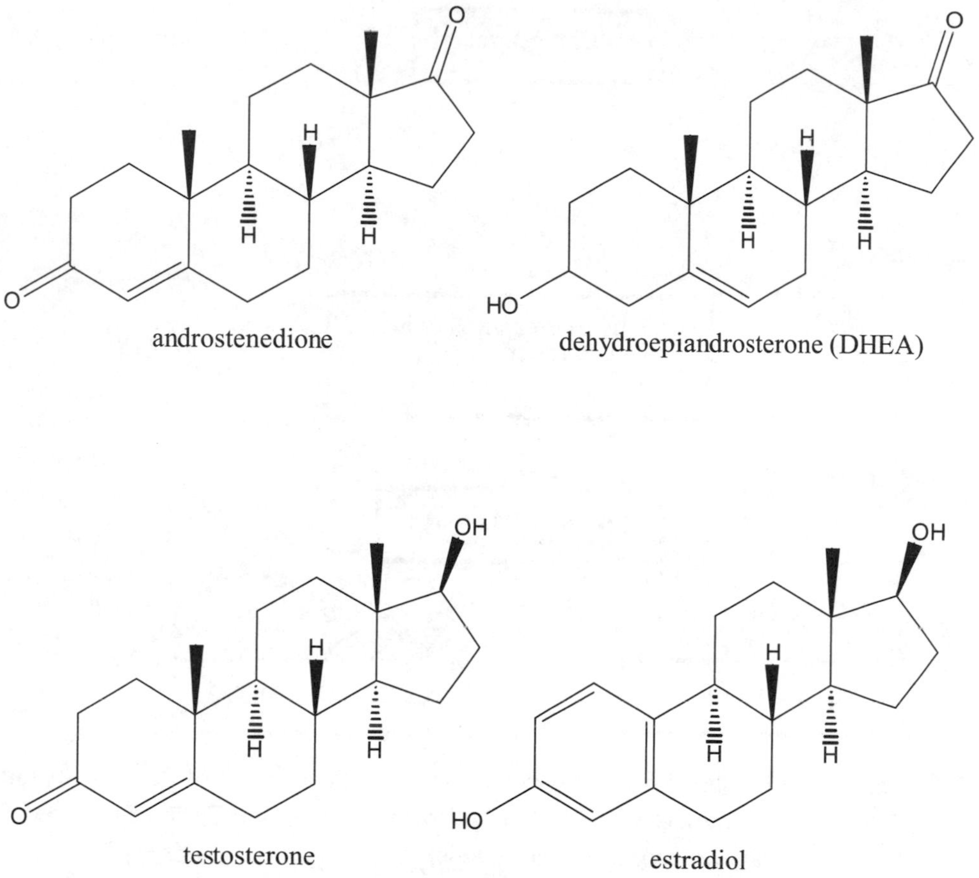

FIGURE 4-2 Molecular Structures of Androstenedione, DHEA, Testosterone, and 17β-estradiol

recovered in the urine after 24 hours. The most abundant metabolites were glucuro- and sulfoconjugates of DHEA, androsterone, and etiocholanolone. Their results also suggested that there was some conversion of the supplemental DHEA to testosterone. Here they used deuterium-labeled DHEA and based their conclusions on the subsequent identification and quantification of deuterium-labeled testosterone. As DHEA is banned in many professional sports and by the IOC, they also suggested that a concentration threshold of 300 mcg/liter of urine of DHEA glucuronide might be used in screening for DHEA. However, a single replacement dose can only be detected during 8 hours that follow ingestion.

DHEA is really a prohormone as it can be converted to another steroid, androstenedione, which itself is one chemical reaction shy of testosterone (see Figure 4-3). Some androstenedione is formed in the adrenal glands, and some testosterone can subsequently be formed in the adrenals as well. However, for the most part these hormones are formed in other tissue. Steroid sulfatase is needed to convert DHEAS to DHEA and then 3β-HSD, as mentioned above, as well as 17β-hydroxysteroid dehydrogenase (17β-HSD). One

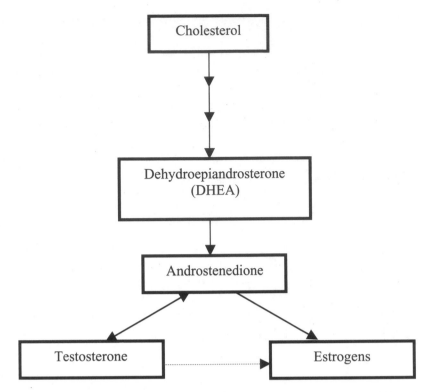

FIGURE 4-3 Simplified Reaction Pathway for the Production of Popular Steroid Substances (DHEA and Androstenedione) and Derived Hormones (Testosterone and Estrogens)

important consideration is the aromatase enzyme that can either convert androstenedione or testosterone to estrogen molecules.

Many types of tissue produce these converting enzymes, including the gonads (i.e., testis and ovaries), liver, kidneys, endometrium, and others.[171-173] Thus, the conversion of DHEA and DHEAS to active steroid molecules can be regulated at the tissue level. The gonads (i.e., testis and ovaries) produce active steroid hormones from cholesterol and release them into the blood. Interestingly, while skeletal muscle fibers contain aromatase and 3β-HSD they lack 17β-HSD, which is needed to convert androstenedione to testosterone. This suggests that muscle can make estrogens but not testosterone. Scientists can assess the efficacy of DHEA and androstenedione supplementation by measuring serum testosterone levels without the need for muscle biopsy.

Aromatase conversion of androstenedione and possibly DHEA may be a consideration in obese males as their estrogen levels tend to be elevated, presumably by aromatization in adipose tissue. Therefore, special consideration should be applied to DHEA and androstenedione supplementation in obese men attempting to increase muscularity.[174] Furthermore, some supplement manufacturers advise their clients to co-supplement androstenedione with the flavonoids chysin and daidzein, which are purported to inhibit aromatization. However, a recent investigation[175] showed that this may not work.

Wallace and colleagues[176] set out to compare the effects of 12 weeks of supplementation of androstenedione versus DHEA on body composition, strength, and related hormones in middle-aged men. Here 40 healthy, trained males were used who had an average age of 48 and an average weight of 80 kg. Supplements of 50 mg were given two times daily. The results showed a small increase in LBM and mean strength in both the androstenedione and DHEA groups, although these changes were not significantly different from those of a placebo group. In the DHEA group there was an increase in DHEAS levels over the placebo group. No adverse side effects were reported during the supplementation trial. The researchers concluded that supplementation with 100 mg daily of either androstenedione or DHEA does not independently elicit a statistically significant increase in LBM, strength, or testosterone levels in healthy adult men over a 12-week supplemental period.

Brown and colleagues[177] investigated the effects of acute DHEA supplementation on serum steroid hormones and chronic DHEA intake on adaptations to resistance training. They recruited 10 young men with an average age of 23 and provided them with 50 mg of DHEA. Blood samples revealed that serum androstenedione concentrations increased by 150% within 1 hour. However, there was no change in serum testosterone and estrogen concentrations.

In a second phase of the study, men of the same age participated in a whole body resistance-training program for 8 weeks and ingested DHEA (150 mg/day) or placebo. While serum androstenedione concentrations were significantly increased in the DHEA supplemented groups at certain points, free and total testosterone, estrone, estradiol, estriol, lipids, and liver transaminases were unaffected by supplementation and training. Also, strength and LBM were not enhanced in comparison to the placebo group.

Rasmussen and colleagues[178] conducted a study to assess whether 5 days of oral androstenedione supplementation at 100 mg daily would lead to increased skeletal muscle anabolism in six healthy young men. They measured muscle protein kinetics using a three-compartment model that involved the infusion of labeled phenylalanine, blood sampling from femoral artery and vein, and muscle biopsies. Androstenedione supplementation did not change plasma testosterone and luteinizing hormone concentrations, but plasma androstenedione and estradiol concentrations were significantly increased. Also, androstenedione did not positively affect muscle protein synthesis and breakdown, nor did it impact phenylalanine net balance across the leg. The researchers concluded that oral androstenedione does not increase plasma testosterone concentrations and has no anabolic effect on muscle protein metabolism in young men with normal gonadal function.

Leder and colleagues[179] also performed a study involving oral administration of androstenedione in 42 healthy men aged 20 to 40 years. Here subjects were provided either a placebo or oral androstenedione in doses of 100 mg/day or 300 mg/day. The researchers obtained several blood samples over the course of the measurement days and were able to develop hormone curves. Based on frequent blood samples, the researchers reported that the 300 mg dosage resulted in a significant increase in the mean area under the curves for both testosterone (24%) and estradiol (128%) in the serum of the participants. Responses differed significantly in individuals as well.

In another study, Ballantyne and coinvestigators[180] provided androstene-dione supplements (200 mg/day for 2 days) to males to judge their impact on hormones in conjunction with heavy resistance exercise. They reported that the supplement elevated plasma androstenedione two to three fold and luteinizing hormone approximately 70%, but did not alter testosterone concentration. Also, though the exercise elevated testosterone levels, there was no enhancing effect of the supplement upon testosterone levels above the exercise stimulus. However, exercise while supplementing did significantly elevate plasma estradiol, by approximately 83% for 90 minutes.

King and colleagues[181] also investigated whether 100 mg of androstene-dione altered blood testosterone levels in untrained young men, as well as whether 300 mg of androstenedione for 8 weeks enhanced the early training effects in previously untrained young men. The participants were normo-testosterogenic men and were not taking any nutritional supplements or androgenic/anabolic steroids. The researchers reported that serum free and total testosterone concentrations were not affected by short-term or long-term androstenedione supplementation. However, serum estradiol concentration was increased in the androstenedione group after the second, fifth, and eighth weeks. Serum estrone levels were also significantly increased after the second and fifth weeks of androstenedione supplementation.

In addition, supplementation did not result in enhanced gains in LBM or Type II muscle fiber cross-sectional area or reductions in body fat. And androstenedione supplementation was reported to reduce serum HDL cholesterol concentration after the second week, and remained low after the fifth and eighth week of training and supplementation. The results of this study suggest that androstenedione supplementation at this level does not increase serum testosterone concentrations. The data also suggest that supplementation does not enhance skeletal muscle adaptations to resistance training in normotestosterogenic untrained young men, and may impact an important risk factor for heart disease. Similar results on HDL were observed elsewhere.[182]

The result of a testosterone use screening by organizations such as the IOC and NCAA is "positive" when the urinary ratio of testosterone to epi-testosterone (T/E), an inactive synthetic byproduct, exceeds 6:1. Because of the potential for DHEA to be converted to testosterone, or perhaps influence testosterone metabolism, Bosy and colleagues[183] investigated the effects of daily supplementation of 50 mg of DHEA for 30 days on the T/E ratio. Urinary samples were collected before ingestion and 2 to 3 hours after ingestion and the T/E results were compared to an average baseline generated from three urine samples obtained before the participants began the supplement regimen.

Researchers reported that DHEA at this dose for this period of time had minimal effect on urine T/E ratios, and probably would not result in a positive screen for testosterone abuse. However, in a single-person experiment, 250 mg of DHEA did increase the T/E ratio by 40% relative to the predose value. Another study[184] indicated more clear disturbances in the T/E ratio with DHEA supplementation. Therefore, athletes using DHEA in sports where its use is not banned should understand that there might be the potential for a false positive test for steroid use.

At this time the efficacy of DHEA and androstenedione as testosterone-raising supplements is highly questionable, and marred by physiological considerations. First, DHEA and androstenedione do not appear to predictably elevate serum testosterone levels[175,176,179,180,182] in younger or middle-aged men.[185] Second, aromatization to estrogens appears to occur with supplementation.[179,181] Last, lowering HDL increases heart disease risk.[182,185]

EPHEDRA (MA HUANG)

Ma Huang is a Chinese herb that has been used for thousands of years to treat conditions such as asthma. The effects of ephedra are generally attributed to the alkaloid ephedrine, which is a sympathomimetic substance. Therefore, ephedrine may produce CNS stimulation, vasoconstriction, elevated blood pressure, bronchodilation, and cardiac stimulation. Because of this, ephedrine and other sympathomimetics are banned by the IOC and other organizations.

In the 1972 Olympic games, American gold medalist Rick Demont had to return his medal and was disqualified from further competition after testing positive for ephedrine.[186] He consumed ephedrine as a component of a prescribed anti-asthma drug. Obviously, athletes must be very cautious about ephedrine, as they may ingest it unknowingly as part of various antiasthmatic, cold, or cough medications. For instance, the urine of a Dutch professional cyclist was found to be positive for norpseudoephedrine during a test for doping.[187] The cyclist had consumed a liquid herbal food supplement with ephedra listed as an ingredient. Interestingly, chemical analysis revealed that the levels of norpseudoephedrine were hundreds of times higher than those of ephedrine in several batches of the herb supplement. Researchers pointed out that increased awareness and regulation of "banned" ingredients in herbal supplements is warranted.

While some may ingest ephedrine and related substances unknowingly, others use these substances in an attempt to promote greater fat utilization and general leanness. Because ephedrine has CNS effects, there may be potential for psychological or physiological addiction with chronic use, as well as with "self prescription" of ephedrin. Gruber and Pope[188] recently assessed 36 female athletes who reported ephedrine use for years at high doses. Most of the women had experienced at least some adverse effects, and 19% displayed frank ephedrine dependence at the time of the interview. The researchers also stated that eating disorders and distorted body images seemed to be prevalent among these women.

The ergogenic potential of ephedrine requires comprehensive investigation. Over 20 years ago Sidney and Lefcoe[189] reported that while ephedrine

(24 mg) increased heart rate and blood pressure during exercise, it did not lead to enhanced muscle strength, endurance, power, or VO$_2$max. Hand-eye coordination was not improved either. Some of the reviews[190,191] of ergogenic agents that followed describe ephedrine as ineffective as an ergogenic aid. For instance, a recent study by Bell and colleagues[191] suggests that ephedrine at a level of 1 mg/kg body weight does not improve endurance performance by itself. However, when ephedrine is combined with caffeine there is an improvement,[192] and the possible synergy of these substances allows for reduced levels of supplements.[193] This reduces the potential for side effects such as vomiting during exercise trials involving higher levels of ephedrine and caffeine.[193]

Clearly, more research is needed regarding ephedrine use and athletic performance. Since ephedrine is a banned substance, many researchers have not pursued such research. Ephedrine is very popular with recreational athletes and people who do not exercise in an attempt to enhance metabolism and general body leanness. These users don't always realize that ephedrine may not be the only stimulant in a supplement. Thus, participants may unknowingly increase their intake of ephedrine.

Supplements such as Ripped Fuel and Metabolift also contain guarana extract, which contains caffeine-like substances. The effects of these supplements should be taken very seriously. Furthermore, several deaths have been attributed to toxicity of ephedra and other sympathomimetic drugs, which is of concern to the FDA.

GLUTAMINE

The nonessential amino acid glutamine has become extremely popular in the bodybuilding community.[1,194,195] Glutamine is the most abundant amino acid in the pool of skeletal muscle cells and in plasma.[196] It seems to be especially important for cells demonstrating rapid turnover, such as leukocytes, where it serves in nucleotide synthesis as well as providing energy.

Plasma glutamine levels are known to decrease after a strenuous bout of exercise, and chronic training may have a cumulative effect.[195] The lowered plasma glutamine levels associated with overtraining syndrome (OTS) may endure for weeks. This may render an athlete more susceptible to microbial infection after an intense and prolonged exercise bout (e.g., marathon, triathlon) or a series of daily bouts (e.g., heavy daily training, cycling tours).[196-200] Interestingly, Bassit and coinvestigators[201] reported that BCAA supplementation could limit plasma glutamine reductions following an endurance bout (e.g., Olympic distance triathlon) as well as inhibit the reduction of interleukin-1 (IL-1) production that occurred in a nonsupplemented group.

In addition to glutamine's potential to help with impaired immune function associated with exercise, it has become one of the most highly touted supplements, purported to improve positive protein balance in skeletal muscle. Rennie and colleagues[202] describe the effects of glutamine in skeletal muscle, which include the stimulation of protein synthesis which occurs in the absence or presence of insulin (response being greater with insulin).

Furthermore, they say that sodium-dependent glutamine transporter is highly associated with the muscle glutamine content in the free amino acid pool.[202,203] This transporter may be inducible/repressible during periods of metabolic stress, which would dictate net glutamine directional flux between skeletal muscle and the plasma.

As with many supplements today, glutamine marketing and use have been ahead of research efforts addressing its efficacy. Is there research at this time to support that ingesting glutamine protects or augments immune function and/or muscle mass? And, if so, at what dose (i.e., g/kg LBM)? With regard to improving immune status or decreasing OTS related immunosuppression, a few recent reviews[194,195] have stated that the evidence supporting glutamine supplementation is weak or at the best equivocal. These thoughts were also shared by Nieman[199] in another review article.

Evidence for muscle mass augmentations in weight trainers is also limited. Zachwieja and colleagues[204] infused glutamine plus an amino acid mixture (0.4 g/kg body weight for 14 hours) into young men and women and estimated fractional protein synthesis rate via labeled leucine metabolism. The participants were given a high protein diet (1.5 g/kg body weight) and the trial occurred in a post-absorptive state. Mixed muscle protein synthesis was estimated to be elevated by 48% in response to the amino acid mixture infusion. However, this rate was not augmented by the addition of glutamine.

Mittendorfer and co-workers[205] measured glutamine kinetics using labeled glutamine in healthy subjects in the postabsorptive state. The glutamine complemented an amino acid mixture which was provided either alone or with additional glucose. While arterial glutamine levels rose by 20% with and without glucose, free glutamine levels in leg muscle remained unchanged (amino acids alone) or were decreased (amino acids plus glucose). The decrease in glutamine concentration associated with the addition of glucose was attributed to less protein breakdown and glutamine production, thus reducing the free glutamine intramuscular pool.

In summary, it is difficult to advocate the use of glutamine as an ergogenic aid. Certainly there is compelling theoretical reason to believe that supplementation may provide some immunoprotection and may increase positive muscle protein balance in weight trainers. However, the research has been less than convincing with regard to immunoprotection, and far from complete with regard to muscle protein metabolism.

GLYCEROL

Glycerol may be an ergogenic aid for two reasons. First, it is a substrate for gluconeogenesis, and thus may become an important supportive euglycemic mechanism late in endurance bouts.[1] Second, supplemented glycerol distributes evenly throughout body fluid and provides an osmotic influence, which could assist hyperhydration efforts prior to exercise in the heat. This would be especially beneficial in sports where even conscientious water intake typically fails to match water losses from perspiration. While the first possibility has been generally dismissed because of the slow rate of glycerol conversion to glucose, the second ergogenic possibility has received some support via research findings.

Dehydration (i.e., hypohydration) during exercise is known to reduce athletic performance.[206-210] Hyperhydration may prevent dehydration. However, the rapid diuretic effect of water consumption alone has often negated the potentially beneficial effect of hyperhydration. With this in mind, researchers began to seek an osmotically active substance to consume prior to exercise to enhance water retention. Glycerol has been suggested to have just such an effect.

For instance, Lyons and colleagues[211] reported that glycerol-induced hyperhydration just before moderate exercise was more effective than water-induced hyperhydration in reducing the thermal stress associated with the heat. Here glycerol was provided at 1 g/kg + 21.4 mL H_2O/kg body weight. Elsewhere, researchers[212] reported that ingestion of 1.2 g of glycerol/kg with 26 mL H_2O/kg body weight extended cycling time till exhaustion at 65% VO_2max in a neutral laboratory environment. The researchers also noted a lower heart rate.

It would seem that glycerol-aided hyperhydration might have ergogenic potential. However, some researchers argue that if an athlete is able to maintain euglycemia during exercise, hyperhydration probably doesn't provide a meaningful advantage.[213] Yet, it would seem that glycerol could indeed promote sustained hyperhydration states.[214,215] Most of the related research to date has involved an isolated exercise bout. However, questions remain about the application of glycerol when several exercise bouts are performed over a few days or within the same day when sweating will be copious.

While not as "mainstream" as some other supplements, glycerol is available commercially. Manufacturers typically recommend 1 g/kg body weight with an additional 1.5 L of water taken 60–120 minutes prior to exercise. Athletes need to experiment with glycerol during training, as some have reported cramping and bloating.[216,217]

β-HYDROXY-β-METHYLBUTYRATE (HMB)

β-hydroxy-β-methylbutyrate (HMB) is a metabolite of the essential amino acid leucine, although its physiological significance is still unidentified.[1] It is available to consumers as an independent supplement or as an ingredient of a combination supplement or sport food. For example, 2.5 g is added to the Met-Rx Protein Plus Bar. HMB has been popularized in the weight training community because it is purported to increase net protein balance by decreasing muscle catabolism associated with heavy resistance training and to promote increases in lean body mass.[1,218,219]

To date, scientific data regarding the efficacy of HMB are limited but somewhat encouraging. Nissen and colleagues[220] provided HMB (1.5 or 3.0 g/day for 3 weeks) to untrained males during supervised strength training sessions (1½ hours, 3 days/week for 3 weeks). Compared to a placebo group, urinary 3-methyl histidine (3-MH) was lower in the HMB supplemented group during the first 2 weeks of exercise, which suggests a lessening of the extent of exercise-induced muscle proteolysis. Enhanced performance was also noted, as the weight lifted by the HMB-supplemented group was greater each week of the study.

The researchers also provided 3 g of HMB daily for 7 weeks to participants who routinely trained for 2-3 hours 6 days/week. Here, fat-free mass and bench press strength increased more in HMB-supplemented subjects than they did in the unsupplemented group for different times in the study. The researchers concluded that supplementation with either 1.5 or 3 g of HMB daily can partly prevent exercise-induced proteolysis and/or muscle damage, and result in larger gains in muscle function associated with resistance training.

HMB (3 g/day) was also reported[221] to increase upper body strength and minimize muscle damage (based on plasma creatine kinase levels) when combined with an exercise program. Here the subjects included both males and females, and training status was varied. Meanwhile, Kreider and colleagues[222] reported that 3 or 6 g of HMB daily provided for 4 weeks to experienced weight lifters failed to reduce protein catabolism or influence changes in body composition and strength relative to a placebo.

INOSINE

Inosine is a nucleoside, and supplemental doses typically range around 5–10 g. Inosine, in the form of inosine monophosphate (IMP) can be used to make adenosine monophosphate (AMP) and guanosine monophosphate (GMP), which in turn can be phosphorylated to the high-energy phosphate molecules ATP and guanosine triphosphate (GTP). Thus, one of the more obvious potential ergogenic effects of inosine supplementation would be enhanced ATP levels in muscle cells, hence increased performance especially during higher intensity efforts.

But most researchers have reported that inosine supplementation does not improve athletic performance.[1,223] For instance, Williams and colleagues[224] provided nine endurance-trained athletes 6 g of inosine for 2 days and measured 3-mile run time, VO$_2$max, RER, and ratings of perceived exertion (RPE). Every athlete also performed a placebo trial and the researchers reported that inosine supplementation did not favorably alter any of the measures and concluded that inosine was not an effective ergogenic aid to enhance athletic performance of an aerobic nature.

Starling and colleagues[225] provided 5 g of inosine (or a placebo) for 5 days to 10 competitive male cyclists who then completed a Wingate Bike Test, a 30-minute self-paced cycling performance bout, and also a constant load, supramaximal cycling spring to fatigue. Following the inosine supplementation, there was no improvement in the Wingate measurements such as peak power, end power, fatigue index, total work completed on the bike tests, and post-test lactate. Although no differences in performance measures were observed during the 30-minute self-paced cycling, when the cyclists received inosine supplements their supramaximal cycling sprint time to fatigue was shorter than in the placebo trial. The researchers concluded that prolonged inosine supplementation did not appear to improve aerobic performance and short-term power production during cycling.

However, they recognized that inosine supplementation might actually have an ergolytic effect under some test conditions. McNaughton and co-workers[226] provided 10 g of inosine to seven trained males for either 5 or 10 days to evaluate its impact on both aerobic and anaerobic performance. The three tests of performance were a 6-second sprint performed five times, a 30-second sprint, and a 20-minute time trial. The researchers reported no performance benefit of inosine supplementation.

It has been speculated that inosine has a performance benefit by increasing the 2,3 diphosphoglycerate (2,3-DPG) in red blood cells, which would shift the oxygen-hemoglobin curve to the left and allow for more unloading of oxygen in muscle tissue. However this was not confirmed by research studies.[1,224-226] Furthermore, blood analysis revealed that uric acid levels may be increased due to inosine supplementation.[225,226] This might raise health issues with regard to long-term supplementation.

MEDIUM CHAIN TRIGLYCERIDES

Medium chain triglycerides (MCT) contain medium chain fatty acids (MCFA), which have 6–12 carbon atoms. Once these fatty acids are liberated by digestive lipases, they are able to diffuse directly into the portal vein and systemically circulate. Thus, MCFA can avoid re-esterification to triglycerides and incorporation into chylomicrons, which would enter the lymphatic circulation.[1] Free MCFA may circulate to tissue such as muscle and cross the mitochondrial inner membrane without the assistance of the carnitine palmitoyl transferase (CPT) system. This might then increase fatty acid availability for oxidation.[1]

As the MCFA derived from MCT would be available for working muscle cells, it has been speculated that MCT supplementation may spare muscle glycogen. Some research[227,228] does indeed suggest that MCT may serve as an energy source during endurance exercise, especially when consumed with carbohydrate. However, the contribution of MCT to total energy expenditure during exercise is still small.[229,230] Even when fat oxidation is increased during exercise in glycogen-compromised athletes, MCTs still fail to make a large contribution to total energy expenditure.[229] In addition, MCT supplementation (i.e., alone or with carbohydrate) has not consistently been shown to alter carbohydrate oxidation or the breakdown and oxidation of muscle glycogen.[230-232]

Addressing the ergogenic potential of MCT, Angus and colleagues[231] reported that carbohydrate ingestion during exercise improves 100-km time trial performance compared with a placebo, but adding MCT does not provide any further performance enhancement. Similarly, when athletes cycled for 2 hours at 63% VO_2max and then performed a simulated 40-km time trial while consuming carbohydrate or carbohydrate plus MCT, there was no performance benefit.[233] One research investigation[228] noted that MCT supplementation alone actually decreased performance in comparison to MCT plus carbohydrate.

MCT is a questionable ergogenic aid. While it seems that MCT can be oxidized for fuel, that may or may not impact the oxidation of carbohydrate—or, more specifically, muscle glycogen. Intensity may be a controlling factor.[227,232] The potential for gastrointestinal discomfort, including diarrhea, in some athletes is a problem with MCT supplements.[234] On review of the available literature, Hawley and colleagues concluded that there is very little convincing scientific evidence to recommend MCT for improving exercise performance.[235]

RIBOSE

Ribose is a five-carbon monosaccharide and a component of nucleotides and (more importantly) ATP. Ribose supplementation is touted as a mechanism for increasing ATP levels in muscle tissue, thus allowing for increased power and strength. Despite the widespread popularity of this supplement, little is known regarding its efficacy in the general population.

VANADIUM

Vanadium is a minor mineral and is probably essential for good nutrition. As a sport supplement, vanadium gained some popularity in the weight training/body building community in the early 1990s but seems to have fallen out of favor. It is thought to enhance lean body mass primarily by increasing the activity of insulin. Therefore, amino acid uptake by muscle would be enhanced in conjunction with protein synthesis.

Studies are limited that test the effects of vanadium as vanadyl sulfate on body composition and performance. Fawcett and co-workers[236] conducted a 12-week weight training study in which some participants received vanadyl sulfate at a level of 0.5 mg/kg body weight daily. Performance measurements included 1-RM and 10-RM for the leg extension and bench press. Body composition was assessed by DEXA (Duel Energy X-Ray Absorptiometry) scans. The investigators reported that, relative to the placebo group, changes in strength and body composition were not enhanced in the vanadium-supplemented group. Thus the researchers concluded that vanadyl sulfate was ineffective as a performance enhancer and anthropometric altering agent. Also, they reported that two of the participants receiving the vanadyl sulfate supplements dropped out of the study due to side effects.

Toxicity studies of vanadium are limited. Supplementation at 13.5 mg/day or 9 mg/day for 6 weeks and 16 months, respectively, was found not to be toxic.[237] However, larger doses have been reported to produce diarrhea, green tongue, gastrointestinal disturbances, and cramps.

There is very little research addressing the ergogenic/metabolic impact of vanadium supplementation. Furthermore, the results of the only study reviewed do not show an ergogenic/metabolic benefit. This conclusion is supported in another review of popular nutrition supplements associated with exercise.[238]

CONCLUSION

For centuries, man has searched for foods and food components that would enhance athletic performance. Today, the production of sport foods and supplements is a multibillion-dollar industry. Numerous chemicals are touted to be ergogenic, including individual elements, amino acids and derivatives, fatty acids, and steroid precursors. These substances claim to improve energy metabolism, protein turnover, mass development, body composition, and strength and power.

However, there are concerns about the effectiveness and safety of ergogenic substances. As well, governing bodies such as IOC and NCAA must decide which ones they will permit athletes to use. Many of these substances (e.g., chromium picolinate, androstenedione, MCT) have not performed as well as expected, and their effects may not be predictable or controllable. Several substances, such as glutamine, ribose, and HMB, are under-researched, so it is difficult to draw conclusions about their effectiveness.

Creatine, on the other hand, has demonstrated its efficacy in many studies. It remains to be seen whether further research will uncover hidden potential among the many and varied substances touted as ergogenic aids.

REFERENCES

1. Wildman REC, Miller BS. Sport Foods, Supplements & Ergogenic Aids. In: *Sport & Fitness Nutrition.* Atlanta, GA: Wadsworth Publishing; 2003.
2. Wildman REC, Medieros DM. Nutrition Supplements and Nutraceuticals. In: *Advanced Human Nutrition.* Boca Raton, FL: CRC Press; 2000:367.
3. Grandjean AC, Hursh LM, Majure WC, et al. Nutrition knowledge and practices of college athletes. *Med Sci Sports Exerc.* 1981;13:82-7.
4. Grandjean AC, Reimers KJ, Ruud JS. Dietary habits of olympic athletes. In: Wolinsky I, ed. *Nutrition in Exercise and Sport.* 3rd ed. Boca Raton, FL: CRC Press; 1998:422.
5. Donati L, Ziegler F, Pongelli G, et al. Nutritional and clinical efficacy of ornithine alpha-ketoglutarate in severe burn patients. *Clin Nutr.* 1999;18:307-11.
6. De Bandt JP, Coudray-Lucas C, Lioret N, et al. A randomized controlled trial of the influence of the mode of enteral ornithine alpha-ketoglutarate administration in burn patients. *J Nutr.* 1998;128:563-9.
7. Jeevanandam M, Petersen SR. Substrate fuel kinetics in enterally fed trauma patients supplemented with ornithine alpha ketoglutarate. *Clin Nutr.* 1999;18:209-17.
8. Isidori A, LoMonaco A, Cappa M. A study of growth hormone release in man after oral adminstration of amino acids. *Curr Med Res Opin.* 1981;7(7):475-81.
9. Suminski RR, Robertson RJ, Goss FL, et al. Acute effect of amino acid ingestion and resistance exercise on plasma growth hormone concentration in young men. *Int J Sports Med.* 1997;7:48-60.
10. Corpas E, Blackman M, Roberson R, et al. Oral arginine-lysine does not increase growth hormone or insulin-like growth factor-I in old men. *J Gerontol.* 1993;48:128-33.
11. Marcell T J, Taaffe DR, Hawkins SA, et al. Oral arginine does not stimulate basal or augment exercise-induced GH secretion in either young or old adults. *J Gerontol A Biol Sci Med Sci.* 1999;54:M395-9.
12. Fogelholm GM, Naveri HK, Kiilavouri KT, et al. Low-dose amino acid supplementation: no effects on serum human growth hormone and insulin in male weightlifters. *Int J Sport Nutr.* 1993;3:291-7.
13. Lambert MI, Hefer JA, Millar RP, et al. Failure of commercial oral amino acid supplements to increase serum growth hormone concentrations in male body-builders. *Int J Sport Nutr.* 1993;3:298-305.
14. Eto B, Le Moel G, Porquet D, et al. Glutamate-arginine salts and hormonal responses to exercise. *Arch Physiol Biochem.* 1995;103:160-4.
15. Ceremuzynski L, Chamiec T, Herbaczynska-Cedro K. Effect of supplemental oral L-arginine on exercise capacity in patients with stable angina pectoris. *Am J Cardiol.* 1997;80:331-3.
16. Bednarz B, Wolk R, Chamiec T, et al. Effects of oral L-arginine supplementation on exercise-induced QT dispersion and exercise tolerance in stable angina pectoris. *Int J Cardiol.* 2000;75:205-10.

17. Maxwell AJ, Ho HK, Le CQ, et al. L-Arginine enhances aerobic exercise capacity in association with augmented nitric oxide production. *J Appl Physiol*. 2001;90:933-8.

18. Colombani PC, Bitzi R, Frey-Rindova P, et al. Chronic arginine aspartate supplementation in runners reduces total plasma amino acid level at rest and during a marathon run. *Eur J Nutr*. 1999;38:263-70.

19. Villalobos C. Mechanisms for the stimulation of rat anterior pituary cells by arginine and other amino acids. *J Physiol (Lond)*. 1997;502(pt 2):421-33.

20. Hagan RD, Upton SJ, Duncan JJ, et al. Absence of effect of potassium-magnesium aspartate on physiologic responses to prolonged work in aerobically trainined men. *Int J Sports Med*. 1982;3:177-81.

21. Maughan RJ, Sadler DJ. The effects of oral supplementation of salts of aspartic acid on the metabolic response to prolonged exhausting exercise in man. *Int J Sports Med*. 1983;4:119-23.

22. deHaan A, van Doorn JE, Westra HG. Effects of potassium + magnesium asparate on muscle metabolism and force development during short intensive static exercise. *Int J Sports Med*. 1985;6:44-9.

23. Trudeau F, Murphy R. Effects of potassium-aspartate administration on glycogen use in the rat during a swimming stress. *Physiol Behav*. 1993;54:7-12.

24. Tuttle JL, Potteiger JA, Evans BW, et al. Effect of acute potassium-magnesium aspartate supplementation on ammonia concentrations during and after resistance training. *Int J Sport Nutr*. 1995;5:102-9.

25. Lancha AH, Recco MB, Abdalla DS, et al. Effect of aspartate, asparagine, and carnitine supplementation in the diet on metabolism of skeletal muscle during a moderate exercise. *Physiol Behav*. 1995;57:367-71.

26. Lancha AH, Santos MF, Palanch AC, et al. Supplementation of aspartate, asparagine, and carnitine in the diet causes marked changes in the ultrastructure of soleus muscle. *J Submicrosc Cytol Pathol*. 1997;29:405-8.

27. Nielsen FH, Hunt CD, Mullen LM, et al. Effect of dietary boron on mineral, estrogen, and testosterone metabolism in postmenopausal women. *FASEB J*. 1987;1:394-7.

28. Green NR, Ferrando AA. Plasma boron and the effects of boron supplementation in males. *Environ Health Perspect*. 1994;102:73-7.

29. Ferrando AA, Green NR. The effect of boron supplementation on lean body mass, plasma testosterone levels, and strength in male bodybuilders. *Int J Sport Nutr*. 1993;3:140-9.

30. Meacham SL, Taper LJ, Volpe SL. Effects of boron supplementation on bone mineral density and dietary, blood, and urinary calcium, phosphorus, magnesium, and boron in female athletes. *Environ Health Perspect*. 1994;102:79-82.

31. Meacham SL, Taper LJ, Volpe SL. Effects of boron supplementation on blood and urinary calcium, magnesium, and phosphorus and urinary boron in athletic and sedentary women. *Am J Clin Nutr*. 1995;61:341-5.

32. Naghii MR. The significance of dietary boron, with particular reference to athletes. *Nutr Health*. 1999;13:31-7.

33. Samman S, Naghii MR, Lyons Wall PM, et al. The nutritional and metabolic effects of boron in humans and animals. *Biol Trace Elem Res*. 1998;66:227-35.

34. Wagenmakers AJ. Nutritional supplements: effects on exercise performance and metabolism. In: Lamb DR, Murray R, eds. *Perspectives in Exercise and Sports Medicine: The Metabolic Basis of Performance and Sport*. Vol 12. Carmel, IN: Cooper Publishing Group; 1999.

35. Wagenmakers AJ, Brookes JH, Coakley JH, et al. Exercise-induced activation of the branched-chain 2-oxo acid dehydrogenase in human muscle. *Eur J Appl Physiol Occup Physiol*. 1989;59:159-67.

36. Wagenmakers AJ, Beckers EJ, Brouns F, et al. Carbohydrate supplementation, glycogen depletion, and amino acid metabolism during exercise. *Am J Physiol*. 1991;260:E883-90.

37. Knapik J, Meredith C, Jones B, et al. Leucine metabolism during fasting and exercise. *J Appl Physiol*. 1991;70:43-7.

38. Wolfe RR, Goodenough RD, Wolfe MH, et al. Isotopic analysis of leucine and urea metabolism in exercising humans. *J Appl Physiol*. 1982;52:458-66.

39. van Hall G, MacLean DA, Saltin B, et al. Mechanisms of activation of muscle branched-chain alpha-keto acid dehydrogenase during exercise in man. *J Physiol*. 1996;494:899-905.

40. Lancha AH, Recco MB, Curi R. Pyruvate carboxylase activity in the heart and skeletal muscles of the rat: evidence for a stimulating effect of exercise. *Biochem Mol Biol Int*. 1994;32:483-9.

41. Lancha AH, Recco MB, Abdalla DS, et al. Effect of aspartate, asparagine, and carnitine supplementation in the diet on metabolism of skeletal muscle during a moderate exercise. *Physiol Behav*. 1995;57:367-71.

42. Paul GL, Gautsch TA, Layman DK. Amino acid and protein metabolism during exercise and recovery. In: Wolinsky I, Driskell J, ed. *Nutrition in Exercise and Sport*. Boca Raton, FL: CRC Press; 1998.

43. Pardridge WM. Blood-brain barrier transport of nutrients. *Nutr Rev*. 1986;44:15-25.

44. Lovenberg WM. Biochemical regulation of brain function. *Nutr Rev*. 1986;44:6-11.

45. van Hall G, Raaymakers JS, Saris WH, et al. Ingestion of branched-chain amino acids and tryptophan during sustained exercise in man: failure to affect performance. *J Physiol*. 1995;486:789-94.

46. Blomstrand E, Andersson S, Hassmen P, et al. Effect of branched-chain amino acid and carbohydrate supplementation on the exercise-induced change in plasma and muscle concentration of amino acids in human subjects. *Acta Physiol Scand*. 1995;153:87-96.

47. Varnier M, Sarto P, Martines D, et al. Effect of infusing branched-chain amino acid during incremental exercise with reduced muscle glycogen content. *Eur J Appl Physiol Occup Physiol*. 1994;69:26-31.

48. Madsen K, MacLean DA, Kiens B, et al. Effects of glucose, glucose plus branched-chain amino acids, or placebo on bike performance over 100 km. *J Appl Physiol*. 1996;81:2644-50.

49. Blomstrand E, Hassmen P, Ekblom B, et al. Administration of branched-chain amino acids during sustained exercise—effects on performance and on plasma concentration of some amino acids. *Eur J Appl Physiol Occup Physiol*. 1991;63:83-8.

50. Mittleman KD, Ricci MR, Bailey SP. Branched-chain amino acids prolong exercise during heat stress in men and women. *Med Sci Sports Exerc*. 1998;30:83-91.

51. Bassit RA, Sawada LA, Bacurau RF, et al. The effect of BCAA supplementation upon the immune response of triathletes. *Med Sci Sports Exerc*. 2000;32:1214-9.

52. Coombes JS, McNaughton LR. Effects of branched-chain amino acid supplementation on serum creatine kinase and lactate dehydrogenase after prolonged exercise. *J Sports Med Phys Fitness*. 2000;40:240-6.

53. Anthony JC, Anthony TG, Kimball SR, et al. Signaling pathways involved in translational control of protein synthesis in skeletal muscle by leucine. *J Nutr*. 2001;131:856S-60S.

54. Costill DL, Dalsky GP, Fink WJ. Effects of caffeine ingestion on metabolism and exercise performance. *Med Sci Sports Exerc*. 1978;10:155-8.

55. Ivy JL, Costill DL, Fink WJ, et al. Influence of caffeine and carbohydrate feedings on endurance performance. *Med Sci Sports Exerc*. 1979;11:6-11.

56. Graham TE, Spriet LL. Caffeine and exercise performance. *Sport Science Exchange*: Gatorade Sports Science Institute. 1996;60:1.

57. Conlee RK. Amphetamine, caffeine and cocaine. In: Lamb DR, Williams MH, eds. *Ergogenics: Enhancement of Performance in Exercise and Sport*. Indianapolis, IN: Brown and Benchmark; 1991.

58. Graham TE, Spriet LL. Performance and metabolic responses to high caffeine dose during prolonged exercise. *J Appl Physiol*. 1991;71:2292-8.

59. Graham TE, Spriet LL. Metabolic, catecholamine and exercise performance responses to varying doses of caffeine. *J Appl Physiol*. 1995;78:867-74.

60. Spriet LL, MacLean DA, Dyck DJ, et al. Caffeine ingestion and muscle metabolism during prolonged exercise in humans. *Am J Physiol*. 1992;262:E891-8.

61. Pasman WJ, VanBaak MA, Jeukendrup AE, et al. The effect of different dosages of caffeine on endurance performance time. *Int J Sports Med*. 1995;16:225-30.

62. Trice I, Haymes EM. Effects of caffeine ingestion on exercise-induced changes during high-intensity, intermittent exercise. *Int J Sport Nutr*. 1995;5:37-44.

63. Collomp K, Ahmaidi S, Audran M, et al. Effects of caffeine ingestion on performance and anaerobic metabolism during the Wingate test. *Int J Sports Med*. 1991;12:439-43.

64. Wiles JD, Bird SR, Hopkins J, et al. Effect of caffeinated coffee on running speed, respiratory factors, blood lactate and perceived exertion during 1500-m treadmill running. *Br J Sports Med*.1992; 26(2):116-20.

65. Williams JH, Signoille JF, Barnes WS, et al. Caffeine, maximal power output and fatigue. *Br J Sports Med*. 1998;229:132-4.

66. Collomp K, Ahmaidi S, Chatard JC, et al. Benefits of caffeine ingestion on sprint performance in trained and untrained swimmers. *Eur J Appl Physiol*. 1992;64:377-80.

67. Anselme F, Collomp K, Mercier B, et al. Caffeine increases maximal anaerobic power and blood lactate concentration. *Eur J Appl Physiol*. 1992;65:188-91.

68. Collomp K, Caillaud C, Audran M, et al. Influence of acute and chronic bouts of caffeine on performance and catecholamines in the course of maximal exercise. *CR Seances Soc Biol Fil*. 1990; 184(1):87-92.

69. Graham TE, Rush JWE, VanSoeren MH. Caffeine and exercise: metabolism and performance. *Can J Appl Physiol*. 1994;2:111-38.

70. VanSoeren MH, Sathasivam P, Spriet LL, et al. Short term withdrawal does not alter caffeine-induced metabolic changes during intensive exercise. *FASEB J*. 1993;7:A518.

71. Weir J, Noakes TD, Myburgh K, et al. A high carbohydrate diet negates the metabolic effect of caffeine during exercise. *Med Sci Sports Exerc*. 1987;19:100-5.

72. Spriet LL. Caffeine and performance. *Int J Sport Nutr*. 1995;5:S54-89.

73. Heinenen OJ. Carnitine and physical exercise. *Sports Med*. 1996;22:109-32.

74. Colombani P, Wenk C, Kunz I, et al. Effects of L-carnitine supplementation on physical performance and energy metabolism of endurance-trained athletes: a double-blind crossover field study. *Eur J Appl Physiol Occup Physiol*. 1996;73:434-9.

75. Vecchiet L, Di Lisa F, Pieralisi G, et al. Influence of L-carnitine administration on maximal physical exercise. *Eur J Appl Physiol Occup Physiol*. 1990;61:486-90.

76. Brass EP, Hiatt WR. The role of carnitine and carnitine supplementation during exercise in man and in individuals with special needs. *J Am Coll Nutr*. 1998;17:207-15.

77. Fagher B, Gederblad G, Erikson M, et al. 1-carnitine and hemodialysis: double blind study of muscle function and metabolism and peripheral nerve function. *Scand J Clin Lab Invest*. 1985;45:169-72.

78. Golper TS, Wolfson M, Ahmad S, et al. Multicenter trial of l-carnitine in hemodialysis patients. Part I: carnitine concentrations and lipid effects. *Kidney Int*. 1990;38:904-11.

79. Ahmad S, Robertson T, Golper TA, et al. Multicenter trial of L-carnitine in hemodialysis patients. Part II: clinical and biochemical effects. *Kidney Int*. 1990;38:912-8.

80. Lancha AH. Supplementation of aspartate, asparagine and carnitine in the diet causes marked changes in the ultrastructure of soleus muscle. *J Submicrosc Cytol Pathol*.1997;29:405-8.

81. Buchman AL, Jenden D, Roch M. Plasma free, phospholipid-bound and urinary free choline all decrease during a marathon run and may be associated with impaired performance. *J Am Coll Nutr*. 1999;18:598-601.

82. Buchman AL, Awal M, Jenden D, et al. The effect of lecithin supplementation on plasma choline concentrations during a marathon. *J Am Coll Nutr*. 2000;9:768-70.

83. Spector SA, Jackman MR, Sabounjian LA, et al. Effect of choline supplementation on fatigue in trained cyclists. *Med Sci Sports Exerc*. 1995;27:668-73.

84. Warber JP, Patton JF, Tharion WJ, et al. The effects of choline supplementation on physical performance. *Int J Sport Nutr Exerc Metab*. 2000;10:170-81.

85. Sachan DS, Hongu N. Increases in VO(2)max and metabolic markers of fat oxidation by caffeine, carnitine, and choline supplementation in rats. *J Nutr Biochem*. 2000;11:521-6.

86. Evans GW, Pouchnik DJ. Composition and biological activity of chromium-pyridine carboxylate complexes. *J Inorg Biochem*. 1993;49:177-87.

87. Amato P, Morales AJ, Yen SS. Effects of chromium picolinate supplementation on insulin sensitivity, serum lipids, and body composition in healthy, nonobese, older men and women. *J Gerontol A Biol Sci Med Sci*. 2000;55(5):260-3.

88. Joseph LJ, Farrell PA, Davey SL, et al. Effect of resistance training with or without chromium picolinate supplementation on glucose metabolism in older men and women. *Metabolism* 1999;48:546-53.

89. Clarkson PM. Effects of exercise on chromium levels: is supplementation required? *Sports Med*. 1997;23:341-9.

90. Andersonm RA. Effects of chromium on body composition and weight loss. *Nutr Rev*. 1998;56:266-70.

91. Lukaski HC. Chromium as a supplement. *Annu Rev Nutr*. 1999;19:279-302.

92. Lukaski IIC, Bolonchik WW, Siders WA, et al. Chromium supplementation and resistance training: effects on body composition, strength, and trace element status of men. *Am J Clin Nutr*. 1996;63:954-65.

93. Trent LK, Theiding-Cancel D. Effects of chromium picolinate on body composition. *J Sports Med Phys Fitness*. 1995;35(4):273-80.

94. Clancy SP, Clarkson PM, DeCheke ME, et al. Effects of chromium picolinate supplementation on body composition, strength, and urinary chromium loss in football players. *Int J Sport Nutr*. 1994;4:142-53.

95. Hallmark MA, Reynolds TH, DeSouza CA, et al. Effects of chromium and resistive training on muscle strength and body composition. *Med Sci Sports Exerc*. 1996;28:139-44.

96. Hasten DL, Rome EP, Franks BD, et al. Effects of chromium picolinate on beginning weight training students. *Int J Sport Nutr*. 1992;2:343-50.

97. Walker LS, Bemben MG, Bemben DA, et al. Chromium picolinate effects on body composition and muscular performance in wrestlers. *Med Sci Sports Exerc*. 1998;30:1730-7.

98. Trent LK, Thieding-Cancel D. Effects of chromium picolinate on body composition. *J Sports Med Phys Fitness*. 1995;35:273-80.

99. Kobla HV, Volpe SL. Chromium, exercise, and body composition. *Crit Rev Food Sci Nutr*. 2000;40:291-308.

100. Evans GW. The effect of chromium picolinate on insulin controlled parameters in humans. *Int J Biosoc Med Res*. 1993;11:163-80.

101. Campbell WW, Joseph LJ, Davey SL, et al. Effects of resistance training and chromium picolinate on body composition and skeletal muscle in older men. *J Appl Physiol*. 1999;86:29-39.

102. Cerulli J, Grabe DW, Gauthier I, et al. Chromium picolinate toxicity. *Ann Pharmacother.*1998;32:428-31.
103. Stearns DM, Wise JP Sr, Patierno S, et al. Chromium (III) picolinate produces chromosome damage in Chinese hamster ovary cells. *FASEB J.* 1995;9:1643-9.
104. Stearns DM, Belbruno JJ, Wetterhahn KE. A prediction of chromium (III) accumulation in humans from chromium dietary supplements. *FASEB J.* 1995;9:1650-7.
105. Karlsson J, Lin L, Sylven C, et al. Muscle ubiquinone in healthy physically active males. *Mol Cell Biochem.* 1996;23:169-72.
106. Braun B, Clarkson PM, Freedson PS, et al. Effects of coenzyme Q10 supplementation on exercise performance, VO2max, and lipid peroxidation in trained cyclists. *Int J Sport Nutr.* 1991;1:353-65.
107. Sniderm IP, Bazzarre TL, Murdoch SD, et al. Effects of coenzyme athletic performance system as an ergogenic aid on endurance performance to exhaustion. *Int J Sport Nutr.* 1992;2:272-86.
108. Laaksonen R, Fogelholm M, Himberg JJ, et al. Ubiquinone supplementation and exercise capacity in trained young and older men. *Eur J Appl Physiol Occup Physiol.* 1995;72:95-100.
109. Porter DA, Costill DL, Zachwieja JJ, et al. The effect of oral coenzyme Q10 on the exercise tolerance of middle-aged, untrained men. *Int J Sports Med.* 1995;16:421-7.
110. Weston SB, Zhou S, Weatherby RP, et al. Does exogenous coenzyme Q10 affect aerobic capacity in endurance athletes? *Int J Sport Nutr.* 1997;7:197-206.
111. Bonetti A, Solito F, Carmosino G, et al. Effect of ubidecarenone oral treatment on aerobic power in middle-aged trained subjects. *J Sports Med Phys Fitness.* 2000;40:51-7.
112. Nielsen AN, Mizuno M, Ratkevicius A, et al. No effect of antioxidant supplementation in triathletes on maximal oxygen uptake, 31P-NMRS detected muscle energy metabolism and muscle fatigue. *Int J Sports Med.* 1999;20:154-8.
113. Ylikoski T, Piirainen J, Hanninen O, et al. The effect of coenzyme Q10 on the exercise performance of cross-country skiers. *Mol Aspects Med.* 1997;18(suppl):S283-90.
114. Vasankari TJ, Kujala UM, Vasankari TM, et al. Increased serum and low-density-lipoprotein antioxidant potential after antioxidant supplementation in endurance athletes. *Am J Clin Nutr.* 1997;65:1052-6.
115. Faff J, Frankiewicz-Jozko A. Effect of ubiquinone on exercise-induced lipid peroxidation in rat tissue. *Eur J Appl Physiol Occup Physiol.* 1997;75(5):413-7.
116. Sinatra ST. Coenzyme Q10: a vital therapeutic nutrient for the heart with special application in congestive heart failure. *Conn Med.* 1997;61(11):707-11.
117. Hofman-Bang C, Rehnqvist N, Swedberg K, et al. Coenzyme Q10 as an adjunctive in the treatment of chronic congestive heart failure: The Q10 Study Group. *J Card Fail.* 1995;1:101-7.
118. Mortensen SA, Vadhanavikit S, Muratsu K, et al. Coenzyme Q10: clinical benefits with biochemical correlates suggesting a scientific breakthrough in the management of chronic heart failure. *Int J Tissue React.* 1990;12:155-62.
119. Soja AM, Mortensen SA. Treatment of chronic cardiac insufficiency with coenzyme Q10, results of meta-analysis in controlled clinical trials. *Ugeskr Laeger.* 1997;159:7302-8.
120. Dodd JR, Zheng T, Christie DL. Creatine accumulation and exchange by HEK293 cells stably expressing high levels of a creatine transporter. *Biochim Biophys Acta.* 1999;1472:128-36.
121. Benzi G. Is there a rationale for the use of creatine either as nutritional supplementation or drug administration in humans participating in a sport? *Pharmacol Res.* 2000;41:255-64.
122. Williams MH, Branch JD. Creatine supplementation and exercise performance: an update. *J Am Coll Nutr.* 1998;17:216-34.
123. Kraemer WJ, Volek JS. Creatine supplementation: its role in human performance. *Clin Sports Med.* 1999;18:651-66.
124. Bolotte CP. Creatine supplementation in athletes: benefits and potential risks. *J La State Med Soc.* 1998;150:325-7.
125. Jacobs I. Dietary creatine monohydrate supplementation. *Can J Appl Physiol.* 1999;24:503-14.
126. Green AL, Simpson EJ, Littlewood JJ, et al. Carbohydrate ingestion augments creatine retention during creatine feeding in humans. *Acta Physiol Scand.* 1996;158:195-202.
127. Green AL, Hultman E, Macdonald IA, et al. Carbohydrate ingestion augments skeletal muscle creatine accumulation during creatine supplementation in humans. *Am J Physiol.* 1996;271:E821-6.
128. Hultman E, Soderlund K, Timmons JA, et al. Muscle creatine loading in men. *J Appl Physiol.* 1996;81:232-7.
129. Rossiter HB, Cannell ER, Jakeman PM. The effect of oral creatine supplementation on the 1000-m performance of competitive rowers. *J Sports Sci.* 1996;14:175-9.
130. Greenwood M, Farris J, Kreider R, et al. Creatine supplementation patterns and perceived effects in select division I collegiate athletes. *Clin J Sport Med.* 2000;10:191-4.
131. Volek JS, Duncan ND, Mazzetti SA, et al. Performance and muscle fiber adaptations to creatine supplementation and heavy resistance training. *Med Sci Sports Exerc.* 1999;31:1147-56.

132. Greenhaff PL. The effect of oral creatine supplementation on skeletal muscle phosphocreatine resynthesis. *Am J Physiol*. 1994;266:E725-30.
133. Mujika I, Padilla S. Creatine supplementation as an ergogenic acid for sports performance in highly trained athletes: a critical review. *Int J Sports Med*. 1997;18:491-6.
134. Mujika I, Chatard JC, Lacoste L, et al. Creatine supplementation does not improve sprint performance in competitive swimmers. *Med Sci Sports Exerc*. 1996;28:1435-41.
135. Greenhaff PL. The nutritional biochemistry of creatine. *Nutr Biochem*. 1997;11:610-8.
136. Burke LM, Pyne DB, Telford RD. Effect of oral creatine supplementation on single-effort sprint performance in elite swimmers. *Int J Sport Nutr*. 1996;6:222-33.
137. Bosco C, Tihanyi J, Pucspk J, et al. Effect of oral creatine supplementation on jumping and running performance. *Int J Sports Med*. 1997;18:369-72.
138. Birch R. The influence of dietary creatine supplementation on performance during repeated bouts of maximal isokinetic cycling in man. *Eur J Appl Physiol Occup Physiol*. 1994;69:268-76.
139. Greenhaff PL, Casey A, Short AH, et al. Influence of oral creatine supplementation on muscle torque during repeated bouts of maximal voluntary exercise in man. *Clin Sci*. 1993;84:565-71.
140. Earnest CP. The effect of creatine monohydrate ingestion on anaerobic power indicies, muscular strength, and body composition. *Acta Physiol Scand*. 1995;153:207-9.
141. Balsom PD, Soderlund K, Sjodin B, et al. Skeletal muscle metabolism during short duration high-intensity exercise: influence of creatine supplementation. *Acta Physiol Scand*. 1995;154:303-10.
142. Becque MD, Lochmann JD, Melrose DR. Effects of oral creatine supplementation on muscular strength and body composition. *Med Sci Sports Exerc*. 2000;32:654-8.
143. Stone MH, Sanborn K, Smith LL, et al. Effects of in-season (5 weeks) creatine and pyruvate supplementation on anaerobic performance and body composition in American football players. *Int J Sport Nutr*. 1999;9:146-65.
144. Kreider RB. Dietary supplements and the promotion of muscle growth with resistance exercise. *Sports Med*. 1999;27:97-110.
145. Mihic S, MacDonald JR, McKenzie S, et al. Acute creatine loading increases fat-free mass, but does not affect blood pressure, plasma creatinine, or CK activity in men and women. *Med Sci Sports Exerc*. 2000;32:291-6.
146. Engelhardt M, Neumann G, Berbalk A, et al. Creatine supplementation in endurance sports. *Med Sci Sports Exerc*. 1998;30:1123-9.
147. Vandebuerie F, Vanden Eynde B, Vandenberghe K, et al. Effect of creatine loading on endurance capacity and sprint power in cyclists. *Int J Sports Med*. 1998;19:490-5.
148. Balsom PD, Harridge SD, Soderlund K, et al. Creatine supplementation per se does not enhance endurance exercise performance. *Acta Physiol Scand*. 1993;149:521-3.
149. Poortmans JR, Francaux M. Adverse effects of creatine supplementation: fact or fiction? *Sports Med*. 2000;30:155-70.
150. Poortmans JR, Francaux M. Long-term oral creatine supplementation does not impair renal function in healthy athletes. *Med Sci Sports Exerc*. 1999;31:1108-10.
151. Schilling BK, Stone MH, Utter A, et al. Creatine supplementation and health variables: a retrospective study. *Med Sci Sports Exerc*. 2001;33:183-8.
152. Wildman REC, Ciliberti L, Sanders C. Preliminary studies in echocardiography in men during creatine loading [thesis]. Lafayette, LA: University of Louisiana; 2002.
153. Labrie F. Intracrinology. *Mol Cell Endocrinol*. 1991;78:C113-8.
154. Labrie F, DuPont A, Belanger A. Complete androgen blockage for the treatment of prostate cancer. In: de Vita VT, Hellman S, Rosenberg SA, eds. *Important Advances in Oncology*. Philadelphia: JB Lippincott; 1985:193-217.
155. Labrie C, Belanger A, Labrie F. Androgenic activity of dehydroepiandrosterone and androsterenedione in the rat ventral prostate. *Endocrinol*. 1988;123:1412-7.
156. Migeon CJ, Keller AR, Lawrence B, et al. Dehydroepiandrosterone and adndrosterone levels in human placenta: effect of age and sex: day-to-day and diurnal variations. *J Clin Endocrinol Metab*. 1957;17:1051-62.
157. Orentreich N, Brind JL, Rizer RL, et al. Age changes and sex differences in serum dehydroepiandrosterone sulfate concentrations throughout adulthood. *J Clin Endocrinol Metab*. 1984;59:551-5.
158. Vermeulen A, Deslypene JP, Schelthout W, et al. Adrenocortical function in old age: response of acute adrenocorticotropin stimulation. *J Clin Endocrinol Metab*. 1982;54:187-91.
159. Barrett-Conner E, Khaw KT, Yen SSC. A prospective study of dehydroepiandrosterone sulfate, mortality and cardiovascular disease. *N Eng J Med*. 1986;315:1519-24.
160. Zumff B, Levin J, Rosenfeld RS, et al. Abnormal 24-hr mean plasma concentrations of dehydroepiandrosterone and dehydroisoandrosterone sulfate in women with primary operable breast cancer. *Cancer Res*. 1981;41:3360-2.

161. Stahl F, Schnorr D, Pilz C, et al. Dehydroepiandrosterone (DHEA) levels in patients with prostatic cancer, heart diseases and under surgery stress. *Exp Clin Endocrinol*. 1992;99:68-70.

162. Neville AM, O'Hare MJ. *The Human Adrenal Cortex. Pathology and Biology-An Integrated Approach.* Berlin, Germany: Springer-Verlag; 1982.

163. Murray RK, Granner DK, Mayes PA, et al. *Harper's Biochemistry*. San Mateo, CA: Appleton & Lange; 1988.

164. Dunn JF, Nisula BC, Rodbard D. Transport of steroid hormones: binding of 21 endogenous steroids to both testosterone-binding globulin and corticosteroid-binding globulin in human plasma. *J Clin Endocrinol Metab*. 1981;53(1):58-68.

165. Plager JE. The binding of androsterone sulfate, etiocholanolone sulfate, and dehydroisoandrosterone sulfate by human plasma protein. *J Clin Invest*. 1965;44:1234-9.

166. Wang D, Bulbrook RD. Binding of the sulfate esters of dehydroepiandrosterone, testosterone, 17-acetoxypregnenolone and pregnenolone in the plasma of man, rabbit, and rat. *J Endocrinol*. 1967;39:405-13.

167. Belenger A, Brochu M, Clinche J. Levels of plasma steroid glucoronides in intact and castrasted men with prostatic cancer. *J Clin Endocrinol Metab*. 1986;62:812-5.

168. Labrie F, Belanger A, DuPont A, et al. Science behind total androgen blockade: from gene to combination therapy. *Clin Invest Med*. 1993;16:487-504.

169. Moghissi E, Ablan F, Horton R. Origin of plasma androstanediol glucuronide in men. *J Clin Endocrinol Metab*. 1984;59:417-21.

170. Dehennin L, Ferry M, Lafarge P, et al. Oral administration of dehydroepiandrosterone to healthy men: alteration of the urinary androgen profile and consequences for the detection of abuse in sport by gas chromatography-mass spectrometry. *Steroids*. 1998;63:80-7.

171. Martel C, Melner MH, Gagne D, et al. Widespread tissue distribution of steroid sulfatase, 3-beta-hydroxysteroid dehydrogenase/delta 5-delta 4-isomerase (3 beta-HSD), 17 beta-HSD 5 alpha-reductase and aromatase activities in the rhesus monkey. *Mol Cell Endocrinol*. 1994;104:103-11.

172. Martel C, Rheaume E, Takahashi M, et al. Distribution of 17 beta-hydroxysteroid dehydrogenase gene expression and activity in rat and human tissues. *J Steroid Biochem Mol Biol*. 1992;41:597-603.

173. Andersson S, Geissler WM, Pate S, et al. The molecular biology of androgenic 17 beta-hydroxysteroid dehydrogenases. *J Steroid Biochem Mol Biol*. 1995;53:37-9.

174. Kley HK, Deselaers T, Peerenboom H, et al. Enhanced conversion of androstenedione to estrogens in obese males. *J Clin Endocrinol Metab*. 1980;51:1128-32.

175. Brown GA, Vukovich MD, Reifenrath TA, et al. Effects of anabolic precursors on serum testosterone concentrations and adaptations to resistance training in young men. *Int J Sport Nutr Exerc Metab*. 2000;10:340-59.

176. Wallace MB, Lim J, Cutler A, et al. Effects of dehydroepiandrosterone vs androstenedione supplementation in men. *Med Sci Sports Exerc*. 1999;31:1788-92.

177. Brown GA, Vukovich MD, Sharp RL, et al. Effect of oral DHEA on serum testosterone and adaptations to resistance training in young men. *J Appl Physiol*. 1999;87:2274-83.

178. Rasmussen BB, Volpi E, Gore DC, et al. Androstenedione does not stimulate muscle protein anabolism in young healthy men. *J Clin Endocrinol Metab*. 2000;85:55-9.

179. Leder BZ, Longcope C, Catlin DH, et al. Oral androstenedione administration and serum testosterone concentrations in young men. *JAMA*. 2000;283:779-82.

180. Ballantyne CS, Phillips SM, MacDonald JR, et al. The acute effects of androstenedione supplementation in healthy young males. *Can J Appl Physiol*. 2000;25:68-78.

181. King DS, Sharp RL, Vukovich MD, et al. Effect of oral androstenedione on serum testosterone and adaptations to resistance training in young men: a randomized controlled trial. *JAMA*. 1999;281:2020-8.

182. Broeder CE, Quindry J, Brittingham K, et al. The Andro Project: physiological and hormonal influences of androstenedione supplementation in men 35 to 65 years old participating in a high-intensity resistance training program. *Arch Intern Med*. 2000;160:3093-104.

183. Bosy TZ, Moore KA, Poklis A. The effect of oral dehydroepiandrosterone (DHEA) on the urine testosterone/epitestosterone (T/E) ratio in human male volunteers. *J Anal Toxicol*. 1998;22:455-9.

184. Johnson R. Abnormal testosterone: epitestosterone ratios after dehydroepiandrosterone supplementation. *Clin Chem*. 1999;45:163-4.

185. Brown GA, Vukovich MD, Martini ER, et al. Endocrine responses to chronic androstenedione intake in 30- to 56-year-old men. *J Clin Endocrinol Metab*. 2000;85:4074-80.

186. DeMeersman R, Getty D, Schaefer DC. Sympathomimetics and exercise enhancement: all in the mind? *Pharmacol Biochem Behav*. 1987;28:361-5.

187. Ros JJ, Pelders MG, De Smet PA. A case of positive doping associated with a botanical food supplement. *Pharm World Sci*. 1999;21:44-6.

188. Gruber AJ, Pope HG Jr. Ephedrine abuse among 36 female weightlifters. *Am J Addict.* 1998;7:256-61.
189. Sidney KH, Lefcoe NM. The effects of ephedrine on the physiological and psychological responses to submaximal and maximal exercise in man. *Med Sci Sports.* 1977;9:95-9.
190. Smith DA, Perry PJ. The efficacy of ergogenic agents in athletic competition. Part II: other performance-enhancing agents. *Ann Pharmacother.* 1992;26:653-9.
191. Bell DG, Jacobs I, Zamecnik J. Effects of caffeine, ephedrine and their combination on time to exhaustion during high-intensity exercise. *Eur J Appl Physiol Occup Physiol.* 1998;77:427-33.
192. Bell DG, Jacobs I. Combined caffeine and ephedrine ingestion improves run times of Canadian Forces Warrior Test. *Aviat Space Environ Med.* 1999;70:325-9.
193. Bell DG, Jacobs I, McLellan TM, et al. Reducing the dose of combined caffeine and ephedrine preserves the ergogenic effect. *Aviat Space Environ Med.* 2000;71:415-9.
194. Wagenmakers AJ. Amino acid supplements to improve athletic performance. *Curr Opin Clin Nutr Metab Care.* 1999;2:539-44.
195. Williams MH. Facts and fallacies of purported ergogenic amino acid supplements. *Clin Sports Med.* 1999;18:633-49.
196. Walsh NP, Blannin AK, Robson PJ, et al. Glutamine, exercise and immune function: links and possible mechanisms. *Sports Med.* 1998;26:177-91.
197. Antonio J, Street C. Glutamine: a potentially useful supplement for athletes. *Can J Appl Physiol.* 1999;24:1-14.
198. Rohde T, Krzywkowski K, Pedersen BK. Glutamine, exercise, and the immune system: is there a link? *Exerc Immunol Rev.* 1998;4:49-63.
199. Nieman DC. Nutrition, exercise, and immune system function. *Clin Sports Med.* 1999;18:537-48.
200. Rowbottom DG, Keast D, Morton AR. The emerging role of glutamine as an indicator of exercise stress and overtraining. *Sports Med.* 1996;21:80-97.
201. Bassit RA, Sawada LA, Bacurau RF, et al. The effect of BCAA supplementation upon the immune response of triathletes. *Med Sci Sports Exerc.* 2000;32:1214-9.
202. Rennie MJ, Tadros L, Khogali S, et al. Glutamine transport and its metabolic effects. *J Nutr.* 1994;124:1503-8S.
203. Rennie MJ, MacLennan PA, Hundal HS, et al. Skeletal muscle glutamine transport, intramuscular glutamine concentration, and muscle-protein turnover. *Metabolism.* 1989;38:47-51.
204. Zachwieja JJ, Witt TL, Yarasheski KE. Intravenous glutamine does not stimulate mixed muscle protein synthesis in healthy young men and women. *Metabolism.* 2000;49:1555-60.
205. Mittendorfer B, Volpi E, Wolfe RR. Whole body and skeletal muscle glutamine metabolism in healthy subjects. *Am J Physiol Endocrinol Metab.* 2001;280:E323-33.
206. Sawka MN, Latzka WA, Matott RP, et al. Hydration effects on temperature regulation. *Int J Sports Med.* 1998;19:S108-10.
207. Senay LC. Temperature regulation and hypohydration: a singular view. *J Appl Physiol.* 1979;47:1-7.
208. Hargreaves M, Febbraio M. Limits to exercise performance in the heat. *Int J Sports Med.* 1998;19:S115-6.
209. Naghii MR. The significance of water in sport and weight control. *Nutr Health.* 2000;14:127-32.
210. Latzka WA, Montain SJ. Water and electrolyte requirements for exercise. *Clin Sports Med.* 1999;18:513-24.
211. Lyons TJ, Gillingham KK, Teas DC, et al. Effects of glycerol-induced hyperhydration prior to exercise in the heat on sweating and core temperature. *Med Sci Sports Exerc.* 1990;22:477-83.
212. Montner P, Stark DM, Riedesel ML, et al. Pre-exercise glycerol hydration improves cycling endurance time. *Int J Sports Med.* 1996;17:27-33.
213. Latzka WA, Sawka MN. Hyperhydration and glycerol: thermoregulatory effects during exercise in hot climates. *Can J Appl Physiol,* 2000;25:536-45.
214. Koenigsberg PS, Martin KK, Hlava HR, et al. Sustained hyperhydration with glycerol ingestion. *Life Sci.* 1995;57:645-53.
215. Riedesel ML, Allen DY, Peake GT, et al. Hyperhydration with glycerol solutions. *J Appl Physiol.* 1987;63:2262-8.
216. Wagner DR. Hyperhydrating with glycerol: implications for athletic performance. *J Am Diet Assoc.* 1999;99:207-12.
217. Sawka MN, Montain SJ, Latzka WA. Hydration effects on thermoregulation and performance in the heat. *Comp Biochem Physiol A Mol Integr Physiol.* 2001;128(4):679-90
218. Kreider RB. Dietary supplements and the promotion of muscle growth with resistance exercise. *Sports Med.* 1999;27:97-110.
219. Mero A. Leucine supplementation and intensive training. *Sports Med.* 1999;27:347-58.
220. Nissen S, Sharp R, Ray M, et al. Effect of leucine metabolite β-hydroxy-β-methylbutyrate on muscle metabolism during resistance training. *J Appl Physiol.* 1996;81:2095-104.

221. Panton LB, Rathmacher JA, Baier S, et al. Nutritional supplementation of the leucine metabolite beta-hydroxy-beta-methylbutyrate (hmb) during resistance training. *Nutrition.* 2000;16:734-9.
222. Kreider RB, Ferreira M, Wilson M, et al. Effects of calcium beta-hydroxy-beta-methylbutyrate (HMB) supplementation during resistance-training on markers of catabolism, body composition and strength. *Int J Sports Med.* 1999;20:503-9.
223. Williams MH. Ergogenic and ergolytic substances. *Med Sci Sports Exerc.* 1992;24:S344-8.
224. Williams MH, Kreider RB, Hunter DW, et al. Effect of inosine supplementation on 3-mile treadmill run performance and VO2 peak. *Med Sci Sports Exerc.* 1990;22:517-22.
225. Starling RD, Trappe TA, Short KR, et al. Effect of inosine supplementation on aerobic and anaerobic cycling performance. *Med Sci Sports Exerc.* 1996;28:1193-8.
226. McNaughton L, Dalton B, Tarr J. Inosine supplementation has no effect on aerobic or anaerobic cycling performance. *Int J Sport Nutr.* 1999;9:333-44.
227. Jeukendrup AE, Saris WH, Schrauwen P, et al. Metabolic availability of medium-chain triglycerides coingested with carbohydrates during prolonged exercise. *J Appl Physiol.* 1995;79:756-62.
228. Van Zyl CG, Lambert EV, Hawley JA, et al. Effects of medium-chain triglyceride ingestion on fuel metabolism and cycling performance. *J Appl Physiol.* 1996;80:2217-25.
229. Jeukendrup AE, Saris WH, Van Diesen R, et al. Effect of endogenous carbohydrate availability on oral medium-chain triglyceride oxidation during prolonged exercise. *J Appl Physiol.* 1996;80:949-54.
230. Massicotte D, Peronnet F, Brisson GR, et al. Oxidation of exogenous medium-chain free fatty acids during prolonged exercise: comparison with glucose. *J Appl Physiol.* 1992;73:1334-9.
231. Angus DJ, Hargreaves M, Dancey J, et al. Effect of carbohydrate or carbohydrate plus medium-chain triglyceride ingestion on cycling time trial performance. *J Appl Physiol.* 2000;88:113-9.
232. Horowitz JF, Mora-Rodriguez R, Byerley LO, et al. Preexercise medium-chain triglyceride ingestion does not alter muscle glycogen use during exercise. *J Appl Physiol.* 2000;88:219-25.
233. Goedecke JH, Elmer-English R, Dennis SC, et al. Effects of medium-chain triaclyglycerol ingested with carbohydrate on metabolism and exercise performance. *Int J Sport Nutr.* 1999;9:35-47.
234. Jeukendrup AE, Thielen JJ, Wagenmakers AJ, et al. Effect of medium-chain triacylglycerol and carbohydrate ingestion during exercise on substrate utilization and subsequent cycling performance. *Am J Clin Nutr.* 1998;67:397-404.
235. Hawley JA, Brouns F, Jeukendrup A. Strategies to enhance fat utilization during exercise. *Sports Med.* 1998;25:241-57.
236. Fawcett JP, Farquhar SJ, Walker RJ, et al. The effect of oral vandyl sulfate on body composition and performance in weight-training athletes. *Int J Sport Nutr.* 1996;6:382-90.
237. Nielsen FH. Other trace elements. In: Ziegler EE, Filer LJ Jr, eds. *Present Knowledge in Nutrition.* 7th ed. Washington, DC: International Life Sciences Institute; 1996.
238. Kreider RB. Dietary supplements and the promotion of muscle growth with resistance exercise. *Sports Med.* 1999;27:97-110.

CHAPTER 5

HERBAL MEDICINES AS NUTRITIONAL SUPPLEMENTS

Kenneth Euler and Louis Williams

Herbal remedies have been used for centuries to treat and prevent disease, but these "old fashioned" dietary supplements are more popular than ever before. Each year, more than 60 million Americans (roughly 1/3 of the adult population) use herbal preparations to supplement or substitute for traditional over-the-counter (OTC) drugs. Sales of herbal medicines and botanicals are skyrocketing, and are projected to increase exponentially in the next few years. According to the Consumer Healthcare Products Association, retail sales of dietary supplements reached $11.3 billion in 2000, compared to $3.9 billion in 1998.

As more patients turn to alternative and complementary medicines to help cure or prevent disease,[1,2] trying an herbal supplement becomes an increasingly appealing option. Why are so many seeking less conventional treatments? Perhaps some people have lost faith in mainstream medicine, especially if it has failed them in the past. An herbal product may offer new hope of a cure. Others may think any "natural" treatment is inherently safer or better than one produced by a pharmaceutical company or high-tech manufacturing facility.

And unlike pharmaceutical companies, herbal manufacturers don't have to provide evidence to support their claims, supply information about their products' contents or side effects, or prove that their products are safe or effective.[3] As a result, herbal preparations are widely advertised, via television, magazines, newspapers, and especially on the Internet. As more people become interested in herbal treatments, they are demanding answers to their questions about safety and efficacy, and expert sources are lacking.

Pharmacists, with their educational background and accessibility to the public, are in an excellent position to provide guidance about the uses and effects of herbal preparations. As clinicians start to think of herbs as viable therapeutic options, the distinction between herbs and OTC drugs is becoming blurred. More herbal supplements next to OTC drugs on pharmacy shelves means more people will turn to pharmacists for advice.

The pharmacist needs to know what information is available on herbal preparations, who prepares it, and how is it disseminated. This chapter categorizes some common nutritional herbs by their uses and reports on their effectiveness. A brief history of the regulation of herbal supplements in the United States is also included.

EVOLUTION OF FOOD AND DRUG REGULATIONS IN THE UNITED STATES

Legislation Leading to Regulation of Herbal Supplements

The Food and Drug Administration (FDA) is the federal agency that oversees marketing and sale of foods, drugs, and dietary supplements. The FDA, part of the Department of Health and Human Services (HHS), enforces pure food and drug laws and ensures that foods are safe to consume and drugs are safe, reliable, and effective.[4]

The United States Pharmacopoeia, created in 1820, was the first agency to clearly define, monograph, and describe drugs, and this regulatory process remained in effect throughout most of the 19th century.[5] Herbals were treated as legitimate medicines; for example, it was perfectly legal to label ginseng a stimulant and a useful drug for stomach complaints.

The food and drug laws of today evolved in response to historical events and the needs of American consumers. Milestone laws have influenced how the FDA classifies and regulates herbal supplements.

Early in the 20th century, investigators discovered grossly unsanitary conditions in the meatpacking industry. Their exposure prompted the passage of the Pure Food and Drug Act in 1906. Designed to protect the public from adulterated foods, the law specified the conditions under which foods or drugs could be considered mislabeled or adulterated and provided for enforcement action in cases of noncompliance.[2,6,7] The Pure Food and Drug Act did not address food and drug safety and efficacy issues.

In 1937, over 100 people died from acute kidney failure after consuming a tainted elixir of sulfanilamide. (The elixir contained 8.8% drug in a 72% solution of diethylene glycol, a liquid used as an antifreeze that is poisonous when ingested.) The tragedy brought renewed focus to the issue of drug

---

Milestone Laws in FDA History

1906 — The **Pure Food and Drug Act** prohibits interstate commerce on misbranded and adulterated foods. This law prevents quacks from making medical claims about worthless and even dangerous cure-all preparations and foreshadows more stringent regulations.

1938 — The **Food, Drug, and Cosmetic Act** requires that drugs are shown to be safe before marketing, authorizes factory inspections, and legislates harsher penalties for drug misbranding.

1951 — The **Durham-Humphrey Amendment** defines prescription drugs and says they can only be sold with authorization from a licensed practitioner. Over-the-counter drugs could be purchased and used without direct medical supervision.

1958 — The FDA publishes the first list of drugs **Generally Recognized as Safe**, consisting of over 200 substances.

1962 — The **Kefauver-Harris Amendments** say that drugs marketed in the U.S. after 1962 must be proven safe and effective. The law was retroactive for drugs marketed between 1938 and 1962; drugs marketed prior to 1938, including herbals, were grandfathered.

1994 — The **Dietary Supplement Health and Education Act** defines dietary supplements and classifies them as foods. It also authorizes the FDA to supervise manufacturing practices for supplements and establishes specific labeling requirements.

---

safety and resulted in the passage of the Federal Food, Drug, and Cosmetic Act in 1938. This Act is the basis for today's food and drug laws.[4,8] It provided standards of quality for foods and required proof of drug safety before marketing. It also regulated medical devices, cosmetics, and facility inspections by the FDA. All drugs already on the market, including herbal preparations, were grandfathered and did not have to go through a new approval process.

The Durham-Humphrey Amendment of 1951 defined the differences between prescription and OTC drugs. Prescription drugs are those used under the supervision of licensed practitioners, and can be sold only with their authorization. OTC drugs can be purchased and used without medical supervision.

Ten years later, another tragic event resulted in even more stringent regulation. The sedative thalidomide, marketed by a German chemical firm, was shown to be a potent teratogen resulting in deformities to 35% of babies whose mothers took the drug during a critical phase of their pregnancies.[9-11] (The drug was never approved for use in the U.S.) The Kefauver-Harris Amendments, enacted in 1962, said drugs could not be marketed in the U.S. unless they had been proven safe and effective. This law was retroactive and applied to drugs introduced to the market between 1938 and 1962.

Herbal medicines were grandfathered as drugs, solely because their documented use in most cases dated before 1938. The FDA put them in regulatory limbo to be sold as foods.

To implement the new regulations, 17 OTC drug evaluation panels were formed. Each panel was responsible for one therapeutic class of drugs. Since about 300 chemical constituents existed in over 7000 drug formulations (some old and some just approved), their task was unwieldy.

Most herbal products, not subject to the new laws, were considered immune from proof of effectiveness requirements. To provide some regulation, the FDA said a drug's claims of efficacy had to be in accordance with the findings of the evaluation panels. An herbal product could only be sold if no claims were made on the label or accompanying literature concerning the product's value in preventing or treating disease.

Further regulation resulted from a study on OTC drugs released in 1990. In the study the FDA established three categories of drugs: Category I was for drugs considered safe and effective, Category II was for drugs considered unsafe and ineffective, and Category III included drugs for which insufficient evidence existed to establish safety and efficacy.[12] Herb-containing OTC drug products were evaluated to be placed in a category. For example, cascara bark containing laxatives was placed in Category I, while peppermint oil containing digestive aid drug products was placed in Category III.

In addition, the FDA added herbs to their list of substances "Generally Recognized as Safe." About 250 herbs made the list based on their use as food additives (flavoring aids and spices).[13] But this classification did not distinguish between culinary herbs and those used medicinally—for example, as digestive aids or to prevent motion sickness.

Dietary Supplement Health and Education Act

As the decade of the '90s proceeded, the popularity of herbal supplements grew. People became convinced that such supplements could play a part in leading a healthy life and demanded up-to-date, accurate information. The Dietary Supplement Health and Education Act (DSHEA) sought to meet the public's demands by further defining supplements as foods, establishing specific labeling requirements, and providing a framework for regulation.

DSHEA came about because the FDA wanted to regulate herbs as drugs, requiring the herbal manufacturing industry to provide proof of their products' safety and efficacy. Industry and consumer groups argued that these products should be considered foods or nutritional supplements which support good health, and should be exempt from FDA regulation as long as they adhered to structure/function labeling requirements. DSHEA was enacted as a result, passed by the 103rd Congress on October 7, 1994, and signed into law by President Clinton on October 25, 1994.[14-16]

DSHEA defines dietary supplements as "dietary substances for use by man to supplement the diet by increasing total dietary intake." The composition of dietary supplements may include herbs or other botanicals, vitamins, minerals, and amino acids in any concentrate, metabolite, constituent, extract, or combination of ingredients.

The Dietary Supplement Health and Education Act

The Dietary Supplement Health and Education Act defines dietary supplements as foods and requires that they carry nutrition labeling. Other provisions of the bill include:

❑ Establishes a new framework for assuring safety (burden of proof on the FDA).

❑ Outlines guidelines for literature displayed where nutritional supplements are sold.

❑ Provides for use of claims and nutritional support statements.

❑ Requires that ingredients be listed on labels.

❑ Grants FDA authority to establish good manufacturing practice regulations.

❑ Requires formation of a Commission on Dietary Supplement Labels and an Office of Dietary Supplements within the National Institutes of Health.

Under the law, if a product first marketed as a dietary supplement is later approved as a new drug, it may still be marketed as a supplement unless the Secretary of HHS rules that it is unsafe. On the other hand, if an ingredient is first approved as a new drug (e.g., taxol), it may not be marketed as a dietary supplement.

Dietary supplements may be manufactured in various pharmaceutical dosage forms, such as tablets, capsules, liquids, powders, softgels or gelcaps. They may even be in the form of a conventional food, provided it is "not represented for use as a conventional food" or as the sole item of a meal or diet.

DSHEA also mandated that a Presidential Commission be appointed to decide what information should be provided on dietary supplements, how best to present it, and what requirements apply to supplement labels. The seven-member Commission is formed of unbiased people who have knowledge of supplements through their involvement in manufacturing, their scientific backgrounds, or their careers in traditional herbal medicine, pharmacognosy, medical botany, or other related sciences.

The Secretary of HHS and ultimately the FDA were charged with publishing proposed changes in regulations (based on the Commission's recommendations) within 24 months. After that time, unpublished recommendations would automatically become law. Until those changes were proposed, no health claims were allowed for supplements unless an authorized regulation was issued for such claims.[14]

In April 1998, the FDA issued regulations pertaining to dietary supplement labeling. Nutritional support statements, content claims for nutrients, and notification of new ingredients for dietary supplements were part of the regulations. Specific rules were issued for the appearance and content of product labels, as well as definitions for the terms "antioxidant" and "high potency."[17] A revised labeling requirement went into effect in 1999.[18-20]

The Office of Dietary Supplements

DSHEA authorized $5 million to establish the Office of Dietary Supplements (ODS) at NIH. Its mission is to strengthen knowledge and understanding of dietary supplements by evaluating scientific information, to stimulate and support research, to disseminate research results, and to educate the public, fostering an enhanced quality of life and health for the U.S. population.[21] The ODS acts as a principal advisor on supplements to the Secretary of HHS, NIH, Centers for Disease Control and Prevention, and the FDA.

The legislative sponsors of DSHEA felt that the ODS would focus research on dietary supplements. Concerned that the FDA would have an institutional bias against supplements in general yet retain the authority to regulate them, they hoped the new office would allow progress in the areas of scientific research, government policy, and health promotion.[14]

ODS evaluates scientific information and makes it available to the public. In addition, the organization compiles and publishes two Annual Bibliographies of Significant Advances in Dietary Supplement Research in conjunction with the Consumer Healthcare Products Association (CHPA). CPHA is a 119-year old trade organization representing the manufacturers and distributors of national and store brand dietary supplements and nonprescription medicines. Its membership includes over 200 companies involved in the manufacture and distribution of these self-care products and their affiliated services (e.g., raw material suppliers, research testing companies, contract manufacturing companies, advertising agencies, etc.).[22]

The first Annual Bibliography compiled by ODS and CHPA was published in 1999. Editors nominated "flagship" original research papers that appeared in their respective peer-reviewed journals. Over 200 nominations were submitted and the top 25 scientific papers were identified for the collection.[22] A subsequent compilation included journals that published papers on botanicals. This nomination process netted over 450 submissions. Another panel determined the top 25 articles, which were then annotated, compiled, and published in October 2000.

"Consumers are the real beneficiaries of the good, credible science available on dietary supplements. This publication is both a tremendous asset to the industry and a valuable source of information for health care professionals and practitioners, government officials, and anyone else interested in learning more about the benefits of dietary supplement products," commented Michael D. Maves, MD, MBA, CHPA President.[22]

National Center for Complementary and Alternative Medicine

Congress first established the National Center for Complementary and Alternative Medicine (NCCAM) in 1998. Based at NIH, its mission is to stimulate, develop, and support research on complementary and alternative medicine for the benefit of the public health. Those goals were defined more specifically by the White House Commission on Complementary and Alternative Medicine (CAM). This 20-member Commission, formed by Executive

---

Studies on Dietary Supplements and Disease Prevention

ODS has funded many grants to explore the role of dietary supplements in health promotion and disease prevention.[23] Below is a listing of five current projects that brought the total to 20 by the end of 2001. These projects are a good illustration of the range of research in this area.

1. **St. John's wort and Drug Interactions.** The research focuses on the effect of St. John's wort on the metabolism of several widely used medications.
2. **B-vitamins and the Brain.** This project examines the relationship between B-vitamins and cognitive function.
3. **Isolating and Identifying Plant Chemicals.** This study seeks to develop methods for isolating, identifying, and quantifying certain compounds, known as phenolic phytochemicals. These compounds are found in soybean, kale, citrus fruits, and other plants, as well as in clinical laboratory samples of tissue, plasma, and urine. This basic research could lead to the development of innovative methods for analyzing metabolic processes and bioavailability of bioactive food and plant components.
4. **Chromium for Diabetes.** This research's focus is on the role of chromium in improving insulin sensitivity in patients with type-2 diabetes.
5. **Zinc in HIV Disease.** Findings from this study will document the need for supplemental zinc as an inexpensive adjuvant therapy in the treatment of immune-related diseases that occur in drug users.

Source: Reference 24.

Order in March of 2000, addresses the continuing public interest in and use of unconventional health care—including herbal medicine of worldwide origin.

The Commission is focusing on several areas, such as research on CAM practices and products, delivery of and public access to CAM services, and dissemination of reliable information on CAM to health care providers and the general public. Appropriate licensing, education, and training of CAM health care practitioners are also concerns.

The Commission has not released its complete findings, due sometime in 2002.[24] But its interim report to the Secretary of HHS made several preliminary recommendations regarding DSHEA. The CAM felt that immediate action was needed in some areas. Priority items included creating more effective systems for manufacturing practices and reporting adverse events, developing more stringent FDA enforcement of structure/function claims, and exploring programs that ensure quality composition of dietary supplements. Changes in these areas would in effect fully implement DSHEA.

HERBAL SUPPLEMENTS AND THE PHARMACIST

Pharmacists need to understand the interrelations and overlapping missions of NCCAM, ODS, DSHEA, and other relevant agencies. They also need current, updated information on new regulations and procedures governing herbals and nutritional supplements. In addition to the federal laws, some states have begun to regulate the sale of herbal products on their own. For instance, Texas regulates ephedrine or "Herbal Ecstacy"[25]; ephedrine (containing products with less than 400 mg guaifenesin) is now available by prescription only.

It is also important for pharmacists to understand the roles of herbals and nutritional supplements and integrative medicine in their practice. They must be aware of standardization and their own legal and commercial jeopardy.

Pharmacists should be familiar with the common dosage forms for herbs. The crude drugs themselves, consisting of dried and powdered plant material, may be formulated into tablets and capsules. These are assayed and standardized, based on one or more of the plant constituents. Additionally, the dried plant material is packaged for use as a tea (infusion or tisane).

Tablets and capsules can also be prepared from fresh or dried extracts of the herbal plant material. After soaking or steeping in a solvent such as boiling water or a hydroalcoholic solution, the material is macerated or percolated. The resulting liquid, dried and standardized, is processed into tablets and capsules. Liquid extractive may also be concentrated and used to prepare a liquid dosage form, such as a tincture or fluid extract. Alternatively, the fresh plant material is expressed to yield its juice, which is then processed into a liquid or solid dosage form.

The first U.S. publication containing information on commonly used drugs, including medicinal plants, was the *United States Pharmacopeia,* published in 1820.[5] In 1888, another compilation, the *National Formulary,* was published.[27] Since then, drugs listed in either publication or their updated revisions are termed "official," and have the letters USP or NF following their names. The current official publication contains the two compendia *The Pharmacopeia of the United States, 25th Revision* and *The National Formulary, 20th Edition*. The compendia include medicinally important plants, qualitative and quantitative requirements for their active constituents, and assay procedures to determine them.[28]

HERBS AS DIETARY SUPPLEMENTS

The DSHEA legislation classifies herbs as nutritional or dietary supplements. Medicinally used herbs, however, exert some pharmacological effect on the body and therefore, from a medical standpoint, should be considered drugs.

One class of herbs can have an effect on nutrition. Herbal digestive aids play a role in maintaining normal functions of the gastrointestinal tract, and therefore aid in the proper absorption of nutrients. They can act to stimulate the flow of digestive juices, to treat flatulence as carminatives, to treat or prevent nausea and vomiting, to treat indigestion (dyspepsia) and nervous stomach, and to provide additional digestive enzymes.

Little research is being done regarding the use of herbs to treat gastrointestinal problems. Much of the information available is anecdotal, with few scientific studies to validate or disprove the efficacy and safety of herbal use. Several years ago the Federal Republic of Germany established a commission to collect and examine data on herbal remedies. The German Commission E evaluated herbal remedies using information from sources including clinical trials, field studies, reports of single cases, scientific literature, and experts from medical associations. The resultant monographs, translated into English and published by the American Botanical Council as *The Complete German Commission E Monographs*, represents one of the most accurate assessments of the uses of herbs.[26]

Herbs That Can Affect the Gastrointestinal Tract

Three herbs are commonly used for gastrointestinal problems: ginger for nausea and vomiting, and peppermint and chamomile for indigestion (dyspepsia).

Ginger

Ginger NF is the rhizome of *Zingiber officinale* Roscoe (family Zingiberaceae), scraped or unscraped. Known in commerce as unbleached ginger,[28] it contains an oleo-resin (volatile oil and resin). In order to be official[28] it must satisfy a number of standards including the following constituent requirements: the alcohol-soluble extractive contains not more than 0.18% of shogaols and not less than 0.8% of gingerols and gingerdiones; and its volatile oil (not less than 1.8 mL per 100 g rhizome) contains the sesquiterpene hydrocarbons zingiberene, bisabolene, and zingiberol.

Ginger is recommended for treatment of nausea. In *The Complete German Commission E Monographs*, it is used for indigestion (dyspepsia) and for the prevention of motion sickness.[26] Ernst and Pittler evaluated the data from six randomized controlled clinical trials that tested the efficacy of ginger for nausea and vomiting.[29] Five of the six studies suggested that ginger was effective in preventing motion sickness, including seasickness, and in reducing post-operative nausea and vomiting in women following gynecological surgery.

A database examination of treatments for nausea and vomiting indicated that 2 of 20 trials used ginger root.[30] The trials concluded that ginger may be of value, but the evidence is weak. Another study revealed that ginger is effective for relieving the severity of nausea and vomiting in pregnancy.[31] Because the ginger preparations tested were not standardized and methods used to evaluate data were different, the results varied.

Commercially, ginger is available in capsules, each containing 500–530 mg of the dried, powdered rhizome. The recommended dosage for treating nausea and vomiting is 2–4 g daily.[26]

Peppermint

Peppermint NF consists of the dried leaf and flowering top of *Mentha × piperita* L (family Lamiaceae alt Labiatae) containing approximately 1% of volatile oil.[28] The oil, to be official, must contain 50% total menthol, free and as esters, and yield not less than 5% of esters, calculated as menthyl acetate.[28]

The most common use of peppermint leaf, according to *The Complete German Commission E Monographs*, is to treat spastic complaints of the gastrointestinal tract as well as of the gallbladder and bile ducts. Peppermint oil is also suggested to treat catarrhs of the respiratory tract and inflammation of the oral mucosa.[26]

Recent studies have used peppermint oil rather than the leaf. A group of patients undergoing gynecologic surgery were given the oil for postoperative nausea and required less of the traditional antiemetics.[32] When patients suffering from irritable bowel syndrome took an enteric coated peppermint oil formulation, they experienced significant decreases in abdominal pain and related symptoms.[33] An analysis of eight controlled studies of peppermint oil used to treat irritable bowel syndrome indicated that the oil may have beneficial effects, but additional studies were needed.[34]

Fixed combinations of enteric coated peppermint oil (90 mg, 36 mg) and caraway oil (50 mg, 20 mg), given to treat indigestion (dyspepsia) reduced pain enough to be statistically significant.[35] In another study, the combination gave comparable results with cisapride in treating indigestion.[36] Recommended daily dosage is 3–6 g of the leaf and 0.6 mL (750 mg) of the oil.[26]

Chamomile

Chamomile (German chamomile) consists of the dried flower heads of *Matricaria recutita* L (*Matricaria chamomilla* L, *Matricaria chamomilla* L var *courrantiana*, *Chamomilla recutita* L) Rauschert (family Asteraceae alt Compositae). It contains not less than 0.4% of blue volatile oil and not less than 0.3% of apigenin-7-glucoside.[28]

There are several other plant species with the common name chamomile; however, German chamomile is the species most commonly used in the United States. A related plant, Roman chamomile [*Chamaemelum nobile* (L) All (family Asteraceae alt Compositae)], contains different constituents.

The blue volatile oil of chamomile contains terpenoid derivatives such as chamazulene, (–)-α-bisabolol and (–)-α-bisaboloxides A and B. These lipophilic components have limited water solubility and are extracted only to the extent of 10%–15% from the herb into a tea.[37] Flavonoid constituents, such as apigenin-7-glucoside, are more water soluble and more readily extracted.[2]

The Complete German Commission E Monographs indicates that chamomile treats gastrointestinal spasms and inflammatory diseases of the gastrointestinal tract.[26] It is most commonly given in a tea, and water soluble flavonoids may be more responsible for any anti-inflammatory action than terpene derivatives. However, studies have verified the spasmolytic effect of both the lipophilic and hydrophilic components of the herb.[38] The herb has an anti-inflammatory effect on the gastrointestinal tract and may also calm and relax the patient, reducing the tension and anxiety that initially triggered problems. The indicated dosage is about 3 g (prepared as a tea and allowed to steep) three or four times a day.[2]

Other Herbal Digestive Aids

In addition to chamomile and ginger, a number of other herbs have been used to treat indigestion and related digestive complaints. *The Complete German Commission E Monographs* lists over 40 herbs that have been accepted as effective. Included in this group as whole herbs or volatile oils are aniseed, caraway, cinnamon, coriander, dandelion, dill, fennel, and lemon balm.[26]

Some herbs may stimulate the flow of digestive juices to increase the appetite, possibly because they taste bitter. *The Complete German Commission E Monographs* lists 24 herbs as effective in treating loss of appetite.[26] Gentian is the best known of these, although the literature shows little scientific evidence to support its efficacy. Angelica, bitter orange peel, cinchona, cinnamon, coriander, and dandelion may also be effective.

Several plants contain enzymes that may be useful in aiding digestion for people who have decreased digestive enzyme production. Papain USP is a proteolytic enzyme mixture obtained from the milky latex of the unripe fruit of the papaya plant *Carica papaya* L (family Caricaceae),[28] with a requirement upon assay of not less than 6000 units per mg. Other enzymes in crude papain can hydrolyze carbohydrates and fats.

Bromelain is a proteolytic enzyme from the juice of the pineapple plant *Ananas comosus* (L) Merr (family Bromeliaceae).[37] Both enzymes are commercially available in digestive aid products singly and in combination, in quantities varying from 3 to 500 mg per unit dose. Because they degrade in combination with digestive juices, their oral effectiveness is questionable.

Herbal Dietary Supplements with Medicinal Uses

Many other herbs are used medicinally under the legal shelter of the category "nutritional or dietary supplement." Some of the more promising ones have been approved or are under evaluation by the United States Pharmacopeial Convention and are listed in Table 5-1[39] with their currently accepted medicinal actions and therapeutic uses.[2]

Since these herbs have no known nutritional value, they will not be discussed in detail.

Herbs that Act as Antioxidants

Herbs with antioxidant components and properties may be considered nutritional supplements. Chapter 1 in this book discusses the antioxidant trace mineral selenium and the antioxidant vitamins and their analogs, namely, vitamin A or retinol and the carotenoids, vitamin E or α-tocopherol and the other tocopherols, and vitamin C or ascorbic acid. People obtain

TABLE 5-1 Herbal Dietary Supplements Official in the USP25-NF20 or Under Consideration or Development

Common Name	Botanical Name	Medicinal Action, Therapeutic Use
Black Cohosh*	*Actaea racemosa* (L) Nutt or *Cimifuga racemosa* (L) Nutt Fam Ranunculaceae	Estrogenic activity PMS, dysmenorrhea, menopause
Cat's Claw*	*Uncaria tomentosa* (Wild) DC Fam Rubiaceae	Immunostimulant activity
Chastetree*	*Vitex agnus-castus* L Fam Verbenaceae	Dopaminergic activity PMS, dysmenorrhea, menopause
Cranberry†	*Vaccinium oxycoccos* L *V macrocarpon* Ait Fam Ericaceae	Microbial anti-adherence Urinary tract infections
Echinacea angustifolia*	*Echinacea angustifolia* DC Fam Asteraceae	Immunostimulant activity Systemic and topical infections
Echinacea pallida*	*Echinacea pallida* (Nutt) Nutt Fam Asteraceae	Immunostimulant activity Systemic and topical infections
Echinacea purpurea*	*Echinacea purpurea* (L) Moench Fam Asteraceae	Immunostimulant activity Systemic and topical infections
Feverfew†	*Tanacetum parthenium* (L) Schultz-Bip Fam Asteraceae	Migraine headaches
Garlic†	*Allium sativum* L Fam Liliaceae	Antihyperlipidemic activity Inhibits platelet aggregation
Ginkgo†	*Ginkgo biloba* L Fam Ginkgoaceae	Free radical scavengers Cerebral circulatory disorders
Ginseng, American*	*Panax quinquefolius* L Fam Araliaceae	Corticosteroid-like activity Fatigue, weakness, convalescence

Common name	Scientific name / Family	Activity / Indication
Ginseng, Asian†	*Panax ginseng* CA Mey Fam Araliaceae	Corticosteroid-like activity Fatigue, weakness, convalescence
Ginseng, Siberian*	*Eleutherococcus senticosus* (Rupr & Maxim) Maxim Fam Araliaceae	Corticosteroid-like activity Fatigue, weakness, convalescence
Hawthorn*	*Crataegus laevata* (Poir) DC *C monogyna* Jacq emend Lindman Fam Rosaceae	Cardioactive Congestive heart failure
Horse Chestnut*	*Aesculus hippocastanum* L Fam Hippocastanaceae	Reduces lysosomal activity Varicose veins, venous insufficiency
Kava*	*Piper methysticum* G Forst Fam Piperaceae	Anticonvulsant, muscle relaxant Analgesia, sleep inducer
Licorice†	*Glycyrrhiza uralensis* Fisch ex DC *G glabra* L Fam Fabaceae	Anti-ulcer, antitussive, expectorant
Milk Thistle†	*Silybum marianum* (L) Gaertner Fam Asteraceae	Liver protective effect Chronic liver diseases, cirrhosis
Nettles*	*Urtica dioica* L ssp *Dioica* *U urens* Fam Urticaceae	Aquaretic Urinary difficulties
Saw Palmetto†	*Serenoa repens* (Bartram) Small Fam Arecaceae	Anti-inflammatory, spasmolytic Anti-androgenic, benign prostatic hypertrophy
St John's Wort†	*Hypericum perforctum* L Fam Hyperaceae	Antidepressant activity Mental depression
Valerian†	*Valeriana officinalis* L Fam Valerianaceae	Anxiolytic, mild hypnotic Insomnia, sleep disturbances

* Monograph under consideration or development.
† Official in the USP25-NF20.

these vitamins from eating higher plant sources. Chapter 1 also lists the plant and other sources of these vitamins and discusses their antioxidant functions, especially how they react with free radicals and protect unsaturated lipids.

In addition to these vitamins, higher plants or herbs contain other constituents that give them antioxidant properties. These herbs contain polyphenolic compounds of the flavonoid type including flavans and biflavonoids. Specifically, compounds that have an o-dihydroxy-(catechol) moiety in their structures are very effective antioxidants.[40]

Some herbs of the Lamiaceae (mint family) have significant quantities of antioxidant components.[41] Flavonoids, tannins unique to the Lamiaceae and esterified forms of hydroxycinnamic acid such as rosmarinic acid and caffeic acid, are polyphenols commonly found in lemon balm (*Melissa officinalis* L), peppermint (*Mentha × piperita* L), sage (*Salvia officinalis* L), sweet marjoram (*Origanum majorana* L), oregano (*Origanum vulgare* L) and thyme (*Thymus vulgaris* L).[26,42] Laboratory screening of these plants, their extracts, and their main constituents show them to be effective antioxidants. However, there are few data from human studies to determine their clinical usefulness in disease prevention or treatment. A multi-mint antioxidant tea has been recommended to treat arthritis and to slow the effects of aging.[43]

Another herb commonly used for its antioxidant properties is green tea (*Camellia sinensis* [L] Kuntze [family Theaceae]). Often ingested as a tea or in extract form, the herb can also be used topically. It is prepared for commercial use by drying the fresh leaves over mild heat and sometimes steaming them. Both procedures inactivate oxidative enzymes, which could degrade the herb's antioxidant polyphenolic constituents.[2]

Green tea's main constituents are the flavan derivatives (–)-epicatechin, (–)-epicatechin gallate, (–)-epigallocatechin, and (–)-epigallocatechin gallate.[44] Fermentation of the fresh leaves results in black tea, and the catechins are oxidized and dimerized to form biflavonoids, theaflavin, theaflavin-3-gallate, theaflavin-3′-gallate, theaflavin-3,3′-digallate, and their analogs.[44] Some studies have shown green tea constituents to be more effective antioxidants than those in black tea,[2,45] while other studies have shown no difference between the two.[44,46]

Studies have found (–)-epigallocatechin gallate to be the most effective antioxidant in green tea[47-50] and theaflavin-3,3′-digallate the most active component in black tea.[44] When (–)-epigallocatechin gallate reacts with peroxyl radicals, the resultant products include a seven-membered B-ring anhydride and a novel dimer.[51] In addition to the catechin constituents, flavonol glycosides of kaempferol, myricetin, and quercetin have been found in both green and black tea leaves.[52]

The vitamin-like antioxidant properties of tea have been investigated in a number of biological systems, both in vivo and in vitro, in studies of animals and people. The constituents may have an inhibitory effect on free radical-induced oxidative damage to biological substances and tissues[49] as well as a sparing effect on vitamin E.[53] Antioxidant activity has been demonstrated in copper+2-mediated oxidation of low-density lipoproteins (LDL) and other lipoproteins, which may lower the risk of coronary heart

Green Tea and Health

Tea drinking dates back thousands of years. Legend has it that Emperor Shen Nung of the Tang Dynasty (c. 2737 B.C.) watched *Camellia sinensis* leaves drift from the plant into a pot of boiling water, noticed an enticing aroma, and sampled the first brew. Japanese priests studying in China brought news of tea's medicinal benefits to their country, and a book espousing tea drinking as a way to maintain health was published in Japan in the early 1200s.

Modern-day Japan has the highest number of smokers in any developed country, yet one of the lowest rates of lung cancer. Is green tea responsible? Yes, say some health experts. Drinking green tea is linked to lower rates of many kinds of cancers, as well as heart disease. It's also said to lower blood pressure and control diabetes, and new research is studying green tea's possible effects in treating the AIDS virus. One Japanese study says swirling tea in your mouth can even prevent cavities.

Green tea is linked to urinary tract health, perhaps because one must drink 10 to 20 cups a day to reap maximum benefits. Since tea contains a significant amount of caffeine, many people choose a green tea extract in capsule form.

Source: Balch, JF. *The Super Antioxidants—Why They Will Change the Face of Healthcare in the 21st Century.* New York: M. Evans and Company Inc.; 1998;173-77.

diseases and atherosclerosis,[44,46,54] preserve erythrocyte membrane polyunsaturated fatty acids,[53] and modulate biochemical pathways involved in inflammatory responses.[48] Anticancer effects include decreased oxidative damage to DNA,[55] modulation of cell proliferation,[48] prevention of skin cancer (especially photocarcinogenesis when used either orally or topically),[56] and protection against chronic gastritis and (possibly resultant) stomach cancer.[57]

Another herbal product used for its antioxidant properties is grape seed extract (*Vitis vinifera* L [family Vitaceae]). The extract contains biflavonoid proanthocyanidins, which have not been further defined chemically, and their oligomeric procyanidins or tannins.[58-60] Along with other polyphenolic compounds, the proanthocyanidins have demonstrated significant free radical scavenging abilities in both in vivo and in vitro models.

Mice pretreated with this extract were almost completely protected against drug-induced hepatotoxicity, pulmonary toxicity, cardiotoxicity, nephrotoxicity, and spleenotoxicity, but only partially protected against neurotoxicity (brain).[58] The extract reduced the frequency and intensity of abdominal pain from chronic pancreatitis caused by free radical mediated tissue damage.[61] It protected against free radical-induced lipid peroxidation (including LDL) and reduced coronary artery disease and atherosclerosis.[62] The extract also protected DNA from damage and demonstrated cytotoxicity to various adenocarcinoma cells, while enhancing the viability of normal human gastric mucosal cells.[59]

Pycnogenol, an extract from French maritime pine bark (*Pinus pinaster* Ait [family Pinaceae]), is a complex mixture of polyphenolic components very similar to those in grape seed extract. It consists of monomeric, dimeric, and trimeric flavonoids, procyanidins, catechin, and other phenolic components which appear to act synergistically on several biological systems.[63,64] Tests in human and other studies show pycnogenol is effective in decreasing systolic (but not diastolic) blood pressure;[63] improving retinal vascularization and visual acuity in retinopathy treatment;[65] reducing venous pressure, pain, and subcutaneous edema of the legs when treating chronic venous insufficiency;[66,67] and inhibiting lipogenesis and the accumulation of lipid droplets in adipose tissue.[68] Pycnogenol also shows promise in preventing or treating some vascular or neurodegenerative diseases (such as Alzheimer's) by protecting vascular endothelial cells from beta amyloid-induced injury.[69]

Ginger, as noted in the discussion on digestive aids, contains shogaols and gingerols, which are phenolic compounds with antioxidant activity. Mice fed a ginger extract showed reductions in plasma triglycerides and cholesterol, in the rate of cellular cholesterol biosynthesis, in the capacity to oxidize LDL, and ultimately in the development of atherosclerotic lesions.[70]

Several of the herbs listed in Table 5-1 have actions and uses attributable in part to their antioxidant components and activities. Patients with osteoarthritis were treated with cat's claw and had a significant reduction of pain. This herb is an effective antioxidant, although its anti-inflammatory properties may result from the inhibition of tumor necrosis factor-alpha (TNF-α) and prostaglandin E_2 (PGE$_2$) production.[71] Its action on the cellular immune system may be due to the presence of pentacyclic oxindole alkaloids.[72]

A number of berries, including cranberry, have a scavenging antioxidant activity against superoxide radicals, hydrogen peroxide, hydroxyl radicals, and singlet oxygen—which means the constituents react with the radicals and prevent their damaging actions. Polyphenolic components (such as the flavonol quercetin) and polymeric proanthocyanidins give the herb its antioxidant properties.[73] Cranberry also treats or prevents urinary tract infections, possibly because it contains sugar fructose as well as the proanthocyanidins.[2]

In one study, an elderberry extract contained four anthocyanin glucosides which were incorporated into the plasma membrane and cytosol of endothelial cells. The reinforced cells protected against oxidative chemical stresses such as hydrogen peroxide and ferrous sulfate/ascorbic acid.[74]

Smokers who were treated with red ginseng showed increases in plasma antioxidant concentrations. Concurrent decreases in the smokers' plasma levels of 8-hydroxyguanosine and carbonyl content indicated inhibition of DNA damage.[75]

An examination of a hawthorn fruit extract found that several antioxidant phenolic compounds were effective in inhibiting copper-2 mediated LDL oxidation and in preventing peroxy free radical-induced oxidation of α-tocopherol in LDL. These actions may be responsible for the cardiovascular protective and hypocholesterolemic effects of hawthorn. Compounds present in the extract of the fruits were hyperoside, isoquercitrin, epicatechin, chlorogenic acid, quercetin, rutin, and protocatechuic acid.[76]

Milk thistle contains silymarin, a mixture of several flavone derivatives of which the most important is silybin.[2] The silymarin complex has been an effective antioxidant in preventing liver damage caused by free radical-induced lipid peroxidation and the resultant liver fibrosis.[77] Another silymarin component, silibinin, has an inhibitory effect on LDL oxidation in vitro, and may be a useful tool in the prevention and therapy of atherosclerosis.[78] Silymarin complex also protects against several skin tumor promoters by impairing epidermal growth factor receptors, which results in significant inhibition of DNA synthesis and cell growth.[79]

CONCLUSION

Herbal supplements continue to show great potential in prevention and treatment of disease. Consumers are increasingly attracted to these preparations, but they also want accurate information about their use. Pharmacists can be a valuable resource, offering guidance about the effectiveness and safety of herbal therapies.

Studies of herbal antioxidants and digestive aids are documenting the efficacy of herbal treatments. More research is needed to evaluate the many and varied uses of herbal supplements.

REFERENCES

1. LaValle JB, Hawkins E. Herb-OTC drug interactions. *Retail Pharmacy News.* June 2000:19-22.
2. Tyler VE, Robbers JE. *Tyler's Herbs of Choice: The Therapeutic Use of Phytomedicinals.* New York: Haworth Herbal Press; 1999.
3. Fetrow CW, Avila JR. *The Complete Guide to Herbal Medicines.* Springhouse, PA: Springhouse Corporation; 2000.
4. About the Food and Drug Administration Organization. The Food and Drug Administration (FDA) Web site. Available at: http://www.fda.gov/. Accessed December 7, 2001.
5. The History of the United States Pharmacopeia. United States Pharmacopeia Revision XIII. April 1, 1947; xvii-xli. Washington DC: United States Pharmacopeial Convention; 1940.
6. Ziporyn T. The Food and Drug Administration: How "those regulations" came to be. *JAMA.* 1985;254:2037-46.
7. Harlow DR. The FDA's OTC drug review: the development and an analysis of some aspects of the procedure. *Food, Drug, Cosmetic Law Journal.* 1977;32:248-74.
8. Leech PN, ed. Elixir of Sulfanilamide-Massengill. *JAMA.* 1937;109:1531-9.
9. Krantz JC Jr. New drugs and the Kefauver-Harris Amendment. *Journal of New Drugs.* 1966;6(2):77-9.
10. Smithells RW, Newman CG. Recognition of thalidomide defects. *J Med Genet.* 1992;29:716-23.
11. Lary JM, Daniel KL, Erickson JD, et al. The return of thalidomide: can birth defects be prevented? *Drug Saf.* 1999;21:161-9.
12. Blumenthal M. FDA Declares 258 OTC ingredients ineffective. *HerbalGram.* 1990;23:32-3,49.
13. Winter R. *A Consumers Dictionary of Food Additives.* Rev ed. New York: Crown Publishers, Inc; 1984.
14. Blumenthal M. Congress passes Dietary Supplement Health and Education Act of 1994. *HerbalGram.* 1994;32:18-20.
15. Israelsen LD. Phytomedicines: the greening of modern medicine. *J Altern Complement Med.* 1995;1:245-8.
16. Blumenthal M, Steele E. DSHEA at five years: a review of structure function claims. *HerbalGram.* 1999;47:38-9.
17. Federal Register. April 29, 1998; 63(82):23623-32.
18. Israelsen LD, Blumenthal M. FDA issues final rules for structure/function claims for dietary supplements under DSHEA. *HerbalGram.* 2000;48:32-8.

19. Federal Register. January 6, 2000; 65(4):999-1050.
20. Food and Drug Administration (FDA) final ruling defining the types of statements that can be made concerning the effect of a dietary supplement on the structure or function of the body. The Food and Drug Administration (FDA) Web site. Available at: http://www.fda.gov/OHRMS/DOCKETS/98fr/oc99257.pdf. Accessed December 8, 2001.
21. Barrett S. Supplement bill passes. *Nutrition Forum.* 1995;12:9-10.
22. Consumer Healthcare Products Association/National Institues of Health (CHPA/NIH) bibliography touts significant advancements in science supporting use of dietary supplements. The Consumer Healthcare Products Association (CHPA) Web site. Available at: http://www.chpa-info.org/. Accessed December 8, 2001.
23. NIH Office of Dietary Supplements Announces Research Awards. The National Institutes of Health (NIH) Web site. Available at: http://ods.od.nih.gov/news/releases/reap_2001.html. Accessed December 7, 2001.
24. White House Commission on Complementary and Alternative Medicine Policy. The Health and Human Services (HHS) Web site. Available at: http://www.whccamp.hhs.gov/. Accessed December 2, 2001.
25. Political news online. Texas classifies ephedrine as a dangerous drug. Herb World News Online: Herb Research Foundation. Available at: http://www.herbs.org/current/ephtexas.html. Accessed December 7, 2001.
26. Blumenthal M, ed. *The Complete German Commission E Monographs: Therapeutic Guide to Herbal Medicines.* Boston: Integrative Medicine Communications; 1998.
27. *The National Formulary.* Washington, DC. American Pharmaceutical Association; 1988.
28. *The Pharmacopeia of the United States, 25th Revision, and The National Formulary, 20th Edition.* Rockville, MD: United States Pharmacopeial Convention, Inc; 2002.
29. Ernst E, Pittler MH. Efficacy of ginger for nausea and vomiting: a systematic review of randomized clinical trials. *Br J Anaesth.* 2000; 84(3):367-71.
30. Jewell D, Young G. Interventions for nausea and vomiting in early pregnancy. *Cochrane Database Syst Rev.* 2000;2:CD000145.
31. Vutyavanich T, Kraisarin T, Ruangsri R. Ginger for nausea and vomiting in pregnancy: randomized double-masked, placebo-controlled trial. *Obstet Gynecol.* 2001;97(4):577-82.
32. Tate S. Peppermint oil: a treatment for post-operative nausea. *J Adv Nurs.*1997;26(3):543-9.
33. Liu JH, Chen GH, Yeh HZ, et al. Enteric-coated peppermint-oil capsules in the treatment of irritable bowel syndrome: a prospective, randomized trial. *J Gastroenterol.*1997; 32(6):765-8.
34. Pittler MH, Ernst E. Peppermint oil for irritable bowel syndrome: a critical review and metaanalysis. *Am J Gastroenterol.* 1998; 93(7):1131-5.
35. Friese J, Kohler S. Peppermint oil-caraway oil fixed combination in non-ulcer dyspepsia: comparison of the effects of enteric preparations. *Pharmazie.* 1999; 54(3):210-5.
36. Madlisch A, Heydenreich CJ, Wieland V, et al. Treatment of functional dyspepsia with a fixed peppermint oil and caraway oil combination preparation as compared to cisapride: a multicenter, reference-controlled double-blind equivalence study. *Arzneimittelforschung.* 1999;49(11):925-32.
37. Tyler VE, Brady LR, Robbers JE. *Pharmacognosy.* 9th ed. Philadelphia: Lea & Febiger; 1988.
38. Achterrath-Tuckermann U, Kunde R, Flaskamp E, et al. Pharmacological investigations with compounds of chamomile. V. Investigations on the spasmolytic effect of compounds of chamomile and Kamillosan on the isolated guinea pig ileum. *Planta Med.* 1980;39(1):38-50.
39. Status of *USP-NF* Botanical Monograph Development. Available at: http://www.usp.org/dietary/availability/htm. Accessed September 20, 2001.
40. Osawa T. Phenolic antioxidants in dietary plants as antimutagens. *ACS Symp Ser.* 1992;507:135-49.
41. Nakatani N. Phenolic antioxidants from herbs and spices. *Biofactors.* 2000;13(1-4):141-6.
42. Triantaphyllou K, Blekas G, Boskou D. Antioxidative properties of water extracts obtained from herbs of the species Lamiaceae. *Int J Food Sci Nutr.* 2001;52(4):313-7.
43. Duke JA. *The Green Pharmacy.* Emmaus, PA: Rodale Press; 1997.
44. Leung LK, Su YL, Chen RY, et al. Theaflavins in black tea and catechins in green tea are equally effective antioxidants. *J Nutr.* 2001;131(9):2248-51.
45. Langley-Evans SC. Antioxidant potential of green and black tea determined using the ferric reducing power (FRAP) assay. *Int J Food Sci Nutr.* 2000;51(3):181-8.
46. Hodgson JM, Proudfoot JM, Croft KD, et al. Comparison of the effects of black and green tea on in vitro lipoprotein oxidation in human serum. *J Sci Food Agric.* 1999;79(4):561-6.
47. Yang FJ, Oz HS, Barve S, et al. The green tea polyphenol (–)-epigallocatechin-3-gallate blocks nuclear factor-kappa B activation by inhibiting I kappa B kinase activity in the intestinal epithelial cell line IEC-6. *Mol Pharmacol.* 2001;60(3):528-33.

48. Katiyar SK, Elmets CA. Green tea polyphenolic antioxidants and skin photoprotection. *Int J Oncol.* 2001;18(6):1307-13. Review.

49. Ma LP, Liu ZQ, Zhou B, et al. Inhibition of free radical induced oxidative hemolysis of red blood cells by green tea polyphenols. *Chinese Sci Bull.* 2001;45(22):2052-6.

50. Mukhtar H, Ahmad N. Green tea in chemoprevention of cancer. *Toxicol Sci.* 1999;52(2)(suppl S):111-7.

51. Valcic S, Muders A, Jacobsen NE, et al. Antioxidant chemistry of green tea catechins: identification of products of the reaction of (−)-epigallocatechin gallate with peroxyl radicals. *Chem Res Toxicol.* 1999;12(4):382-6.

52. Wang HF, Helliwell K. Determination of flavonols in green and black tea leaves and green tea infusions by high-performance liquid chromatography. *Food Res Int.* 2001;34(2-3):223-7.

53. Pietta PG. Flavonoids as antioxidants. *J Nat Prod.* 2000; 63(7):1035-42.

54. Yang TTC, Koo MWL. Inhibitory effect of Chinese green tea on endothelial cell-induced LDL oxidation. *Atherosclerosis.* 2000;148(1):67-73.

55. Benzie IFF, Szeto YT, Strain JJ, et al. Consumption of green tea causes rapid increase in plasma antioxidant power in humans. *Nutr Cancer.* 1999;34(1):83-7.

56. Ahmad N, Mukhtar H. Cutaneous photochemoprotection by green tea: a brief review. *Skin Pharmacol Appl Skin Physiol.* 2001;14(2):69-76.

57. Setiawan VW, Zhang ZF, Yu GP, et al. Protective effect of green tea on the risks of chronic gastritis and stomach cancer. *Int J Cancer.* 2001; 92(4):600-4.

58. Bagchi D, Ray SD, Patel D, et al. Protection against drug- and chemical-induced multi-organ toxicity by a novel IH636 grape seed proanthocyanidin extract. *Drugs Exp Clin Res.* 2001; 27(1): 3-15.

59. Bagchi D, Bagchi M, Stohs SJ, et al. Free radicals and grape seed proanthocyanidin extract: importance in human health and disease prevention. *Toxicology.* 2000;148(2-3):187-97.

60. Tebib K, Rouanet JM, Besancon P. Antioxidant effects of dietary polymeric grape seed tannins in tissues of rats fed a high cholesterol vitamin E-deficient diet. *Food Chem.* 1997;59(1):135-41.

61. Banerjee B, Bagchi D. Beneficial effects of a novel IH636 grape seed proanthocyanidin extract in the treatment of chronic pancreatitis. *Digestion.* 2001;63(3):203-6.

62. Nuttall SL, Kendall MJ, Bombardelli E, et al. An evaluation of the antioxidant activity of a standardized grape seed extract, Leucoselect. *J Clin Pharm Ther.* 1998;23(5):385-9.

63. Hosseini S, Lee J, Sepulveda RT, et al. A randomized, double-blind, placebo-controlled, prospective, 16-week crossover study to determine the role of Pycnogenol in modifying blood pressure in mildly hypertensive patients. *Nutr Res.* 2001;21(9):1251-60.

64. Park YC, Rimbach G, Saliou C, et al. Activity of monomeric, dimeric, and trimeric flavonoids on NO production, TNF-alpha secretion, and NF-kappa B-dependent gene expression in RAW 264.7 macrophages. *FEBS Lett.* 2000; 465(2-3):93-7.

65. Spadea L, Balestrazzi E. Treatment of vascular retinopathies with Pycnogenol. *Phytother Res.* 2001;15(3):219-23.

66. Petrassi C, Mastromarino A, Spartera C. Pycnogenol in chronic venous insufficiency. *Phytomedicine.* 2000;7(5):383-8.

67. Arcangeli P. Pycnogenol in chronic venous insufficiency. *Fitoterapia.* 2000;71(3):236-44.

68. Hasegawa N. Inhibition of lipogenesis by pycnogenol. *Phytother Res.* 2000;14(6):472-3.

69. Liu FJ, Lau BHS, Peng QL, et al. Pycnogenol protects vascular endothelial cells from beta-amyloid-induced injury. *Biol Pharm Bull.* 2000;23(6):735-7.

70. Fuhrman B, Rosenblat, Hayek T, et al. Ginger extract consumption reduces plasma cholesterol, inhibits LDL oxidation and attenuates development of atherosclerosis in atherosclerotic apolipoprotein E-deficient mice. *J Nutr.* 2000;130(5):1124-31.

71. Piscoya J, Rodriguez Z, Bustmante SA, et al. Efficacy and safety of freeze-dried cat's claw in osteoarthritis of the knee: mechanisms of action of the species Uncaria guaiansis. *Inflamm Res.* 2001;50(9):442-8.

72. Reinhard KH. Uncaria tomentosa (Willd) DC: Cat's claw, Una de Gato, or Saventaro. *J Altern Complement Med.* 1999;5(2):143-51.

73. Wang SY, Jiao HJ. Scavenging capacity of berry crops on superoxide radicals, hydrogen peroxide, hydroxyl radicals, and singlet oxygen. *J Agric Food Chem.* 2000;48(11):5677-84.

74. Youdim KA, Martin A, Joseph JA. Incorporation of the elderberry anthocyanins by endothelial cells increases protection against oxidative stress. *Free Radic Biol Med.* 2000;29(1):51-60.

75. Lee BM, Lee SK, Kim HS. Inhibition of oxidative DNA damage, 8-OHdG, and carbonyl contents in smokers treated with antioxidants (vitamin E, vitamin C, beta-carotene, and red ginseng). *Cancer Lett.* 1998;132(1-2):219-27.

76. Zhang ZS, Chang Q, Zhu M, et al. Characterization of antioxidants present in hawthorn fruits. *J Nutr Biochem.* 2001;12(3):144-52.

77. Halim AB, El-Ahmady C, Hassab-Allah S, et al. Biochemical effect of antioxidants on lipids and liver function in experimentally induced liver damage. *Ann Clin Biochem.* 1997;34(pt 6):656-63.
78. Locher R, Suter PM, Weyhenmeyer R, et al. Inhibitory action of silibinin on low density lipoprotein oxidation. *Arzneimittelforschung.* 1998;48(3):236-9.
79. Ahmad N, Gali H, Javed S, et al. Skin cancer chemopreventive effects of a flavonoid antioxidant silymarin are mediated via impairment of receptor tyrosine kinase signaling and perturbation in cell cycle progression. *Biochem Biophys Res Commun.* 1998;247(2):294-301.

CHAPTER 6

PEDIATRIC NUTRITION

Imad F. Btaiche, May B. Saba, Kelly P. Popa

Pharmacists can play an integral role in the nutritional care of children in the community and clinical setting alike by promoting better health care and preventing diseases. Assessing children's nutritional status regularly is essential to identify and treat childhood nutritional abnormalities. Nutritional care is age- and disease-specific, especially throughout infancy and adolescence at crucial phases of growth and development.

Infants and children have higher metabolic rates, lower tissue reserves, and greater energy requirements per unit of body weight than adults. Inadequate early nutrition during infancy and childhood may result in growth retardation with learning and behavioral deficits. Nutritional intake and eating habits during the period of growth and development may also affect the state of health later in life.

This chapter reviews the nutritional assessment and nutrient requirements in the pediatric population, the benefits of breastfeeding and human milk, the nutritional management of food hypersensitivities, and special nutritional requirements and restrictions in infants with inborn errors of metabolism. This chapter also discusses enteral and parenteral nutrition in pediatric patients.

PEDIATRIC NUTRITIONAL ASSESSMENT

Nutritional screening of children is an integral part of pediatric health care. The accurate collection and interpretation of nutritional data play an instrumental role in evaluating the child's growth, identifying nutritional problems, and preventing or correcting nutritional deficiencies. Assessing nutritional status is based on subjective and objective information. The assessment encompasses a thorough review of the medical history, diet history, and growth data, including anthropometric measurements, as well as a body protein and fat stores estimate, biochemical assessment, and physical examination.

Medical History

The medical history provides valuable insight into the child's nutritional status and should be obtained with the assistance of parents or caregivers. A medical history includes perinatal history, birth history (birth weight and length, gestational age), presence of acute or chronic illnesses, history of surgical or diagnostic procedures, and drug therapy.

Diet History

An accurate and comprehensive diet history includes an assessment of the following factors:[1]

1. Nutrient intake pattern—development of feeding skills, sucking and swallowing reflex, food habits, food frequency, and restricted diets.
2. Factors that affect nutrient intake—socioeconomic status, psychosocial issues, cultural beliefs, gastrointestinal diseases or resections, bowel habits, eating disorders, dentition, and food allergies or intolerances.
3. Factors that affect caloric and nutrient needs—activity level and acute and chronic diseases.
4. Intake of nutritional supplements—vitamins, minerals, and alternative medicines.
5. Evaluation of any drug-induced nutrient deficiencies.

A 24-hour diet recall helps obtain a rapid estimate of caloric intake, but its reliability is limited to the day being evaluated and on the interview technique. Maintaining a list of food frequency helps in assessing the trends in food consumption and the overall balance in the diet. A 3–5 day diet diary is the most accurate method of diet history. This method accounts for daily variation in intake and eliminates the subjectiveness of diet recall.[2]

Growth Data

Anthropometric measurements—which evaluate the size, weight, and proportions of the human body—are a rapid, noninvasive, and inexpensive method of evaluating nutritional status.[3] This is important because adequate nutrition plays a key role in ensuring age-appropriate growth. For example, term infants usually triple their birthweight by one year of age. Table 6-1 shows weight gain expectations relative to age.[4-5]

Monitoring growth through serial measurements of weight, length or height, and head circumference (children ≤ 3 years of age) is essential to determining a child's own growth curve. Pediatricians plot these measurements on the National Center for Health Statistics, Centers for Disease Control and Prevention (NCHS/CDC) growth charts to evaluate the physical growth of infants, children, and adolescents in the United States. The growth charts consist of curves called "percentiles" that illustrate the distribution of children across the United States according to body measurements. Plotted growth data compare the child to a reference population of healthy children in the United States. Pediatricians use these measurements over time to monitor trends in growth percentiles.

TABLE 6-1 Expected Average Weight
Gain in Infants and Children

Age	Grams per Day
Premature	15–30
0–3 months	24–35
3–6 months	15–21
6–12 months	10–13
1–6 years	5–9
6–10 years	6–11

Source: References 4,5.

Significant deviations in the growth of a child can be related to illness, overnutrition, or undernutrition. Special growth charts are available for premature infants and children with Down's syndrome, Turner's syndrome, myelomeningocele, cerebral palsy, and Prader-Willi syndrome. Alternatively, for premature infants, growth data are plotted with correction for their gestational age up to 2 years.[6]

New growth charts published in the year 2000 have replaced the weight-for-stature charts by including body mass index-for-age for boys and girls between 2 and 20 years of age. The weight-for-stature charts are available as an alternative for children between 2 and 5 years of age who are not evaluated beyond the preschool years. Body mass index (BMI) is calculated using the individual's weight and height [weight (kg)/height (m²)] and is used to assess whether the person's weight is appropriate for their height. BMI is predictive of body fat and can be used to characterize underweight and overweight or to detect risks for obesity.[7]

Body Protein and Fat Stores

Body composition is estimated by measuring the midarm circumference, which is an indicator of muscle mass, and skinfold thickness at the triceps and subscapular sites, which indicate body fat stores.[3,8] These measurements are then compared to percentiles of reference data. In chronic malnutrition, depletion of fat stores at the triceps is common.[9] Subscapular site thickness indicates truncal fat stores and reflects long-term nutritional status. Limitations of this method include errors related to the observer, instrument, patient's position, and fluid status. Skinfold measurements should be interpreted with caution in small children because even small variations can account for significant differences between percentiles.[8]

Biochemical Data

Biochemical assessment of nutritional status relies on the laboratory measurement of serum visceral proteins, such as albumin, prealbumin, retinol-binding protein, and transferrin; vitamin and mineral concentrations; and hematological indices such as those that relate to iron status. As detailed in

Components of Pediatric Nutritional Assessment
❑ Medical history
❑ Diet history
❑ Growth data
❑ Body protein and fat stores
❑ Biochemical data
❑ Physical examination

TABLE 6-2 Serum Proteins Used in Assessment of Nutritional Status

Serum Protein	Half-life (days)	Serum Reference Range* (age)	Factors that Increase Levels	Factors that Decrease Levels
Albumin (g/dL)	20	2.6–3.6 (< 5 days) 3.4–4.2 (1–3 years) 3.5–5.2 (4–6 years) 3.7–5.6 (7–19 years)	Dehydration Steroids Insulin	Edema, Cirrhosis, Sepsis, Nephrotic syndrome, Burns, Stress, Trauma, Congestive heart failure, Inadequate nutrition, Neoplasms
Prealbumin (mg/dL) (Transthyretin)	2	6–21 (< 5 days) 14–30 (1–5 years) 15–33 (6–9 years) 20–36 (10–13 years) 22–45 (14–19 years)	Renal dysfunction	Cirrhosis, Hepatitis, Stress, Surgery, Cystic fibrosis, Hyperthyroidism, Inflammation
Transferrin (g/L)	10	1.43–4.46 (≤ 5 days) 2.18–3.47 (1–3 years) 2.08–3.78 (4–6 years) 2.25–3.61 (7–9 years) 2.24–4.42 (10–13 years) 2.33–4.44 (14–19 years)	Iron deficiency Blood loss Pregnancy Estrogens	Cirrhosis, Iron, Nephrotic syndrome, Burns, Enteropathies, Testosterone, Steroids, Chronic infection
Retinol-binding protein (mg/dL)	0.5	0.8–4.5 (≤ 5 days) 1–7.6 (1–5 years) 2–7.8 (6–9 years) 1.3–9.9 (10–13 years) 3–9.2 (14–19 years)	Renal dysfunction Vitamin A	Vitamin A deficiency, Cirrhosis, Hepatitis, Stress, Surgery, Cystic fibrosis, Hyperthyroidism, Inflammation

* Ranges vary between laboratories.

Source: References 10–13.

Table 6-2, reference ranges for serum proteins are age-dependent. When interpreting their values, it is important to consider their nutritional specificity and sensitivity in relation to the patient's clinical status.[10-13]

Physical Examination

Pediatricians interpret findings from a physical examination in conjunction with the patient's clinical status, medical history, and nutritional parameters.

Caloric Intake Levels

The distribution of caloric intake in normally fed infants is:

❑ 7% to 16% of calories from protein.
❑ 30% to 55% of calories from fat.
❑ The remaining calories from carbohydrates.

Source: Fomon SJ, Filer LJ. Milks and formulas. In: Fomon SJ, ed. *Infant Nutrition.* 2nd ed. Philadelphia: WB Saunders Company; 1974:359-407.

Table 6-3 lists physical findings related to specific nutritional deficiencies or excesses.[14]

CALORIC AND PROTEIN REQUIREMENTS

Caloric and protein requirements in normal healthy infants and children are estimated based on the recommended dietary allowances (RDA).[15] In sick infants and children, the requirements may become different and adjustments to the RDA intake levels may be necessary based on the patient's clinical and nutritional status.

In normally fed infants, the distribution of caloric intake is 7%–16% of calories from protein, 30%–55% of calories from fat, and the remaining calories from carbohydrates.[16] In children, 10%–15% of the calories are derived from protein, about 30% from fat, and 50%–60% from carbohydrates.

Table 6-4 outlines the recommended energy requirements for each age group. Special requirements for premature infants will be described throughout this chapter.

HUMAN MILK AND BREASTFEEDING

There is strong evidence that human milk has protective and growth promoting benefits that cannot be replicated with infant formulas.[17] Because of the benefits to the infant and mother, health care professionals should encourage breastfeeding except when specific contraindications exist.[18] Human milk provides enzymatic and immunologic components that have been shown to decrease the incidence of gastrointestinal and respiratory infections and reduce the incidence and severity of diarrhea. Other advantages include improved cognitive development, enhanced maternal-infant bonding, and cost savings.[19]

Human milk properties and biochemical composition vary among individuals depending on maternal diet, stage of lactation, and time into nursing. Colostrum is the milk produced during the first days following delivery and is rich in immunologic factors and proteins. Transition milk begins 1-2 weeks

TABLE 6-3   Clinical Findings on Physical Examination Related
to Nutrient Deficiencies or Excesses

Clinical Findings	Possible Nutrient Deficiency*	Possible Nutrient Excess
Hair		
Flag sign (transverse depigmentation of hair)	Protein	
Easily pluckable hair	Protein	
Sparse hair	Protein, Biotin, Zinc	Vitamin A
Corkscrew hairs and unmerged coiled hairs	Vitamin C	
Nails		
Transverse ridging of nails	Protein	
Skin		
Scaling	Vitamin A, Zinc, Essential fatty acids	Vitamin A
Cellophane appearance	Protein	
Cracking (flaky paint or crazy pavement dermatosis)	Protein	
Follicular hyperkeratosis	Vitamins A, C	
Petechiae (especially perifollicular)	Vitamin C	
Purpura	Vitamins C, K	
Pigmentation, desquamation of sun-exposed areas	Niacin	
Yellow pigmentation-sparing sclerae (benign)		Carotene
Eyes		
Papilledema		Vitamin A
Night blindness	Vitamin A	
Perioral		
Angular stomatitis	Riboflavin, Pyridoxine, Niacin	
Cheilosis (dry, cracking ulcerated lips)	Riboflavin, Pyridoxine, Niacin	
Oral		
Atrophic lingual papillae (slick tongue)	Riboflavin, Niacin, Folate, Protein, Iron, Vitamin B_{12}	
Glossitis	Riboflavin, Niacin, Folate, Pyridoxine, Vitamin B_{12}	
Hypogeusesthesia, Hyposmia	Zinc	
Swollen, retracted, bleeding gums (if teeth are present)	Vitamin C	
Bones and Joints		
Beading of ribs, Epiphyseal swelling, Bowlegs	Vitamin D	
Tenderness (subperiosteal hemorrhage in children)	Vitamin C	

TABLE 6-3 Clinical Findings on Physical Examination Related to Nutrient Deficiencies or Excesses (continued)

Clinical Findings	Possible Nutrient Deficiency*	Possible Nutrient Excess
Neurologic		
Headache		Vitamin A
Drowsiness, Lethargy, Vomiting		Vitamins A, D
Dementia	Vitamin B$_{12}$, Niacin	
Confabulation, Disorientation	Thiamin (Korsakoff's psychosis)	
Ophthalmoplegia	Thiamin, Phosphorus	
Peripheral neuropathy (weakness, paresthesias, ataxia, decreased tendon reflexes, fine tactile sense, vibratory sense, position sense)	Thiamin, Pyridoxine, Vitamin B$_{12}$	Pyridoxine
Tetany	Calcium, Magnesium	
Other Body Systems		
Parotid enlargement	Protein (also consider bulimia)	
Heart failure	Thiamin (wet beriberi), Phosphorus	
Sudden heart failure and death	Vitamin C	
Hepatomegaly	Protein	Vitamin A
Edema	Protein, Thiamin	
Poor wound healing, decubitus ulcers	Protein, Zinc, Vitamin C	

* In this table, protein deficiency is used to signify Kwashiorkor (severe protein malnutrition).
Source: Adapted with permission from reference 14.

TABLE 6-4 Recommended Dietary Allowances for Energy and Protein*

	Age (years)	Energy (kcal/kg)	Protein (g/kg)
Infants	0.0–0.5	108	2.2
	>0.5–1	98	1.6
Children	>1–3	102	1.2
	4–6	90	1.1
	7–10	70	1
Males	11–14	55	1
	15–18	45	0.9
Females	11–14	47	1
	15–18	40	0.8

* Adjustments to these levels of intake may be necessary during illness or under specific disease states.
Source: Reference 15.

Why Breastfeed?

Human milk provides enzymatic and immunologic components that have been shown to decrease the incidence of gastrointestinal and respiratory infections and reduce the incidence and severity of diarrhea. Other advantages include improved cognitive development, enhanced maternal-infant bonding, and cost savings.[19]

after delivery and has increased lactose, fat, and calories. Mature milk begins at about 2 weeks after delivery and continues until about 8 months. Extended lactation beyond 8 months results in lower milk contents of vitamins and minerals.[20]

Breast milk is recommended as the sole food for the first 4–6 months of age. As the preferred feeding for infants, human milk should be initiated shortly after birth and continued for the first 12 months of age.[21] Infants weaned before 12 months of age should receive iron-fortified formula with gradual addition of solid foods in the second half of the first year.[22] Before 6 months of age, vitamin D supplementation may be needed in infants not exposed to adequate sunlight or those born to mothers who are vitamin D deficient. Infants with anemia or low iron stores will need iron supplementation.[19]

Fluoride supplementation is no longer recommended during the first 6 months of life to either breastfed or formula-fed infants. Fluoride is supplemented at 0.25 mg/day for children between 6 months and 3 years of age if the water supply contains <0.3 ppm of fluoride[23] and for infants exclusively fed ready-to-feed formulas.[20]

Breastfeeding is contraindicated in infants with galactosemia, and in infants whose mothers use illegal drugs, have active tuberculosis, are infected with the immunodeficiency virus (HIV), or take medications that are deemed harmful to the infant.[19,24] Women receiving chemotherapy and those living in the United States who are infected with HIV should not breastfeed, since infant formulas are easily available.[25] Specialized formulas are used as alternatives to human milk in infants with galactosemia or other conditions of intolerance to human milk.

INFANT FORMULAS

Iron-fortified infant formulas are used as alternatives or supplements to breastfeeding up to 12 months of age.[26] The Committee on Nutrition of the American Academy of Pediatrics[27] and the Food and Drug Administration[28] have recommended nutrient requirements for infant formulas. The American Academy of Pediatrics has recommended that the manufacturing of low-iron infant formulas containing less than 4 mg/L of iron should be discontinued. In order to maintain adequate iron stores and prevent iron deficiency, infants should only be given formulas fortified with iron at concentrations between 10 and 12 mg/L during the first year of life.[26]

TABLE 6-5 Examples of Formulas for Infants and Children

Formula Type	Products (Manufacturer)	Indications
Cow's milk-based	Enfamil with Iron (MJ) Enfamil LIPIL with Iron (MJ) Similac with Iron (R) Carnation Good Start (NC)	Normal healthy infants
Soy-based	Isomil (R), Prosobee (MJ)	Lactose intolerance, galactosemia
Casein hydrolysates (infants)	Nutramigen (MJ)	Cow's milk and soy protein allergy or intolerance
	Pregestimil (MJ), Alimentum (R)	Cow's milk and soy protein allergy or intolerance, malabsorption
Free amino acids (infants)	Neocate (SHS)	Cow's milk allergy, protein intolerance, malabsorption
Children (1–10 years) standard formula	Pediasure (R), Kindercal (MJ), Nutren Junior (N)	Normally functional gastrointestinal tract
Whey hydrolysates (children)	Peptamen Junior (N), Pro-Peptide for Kids (NM)	Protein intolerance, malabsorption
Free amino acids (children)	Vivonex Pediatric (NN), Neocate One + (SHS)	Cow's milk allergy, protein intolerance, malabsorption
Special diets	Lofenalac (MJ), Phenex-1 (R),	Phenylketonuria
	MSUD Diet Powder (MJ), Ketonex-1 (R)	Maple syrup urine disease
	I-Valex-1 (R)	Isovaleric acidemia
	Propimex-1 (R)	Propionic or methylmalonic acidemia
Modular	ProMod (R), Casec (MJ), Resource Instant Protein Powder (NN)	Protein supplements
	Polycose (R), Moducal (MJ)	Carbohydrate supplements
	Mirolipid (MJ), MCT oil	Fat supplements
	Duocal (SHS)	Carbohydrate and fat supplement

Manufacturer: MJ = Mead Johnson; R = Ross; NC = Nestle Carnation Baby Formulas; SHS = Scientific Hospital Supplies; N = Nestle Clinical Nutrition; NM = Nutrition Medical; NN = Novartis Nutrition.

The standard infant formula concentration is 20 kcal/oz (0.67 kcal/mL), whereas standard premature ready-to-feed infant formulas are 20 or 24 kcal/oz (0.67 or 0.8 kcal/mL). Higher concentrations up to 30 kcal/oz are indicated in infants with fluid restriction or with increased metabolic needs. When high feeding concentrations are used, it is essential to monitor for feeding tolerance, hydration status, fluid and electrolyte disturbances, and renal function.

Infant formulas are classified according to the age group (premature infants, term infants up to 1 year of age) and formula composition (standard cow's milk, soy, protein hydrolysate, and amino acid formulas). Table 6-5 shows examples of infant formulas.

Premature infant formulas are milk-based preparations, modified to account for alterations in digestion and absorption. Details of these formulas are described in the Special Nutritional Requirements of Premature Infants section.

Infant Feeding Formulas

The four main categories of infant feeding formulas include:

❑ Standard cow's milk formulas (such as Enfamil LIPIL with Iron, Similac with Iron, and Carnation Good Start) are used for term infants up to 12 months of age, and are the most common human milk substitutes.

❑ Soy-based formulas (such as Prosobee and Isomil), which are free of lactose and cow's milk proteins, are used for infants with lactose intolerance and galactosemia.

❑ Protein hydrolysate or semi-elemental casein-based formulas (such as Nutramigen, Pregestimil, and Alimentum), are used in infants with cow's milk and soy protein allergy or intolerance. Pregestimil and Alimentum are also used in infants who have significant malabsorption due to gastrointestinal (e.g., short gut syndrome, cystic fibrosis, protracted diarrhea) or hepatobiliary (e.g., cholestasis, biliary atresia) disease.

❑ Amino acid-based or elemental infant formula (such as Neocate) is indicated in infants with cow's milk allergy, protein intolerance, and intractable malabsorption.

Source:

Hall RT, Carroll RE. Infant feeding. *Pediatr Rev.* 2000;21:191-9.

Redel CA, Shulman RJ. Controversies in the composition of infant formulas. *Pediatr Clin North Am.* 1994;41:909-24.

For term infants up to 12 months of age, standard cow's milk formulas (such as Enfamil with Iron, Enfamil LIPIL with Iron, Similac with Iron, and Carnation Good Start) are the most common human milk substitutes used. Protein concentrations in these formulas are 1.4 to 1.6 g/dL, and are approximately 40% higher than in human milk.[29] In cow's milk formulas, lactose is the major carbohydrate source, and fat constitutes approximately 50% of energy. In addition, the butterfat is replaced largely with vegetable oils to enhance digestibility and absorption. Enfamil LIPIL contains the fatty acids docasahexaenoic acid (DHA) and arachidonic acid (ARA) that potentially support brain function and vision development.

Soy-based formulas (such as Prosobee and Isomil) contain purified soy proteins, and a mixture of vegetable oils as the fat source.[30] They are lactose-free, and carbohydrate sources are corn syrup solids, cornstarch, or sucrose.[31] Indications for soy formulas include lactose intolerance, galactosemia, or when parents desire to provide the child with a vegetarian diet. Soy formulas should be avoided in infants with milk protein allergy or intolerance because certain infants with an allergen-induced reaction to cow's milk protein are also intolerant to soy.[30,32] Soy formulas are not recommended to prevent infantile colic or for use in premature infants weighing less than 1800 g.[30,33]

Protein hydrolysate or semi-elemental formulas for infants are casein hydrolysates (such as Nutramigen, Pregestimil, and Alimentum). In these

TABLE 6-6   Terminology Used in Reference to Premature Infants

Terminology	Definition*
Small-for-gestational age (SGA)	< 10th percentile
Appropriate-for-gestational age (AGA)	≥ 10th and ≤ 90th percentile
Large-for-gestational age (LGA)	> 90th percentile
Premature (Preterm) infant	Gestational age < 38 weeks
Term infant	Gestational age 38–42 weeks
Extremely low birth weight (ELBW)	Birth weight < 1000 g
Very low birth weight (VLBW)	Birth weight < 1500 g
Low birth weight (LBW)	Birth weight < 2500 g

* Percentiles are for birth weight for gestational age.
Source: References 36-37.

formulas, proteins are broken down by heat treatment or enzymatic hydrolysis resulting in free amino acids and peptides. Formulas are then fortified with amino acids to compensate for the amino acids lost during manufacturing. Indications for protein hydrolysates include cow's milk and soy protein allergy or intolerance. Pregestimil and Alimentum are also used in infants with significant malabsorption due to gastrointestinal (e.g., short gut syndrome, cystic fibrosis, protracted diarrhea) or hepatobiliary (e.g., cholestasis, biliary atresia) disease.[29] Pregestimil and Alimentum contain medium chain triglycerides (MCT) to improve fat intake in patients with malabsorption syndromes. Protein hydrolysate formulas are lactose-free. Sources of carbohydrates include corn syrup solids, modified cornstarch, sucrose, or glucose.[29,34] Disadvantages of protein hydrolysate formulas include palatability and high cost.

Amino acid-based or elemental formula (such as Neocate) is indicated in infants with cow's milk allergy, protein intolerance, and intractable malabsorption.[35] The protein component is comprised of 100% free amino acids, making it the most hypoallergenic infant formula available. Carbohydrates are from corn syrup solids and fat is from a mixture of vegetable oils. Disadvantages of a free amino acid formula include palatability and high cost.

SPECIAL NUTRITIONAL REQUIREMENTS
OF PREMATURE INFANTS

Premature infants are neonates born before 38 weeks of gestation compared to term infants born at 38–42 weeks of gestation. Table 6-6 shows the classification of newborns in relation to gestational age and birth weight.[36-37]

Premature infants are at risk for nutritional deficiency due to limited reserves, immature physiological systems, and associated diseases of prematurity. The goal of nutritional management of low birth weight (LBW) infants is to provide sufficient amounts of nutrients to simulate at least the intrauterine growth rate.[38] Table 6-7 lists the recommended nutrient intakes for LBW infants.[38-42]

TABLE 6-7 Enteral Nutritional Requirements
for Low Birth Weight Infants

Nutrient	Recommended Intake (amount/100 kcal)
Protein (g)	2.9–3.3
Carbohydrates (g)	9–13
Fat (g)	4.5–6 (400 mg essential fatty acids)
Trace Minerals	
Copper (mcg)	90
Iodine (mcg)	5
Manganese (mcg)	> 5
Zinc (mg)	> 0.5
Iron	1.7–2.5
Water-soluble Vitamins	
Thiamin (mcg)	200
Riboflavin (mcg)	60–600
Niacin (mg)	0.25–5
Pyridoxine (mcg)	35–250 (15 mcg/g protein)
Folic acid (mcg)	21–60
Vitamin B_{12} (mcg)	0.15–0.25
Pantothenic acid (mg)	0.3–1.5
Biotin (mcg)	1.5–5
Vitamin C (mg)	35
Fat-soluble Vitamins	
Vitamin A (IU)	77–1250
Vitamin D (IU)	270
Vitamin E (IU)	> 1.1 (1 IU/g of linoleic acid)
Electrolytes	
Magnesium (mg)	6.6–12.5
Chloride (mg)	59–89
Sodium (mg)	48–67
Potassium (mg)	66–98
Calcium (mg)	175
Phosphorus (mg)	91.5

Source: References 38–42.

Preterm milk composition and milk volume production may be inadequate to nourish the infant.[43] Therefore, human milk fortifiers (such as Similac Human Milk Fortifier or Enfamil Human Milk Fortifier) or selected individual supplements should be added to the milk. Table 6-8 shows examples of preterm infant formulas and their nutritional composition.

Energy

The enteral caloric intake necessary for most LBW infants to achieve satisfactory growth rate is 105–130 kcal/kg/day.[38-44] Daily energy expenditure in LBW infants is estimated as the sum of energy required for resting energy expenditure (50 kcal/kg), growth (25 kcal/kg), intermittent activity (15 kcal/kg), stool losses (12 kcal/kg), occasional cold stress (10 kcal/kg), and specific dynamic action (8 kcal/kg).[45]

Nutritional Needs of Low Birth Weight (LBW) Infants

- ❑ Caloric Requirements— The enteral caloric intake necessary for most LBW infants to achieve satisfactory growth rate is 105–130 kcal/kg/day, and is estimated as the sum of energy required for resting energy expenditure (50 kcal/kg), growth (25 kcal/kg), intermittent activity (15 kcal/kg), stool losses (12 kcal/kg), occasional cold stress (10 kcal/kg), and specific dynamic action (8 kcal/kg).
- ❑ Protein—Protein intake of 2.5–3 g/kg/day appears adequate for most infants. To achieve the intrauterine rate of protein accretion, LBW infants may need up to 3.85 g/kg/day of amino acids.
- ❑ Carbohydrates—There are no absolute requirements for carbohydrates in LBW infants. Carbohydrates make up about half of the nonprotein calories in human milk and infant formulas.
- ❑ Fat—Fat accounts for about 40%–50% of nonprotein calories in human milk.
- ❑ Calcium and Phosphorus—Infants require high calcium and phosphorus intake in order to achieve normal growth and adequate bone mineralization.
- ❑ Iron—Iron is an essential element for growth and development. Because most iron accretion occurs during the third trimester of gestation, premature infants are at higher risk for iron deficiency. Premature infants who are exclusively breastfed or receiving human milk should receive oral iron supplements. Iron-fortified formulas provide the required iron amount for most premature infants.
- ❑ Vitamins—Premature infants have low water-soluble vitamin reserves and increased vitamin requirements. They also need fat-soluble vitamin supplements. Human milk fortifiers, preterm formulas, or multivitamin supplements can help meet these increased vitamin requirements.

Source:

American Academy of Pediatrics, Committee on Nutrition. Nutritional needs of low-birth-weight infants. *Pediatrics.* 1977;60:519-30.

Stekel A, Olivares M, Pizarro F, et al. Absorption of fortification iron from milk formulas in infants. *Am J Clin Nutr.* 1986;43:917-22.

American Academy of Pediatrics, Committee on Nutrition. Iron fortification of infant formulas. *Pediatrics.* 1999;104:119-23.

Proteins

Protein intake of 2.5–3 g/kg/day appears adequate for most infants. To achieve the intrauterine rate of protein accretion, LBW infants may need up to 3.85 g/kg/day of amino acids.[46] The digestibility of proteins in premature infant formulas is improved by using a whey-to-casein ratio of 60:40.[47] Also,

TABLE 6-8   Composition of Preterm Infant Formulas (Nutrient/100 kcal)*

Composition	Product (Manufacturer)			
	Preterm Human Milk + Similac Natural Care 50:50 ratio† (Ross)	Similac Special Care with Iron 24 (Ross)	Similac Neosure (Ross)	Enfamil Premature Formula 24 (MeadJohnson)
Energy (kcal)	100	100	100	100
kcal/mL	0.74	0.8	0.74	0.8
Protein (g)	2.43	2.71	2.6	3
Source	Mature preterm human milk, Non-fat milk, Whey protein concentrate	Non-fat milk, Whey protein concentrate	Non-fat milk, Whey protein concentrate	Non-fat milk, Whey protein concentrate
% of total calories	10	11	10	12
Fat (g)	5.6	5.43	5.5	5.1
Source	Mature preterm human milk, MCT, Soy, Coconut oils	MCT, Soy, Coconut oils	MCT, Soy, Coconut oil, Safflower oil	MCT, Soy, Coconut oils
% of total calories	50	49	49	44
Linoleic acid (mg)	587	700	750	1060
Carbohydrates (g)	10.3	10.6	10.3	11.1
Source	Corn syrup solids, Lactose	Corn syrup solids, Lactose	Corn syrup solids, Lactose	Corn syrup solids, Lactose
% of total calories	41	42	41	44
Vitamins				
Vitamin A (IU)	1105	1250	460	1250
Vitamin D (IU)	83	150	70	270
Vitamin E (IU)	2.9	4	3.6	6.3
Vitamin K (mcg)	7	12	11	8
Thiamin (mcg)	150	250	220	200
Riboflavin (mcg)	371	620	150	300

Vitamin B$_6$ (mcg)	146	250	100	150
Vitamin B$_{12}$ (mcg)	0.33	0.55	0.4	0.25
Niacin (mcg)	2831	5000	1950	4000
Folic acid (mcg)	22	37	25	35
Pantothenic acid (mcg)	1159	1900	800	1200
Biotin (mcg)	20.6	37	9	4
Vitamin C (mg)	28	37	15	20
Choline (mg)	12	10	16	12
Inositol (mg)	13	6	6	17
Electrolytes and Minerals				
Calcium (mg) [mEq]	131 [6.6]	180 [9]	105 [5.2]	165 [8.2]
Phosphorus (mg)	72	100	62	83
Magnesium (mg)	8.6	12	9	6.8
Iron (mg)	0.28	1.8	1.8	1.8
Zinc (mg)	1.05	1.5	1.2	1.5
Manganese (mcg)	7	12	10	6.3
Copper (mcg)	180	250	120	125
Iodine (mcg)	11	6	15	25
Selenium (mcg)	2.3	1.8	2.3	—
Sodium (mg) [mEq]	40 [1.8]	43 [1.9]	33 [1.4]	39 [1.7]
Potassium (mg) [mEq]	109 [2.8]	129 [3.3]	142 [3.6]	103 [2.6]
Chloride (mg) [mEq]	81 [2.3]	81 [2.3]	75 [2.1]	85 [2.4]
Osmolarity (mOsm/L)	251	250	224	270
Renal solute load¶ (mOsm)	23	26.1	24	26.1
Volume (mL)	135	124	134	124

* Composition listed is subject to change by manufacturer.
† Preterm human milk plus fortifier.
¶ Estimated renal solute load = [Protein (g) × 4] + [Na (mEq) + K (mEq) + Cl (mEq)]

many infant formulas contain added taurine (such as Prosobee 20, Pregestimil, Portagen, and Enfamil 24 Premature), an amino acid that primarily conjugates bile acid.[48]

Fat

Fat accounts for about 40%–50% of nonprotein calories in human milk. Premature infants poorly digest and absorb long chain triglycerides (LCTs) due to their reduced pool of bile acids. Since LBW infants better absorb medium chain triglycerides (MCTs) because their digestion and absorption are not dependent on bile acids, preterm infant formulas are enhanced with MCTs to improve fat intake.[38] MCTs do not provide essential fatty acids; thus a portion of the fat is supplied as LCTs. Linoleic acid, which prevents essential fatty acid deficiency, accounts for about 3% of total fat calories in the formulas.[47]

Carbohydrates

There are no absolute requirements for carbohydrates in LBW infants. Carbohydrates make up about half of the nonprotein calories in human milk and infant formulas. Lactose is the sole source of carbohydrates in human milk. Premature milk has about 15% less lactose than mature milk.[47] Although LBW infants may have difficulty digesting lactose due to low lactase activity, glucosidase enzymes appear sufficient for glucose polymer metabolism. Thus, formulas for preterm infants are made with a glucose polymers-to-lactose ratio of approximately 1:1 in order to facilitate carbohydrate digestion.[49] Glucose polymers also help reduce the osmotic load of the formula when compared to lactose and monosaccharides.[38]

Calcium and Phosphorus

Infants require high calcium and phosphorus intake to achieve normal growth and adequate bone mineralization. Since the fetus accrues about 80% of calcium, phosphorus, and magnesium in the last few months of pregnancy, infants born prematurely and fed human milk require adequate supplementation of these minerals for adequate bone mineralization.[42] This supplementation can be achieved by using human milk fortifiers or premature infant formulas.

Iron

Iron is an essential element for growth and development. Because most iron accretion occurs during the third trimester of gestation, premature infants are at higher risk for iron deficiency if they do not receive adequate iron supplementation postnatally.[50-51] With the increased use of iron-fortified infant formulas, however, the incidence of iron deficiency anemia in children has dropped significantly.[52]

To prevent iron deficiency, premature infants who are exclusively breastfed or receiving human milk should receive iron supplementation at an oral dose of 2–4 mg/kg/day, which can be given in the form of drops. Iron-fortified formulas provide the required iron amount for most premature infants.[26]

Vitamins

Premature infants have low water-soluble vitamin reserves and increased vitamin requirements. They also need fat-soluble vitamin supplements. Human milk fortifiers, preterm formulas, or multivitamin supplements can help meet these increased vitamin requirements.

Vitamin D intake at 400 IU/day in fortified human milk and premature infant formulas meets the needs of premature infants and prevents the development of rickets.[53] Vitamin K is important for the synthesis of coagulation factors. To prevent hemorrhagic disease of the newborn, routine vitamin K administration is recommended for all neonates as a single intramuscular dose of 0.5–1 mg within one hour of birth.[54-55] The recommendations for vitamin A intake range from 77–1250 IU/100 kcal. However, because of the potential association between vitamin A deficiency and bronchopulmonary dysplasia, additional supplementation of vitamin A to premature infants at risk for lung disease may be necessary. Additional information about vitamin metabolism and LBW infant requirements can be found in sources outside this text.[56]

SUPPLEMENTAL FOODS FOR INFANTS

Parents should introduce supplemental foods when the infant can sit with support and has good neuromuscular control of the head and neck. At this stage, the infant can indicate a desire for food by opening the mouth and leaning forward, or indicate disinterest or satiety by leaning backward and turning its head away.

The age for introducing supplemental foods will vary, depending on the infant's developmental stage, growth rate, and activity level. Breast milk or iron-containing formulas are the only recommended source of nutrition for infants during the first 4–6 months of life.[57] Iron-fortified single-grain infant cereals mixed with human milk or infant formula are introduced at 4–6 months of age when infants can swallow nonliquid foods. Because it is an unlikely allergen, rice cereal is commonly introduced as the first supplemental food. Dry baby cereal is thinned with breast milk or infant formula and fed from a spoon. Adding cereal to bottles should be avoided, except when medically indicated (in cases such as gastroesophageal reflux disease), because it deprives children of learning to self-feed. Thereafter, single-ingredient foods are started one at a time at 1-week intervals to help identify any food allergies or intolerances.[29] It is important to offer supplemental foods by 6 months of age. Otherwise, the child may have difficulty accepting them later.[58]

At 6–8 months of age, pureed fruits and vegetables are initiated, followed by pureed meats and soft table food at 8 months of age. Fruit juice is introduced when the infant can drink from a cup. Fruit juice should not replace milk or infant formula because excessive juice consumption increases the risk of dental caries, diarrhea, failure to thrive, short stature, and obesity.[20,59]

What Is Food Allergy?

Food allergies refer to clinical symptoms resulting from an inappropriate immune response to specific food proteins or additives. They can be classified as IgE-mediated and non-IgE mediated immune reactions. Food intolerance refers to an adverse reaction that is nonimmune in nature.

Source: Bruijnzeel-Koomen C, Ortolani C, Aas K, et al. Adverse reactions to food: European Academy of Allergology and Clinical Immunology Subcommittee. *Allergy.* 1995;50:623-35.

Whole cow's milk does not provide optimal nutrition for infants during the first year of life and should not be started before 12 months of age. Cow's milk contains low vitamin E, vitamin C, and iron, and has excessive protein, sodium and potassium.[57] Because young children need fat for neurodevelopment, nonfat and reduced-fat milk are not recommended before 2 years of age due to their low caloric density.[60]

FOOD ALLERGIES

Most food reactions occur during the first year of life. This is because food proteins with large molecular weight (10–60 Kd) are more capable of provoking immunological reactions in an immature gut.[61-62] The European Academy of Allergology and Clinical Immunology (EAACI) classifies food-related adverse reactions as toxic and nontoxic reactions. Toxic reactions occur in any individual if a sufficient dose of a toxic compound (e.g., food contaminants) is ingested. Nontoxic reactions depend on individual susceptibility and are the result of immune (food allergy) or nonimmune (food intolerance) mechanisms.[63]

Allergy vs. Intolerance

It is important to differentiate food allergies from food intolerance because many symptoms may overlap in presentation. Food allergies refer to clinical symptoms resulting from an inappropriate immunologic response to specific food proteins or additives. They can be classified as IgE-mediated and non-IgE mediated immune reactions.[63-64] Food intolerance refers to an adverse reaction or abnormal physiologic response to food or food additives that does not involve the immune system. The processes that cause food intolerance may be due to pharmacologic substances in the food (tyramine, histamine, serotonin in food), enzymatic deficiency (lactase deficiency), and idiosyncratic or neuropsychologic (hyperactivity, irritability) responses.[65]

IgE antibodies mediate the majority of food allergies, and their reactions are usually easily identified. IgE-mediated reactions usually appear within minutes to hours of ingesting an allergen. Symptoms may involve the skin, the respiratory system, and the gastrointestinal tract. Anaphylactic shock can occur within a few minutes to hours of ingesting the allergen, requiring immediate medical attention.[66] Skin symptoms are common and present as urticaria and atopic dermatitis. Upper and lower respiratory symptoms may present as tightness of the chest, shortness of breath, cough, rhinitis, angioedema, and wheezing. Gastrointestinal symptoms may include nausea, vomiting, diarrhea, abdominal cramps, oral and perioral pruritus, swelling of the lips, and throat tightness.[67-68]

Non-IgE-mediated reactions may involve IgA, IgG, and IgM antibodies or can be T-cell-mediated. Non-IgE-mediated reactions may take hours and days to develop. However, the role of these antibodies in food allergy is not clearly identified and measuring these antibodies to specific foods has limited usefulness. Some examples of non-IgE-mediated reactions include disorders such as allergic eosinophilic gastroenteritis, enterocolitis, and celiac disease, which are believed to have an immunologic basis.[65,69-70]

Common Food Allergens

Foods that most often cause an allergic reaction in the first year of life are cow's milk, eggs, wheat, peanuts, and soy. Fish, shellfish, peanuts, and tree nuts (such as walnuts and almonds) cause most allergic reactions in older children.[67,71] Some food additives like preservatives, dyes, sweetening agents, pH-adjusting chemicals, and emulsifiers may also trigger an allergic reaction.[64]

Cow's milk allergy (CMA) has become more prevalent since cow's milk formulas have been used as a breast milk substitute early in infancy. Cow's milk formulas contain much higher amounts of protein than breast milk. These proteins are potent allergens and may trigger gastrointestinal (vomiting and diarrhea) and cutaneous (urticaria and atopic dermatitis) reactions. Studies estimate that cow's milk allergy (CMA) occurs in 2% to 3% of infants.[72]

Early introduction of cow's milk may be a risk factor for CMA. In a prospective study of 6209 healthy full term infants, 13% of infants were exclusively breastfed and 87% required supplemental milk while in the maternity hospital. After an 18–34 month follow-up for symptoms suggestive of CMA, the cumulative incidence of CMA was 2.4% in infants fed cow's milk formula, compared to 1.7% and 1.5% for infants fed pasteurized human milk and whey hydrolysate formula, respectively. CMA developed in 2.1% of infants who were exclusively breastfed. The authors concluded that early cow's milk feeding increases the risk of CMA, but exclusive breastfeeding does not eliminate future risk.[73]

Diagnosing Food Allergy

Because the risks of developing food allergy can be related to environmental factors, exposure to allergens, and parental history of allergy, a thorough review of history for a suspected food allergy is crucial for the correct diagnosis. The history should include identification of the food in question, quantity of the food ingested, description of the symptoms, the time between

Common Food Allergens

❑ Foods that most often cause an allergic reaction in the first year of life are cow's milk, eggs, wheat, peanuts, and soy.

❑ Fish, shellfish, peanuts, and tree nuts (such as walnuts and almonds) cause most allergic reactions in older children.

❑ Some food additives like preservatives, dyes, sweetening agents, pH-adjusting chemicals, and emulsifiers may also trigger an allergic reaction.

Source:

Chandra RK. Food hypersensitivity and allergic disease: a selective review. *Am J Clin Nutr.* 1997;66:526S-9S.

Watson WT. Food allergy in children. *Clin Rev Allergy Immunol.* 1995;13:347-59.

Burks AW, Stanley JS. Food allergy. *Curr Opin Pediatr.* 1998;10:588-93.

the ingestion of the food and the onset of symptoms, description of any precipitating factors such as exercise, and form of the food (such as raw versus cooked) ingested.[65,69]

Several tests can confirm the diagnosis of food hypersensitivities. The double-blind placebo-controlled food challenge (DBPCFC) test is the "gold-standard" to confirm the diagnosis of food allergy.[74-76] The patient ingests graded amounts of the substance to be challenged versus placebo and is observed for any signs and symptoms of an allergic reaction. The test is performed a number of times and the response observed for at least 30 minutes. The patient, parents, and investigators performing the challenge are blinded to the administered substance. Only the person who prepared the challenge (such as a dietitian) knows if it is the real food or the placebo. The test is performed at a facility where emergency care is available in case of a severe reaction. The absence of an immediate reaction does not preclude a delayed-type reaction.[77]

If an IgE-mediated food allergy is suspected, skin testing for the presence of antibodies to suspected allergens should be performed. The skin prick test is the most practical and sensitive method to screen for IgE-mediated food allergy. A small drop of the food extract is placed on the skin and then the skin is scratched lightly through the drop using a specialized probe or needle. Food extracts are tested against positive (histamine) and negative (saline) controls. A negative skin test is highly predictive of the absence of IgE-mediated food hypersensitivity.[76,78] A positive skin test with the wheal at least 3 mm greater than the negative control indicates the presence of specific IgE to the food allergen.[79] A DBPCFC test is often needed to confirm positive skin test results.

The radioallergosorbent test (RAST) is another assay used to identify and quantify allergen-specific IgE antibodies in vitro. It is similar to the prick test in its accuracy but is more expensive.[68,71] T-lymphocyte markers have also been used to predict allergic disease. However, their uncertain predictive capacity and high cost limit their use.[80]

Treating Food Allergies

Treating food allergies relies on removing the offending allergen from the diet. If eliminating the offending foods does not result in clinical improvement, then the diagnosis should be reconsidered.[67,71]

Feeding formulas with hydrolyzed proteins reduce the allergenicity of cow's milk proteins. Partially hydrolyzed formulas contain a significant amount of peptides with molecular weights ranging between 8 and 40 Kd,[81] whereas extensively hydrolyzed formulas contain amino acids and peptides with molecular weight less than 1500 Kd.[70] However, no standardized criteria exist for defining peptide molecular weight as hypoallergenic or nonimmunogenic.[62,82]

The American Academy of Pediatrics has defined hypoallergenic formulas as those formulas that do not provoke reactions in 90% of infants and children with documented CMA with 95% confidence, based on prospective randomized double-blind placebo-controlled studies. Extensively hydrolyzed and free amino acid formulas meet these criteria and are considered hypoallergenic.[70] In a study of 28 infants with continued symptoms of protein intolerance (bloody stools, vomiting, diarrhea, irritability, failure to gain weight) while receiving casein hydrolysate formula, changing to an amino acid-based formula led to resolution of symptoms in 25 of the 28 infants.[83] In another study of 16 infants who had adverse reactions to cow's milk protein and persistent symptoms while exclusively receiving extensively hydrolyzed protein formulas, switching to an amino acid-based formula resulted in improvement in eczema, disappearance of noncutaneous symptoms, and weight gain in 13 of the 16 infants.[84]

Although most children with CMA tolerate extensively hydrolyzed formulas,[70,81] this may not always be the case for highly CMA allergic children.[81] In this case, amino acid-based formulas can serve as an alternative.[84] Milk from goats, sheep, or other animals, or partially hydrolyzed formulas are inappropriate substitutes in infants with CMA.[62]

About 14% of infants with IgE-mediated CMA will react to soy, but reports of anaphylactic reactions are rare.[70,85] However, a higher prevalence (25%–60%) of cross-sensitivity exists between soy protein and cow's milk among infants with non-IgE associated syndromes such as enterocolitis and proctocolitis. In these cases, therefore, soy formulas are not recommended and extensively hydrolyzed protein or amino acid-based formulas should be used to avoid similar cross-sensitivity reactions.[70]

Preventing Food Allergies

The role of breastfeeding in preventing food allergy remains controversial.[63] In a long-term follow-up study from birth to age 17, breastfeeding was associated with lower rates of food allergy and eczema at ages 1 and 3, and it protected against respiratory allergy up to age 17.[86] In another study, high-risk infants with a family history of atopy were followed until 5 years of age. Exclusively breastfed infants and those fed with partially hydrolyzed formula had a lower incidence of allergic disease compared to infants fed soy protein formula or conventional cow's milk formula.[87] Although these studies had methodological problems, they suggest that exclusive breastfeeding may protect high-risk infants—especially when common allergens are eliminated from the maternal diet during breastfeeding.[70]

Maternal dietary elimination of cow's milk and eggs during pregnancy does not prevent later appearance of food allergy in children.[80,88] In contrast, maternal dietary restriction of allergenic foods (cow's milk, eggs, fish, peanuts, tree nuts) during breastfeeding has shown to decrease the incidence of hypersensitivity reactions.[89-90] Allergenic proteins ingested by the mother pass into the breast milk and may cause a reaction in the child. Since human milk has many nutritional and immunological functions, the mother should avoid eating high-risk allergenic food instead of stopping breastfeeding. Because it is difficult to adhere to such a prophylactic regimen, investigators recommend prophylaxis in highly motivated mothers and families with a strong history of allergic diseases.[63]

Up to 85% of young children outgrow their food hypersensitivity by 3 years of age.[61,72] Also, children usually outgrow most non-IgE-mediated food allergies with time.[91] Allergies to peanuts, nuts, fish, and shellfish, however, are longer lasting and may not be outgrown. Patients with celiac disease have to avoid gluten for life.[65]

Delaying exposure to potentially allergenic foods may prevent or delay food allergies. Solid foods should be delayed until 6 months of age. Cow's milk should not be introduced before age 1 and eggs until age 2. Highly allergenic foods like peanuts, nuts, and fish should be excluded from the diet of all children for the first 3 years of life.[92-93]

For high-risk infants with food allergy, recommended prophylactic measures include exclusive breastfeeding, maternal avoidance of food allergens, and supplementation with hypoallergenic formulas if necessary.[94] Parents should educate themselves about food allergy, ensure that the child avoids major food allergens, and carefully read product labels to exclude allergenic ingredients. Also, providing psychological and social support to the growing child with allergies is necessary.

Treating Food Allergic Reactions

In the absence of respiratory or cardiovascular symptoms, diphenhydramine may be used for skin reactions.[95] Medications such as corticosteroids, antihistamines, ketotifen, and cromolyn sodium may alleviate the symptoms of food allergy but have minimal efficacy in preventing attack exacerbations.[91] Acute severe reactions such as angioedema, urticaria, respiratory problems, and hypotension should be treated immediately with epinephrine and bronchodilators. Patients with potential anaphylactic reactions should have a prefilled epinephrine syringe and antihistamines available at all times for self-administration.[91] Prefilled epinephrine in 2 mL syringes are available via prescription as EpiPen (0.3 mg) or EpiPen Jr. Auto-Injector (0.15 mg) for intramuscular injection. They should be auto-injected into the outer thigh as soon as the symptoms of anaphylaxis are detected. Antihistamines and steroids are often used to further improve recovery, but never instead of epinephrine.

Valuable educational material on food allergies can be obtained from the Food Allergy Network (Fairfax, Virginia; phone: 800-929-4040; Web site: http://www.foodallergy.org).

INBORN ERRORS OF METABOLISM

Inborn errors are defined as "discontinuous traits resulting from variation in the structure and function of enzymes and protein molecules."[96] This section briefly describes three inherited metabolic diseases out of hundreds of genetic disorders that have a defined biochemical basis. These metabolic diseases are inherited as autosomal recessive disorders known as phenylketonuria (PKU), maple syrup urine disease (MSUD), and organic acidemias and acidurias. They are managed with diet restriction and/or supplementation of specific cofactors. Specific guidelines for nutrition support in inborn errors of metabolism can be found in sources outside this text.[96-97]

Children may develop signs of an inborn error of metabolism at different stages of early life, but the majority of metabolic problems appear during the first few days after birth. Affected infants may have nonspecific signs and symptoms such as poor feeding, vomiting, metabolic acidosis, failure to thrive, neurological symptoms, and elevated blood or urine levels of specific amino acids and organic acids. If a physician suspects that a patient has an inborn error of metabolism, numerous laboratory studies are performed including urinalysis, urine organic acids and reducing substances, serum electrolytes, blood glucose, blood gases, plasma and urine amino acids, urine ketones if there is acidosis or hypoglycemia, and plasma ammonia and lactate.[98-100]

Nutrient requirements for patients with inborn errors of metabolism may differ from those based on the RDA for normal individuals.[97] The goals of providing specialized nutrition to these children include promoting normal growth, preventing or minimizing neurologic impairment, and avoiding metabolic crisis.[101] These goals can be nutritionally achieved by the following interventions:[97,101]

1. Providing high caloric feedings.
2. Restricting specific nutrients to correct the primary imbalance (e.g., restriction of branched chain acids leucine, isoleucine, and valine in MSUD).
3. Providing alternate pathways for metabolism to reduce toxic substrate accumulation (e.g., glycine and carnitine supplementation in isovaleric acidemia).
4. Providing products of a blocked pathway (e.g., arginine in urea cycle disorders).

5. Supplementing certain conditionally essential nutrients (e.g., carnitine in organic acidurias).
6. Replacing deficient cofactors (e.g., vitamin B_{12} in methylmalonic aciduria).
7. Providing additional vitamins to stabilize altered enzymes (e.g., thiamine in MSUD).
8. Supplementing nutrients that are not adequately absorbed or released (e.g., zinc in acrodermatitis enteropathica).

Children with inborn errors of metabolism require frequent monitoring and adjustment of the nutrition prescription. Appropriate therapy is important to ensure normal growth of the infant. Patients and caregivers need to be aware of the signs and symptoms of metabolic crisis and seek immediate medical intervention to avoid any irreversible damage.

Phenylketonuria (PKU)

The classic PKU results from complete or near complete deficiency of the phenylalanine hydroxylase enzyme that is responsible for metabolizing phenylalanine to tyrosine. This deficiency causes phenylalanine and its metabolites to accumulate and cause brain damage. Phenylketonuria is one of the different forms of hyperphenylalaninemia.

Children with classic PKU typically have an unpleasant odor that is described as mousy or musty due to accumulation of phenylacetic acid. Infants with PKU are normal at birth but neurological problems and mental retardation develop gradually. The biochemical assessment of classic PKU shows a plasma phenylalanine concentration of greater than 20 mg/dL, normal plasma concentrations of tyrosine and cofactor tetrahydrobiopterin, and increased urinary concentrations of phenylalanine metabolites.[98]

Maternal PKU embryopathy is a distinct condition that affects children born of mothers with PKU. Therefore, a woman affected with PKU needs to have a phenylalanine restricted diet throughout pregnancy to maintain blood concentrations less than 10 mg/dL.[101]

Treatment of PKU consists of a low phenylalanine diet with adequate intake of tyrosine, which becomes an essential amino acid in patients with PKU. Because phenylalanine is an essential amino acid, patients must maintain serum phenylalanine concentrations of 3–15 mg/dL to avoid deficiency.[98,102] Special nutritional preparations (such as Lofenalac and Phenex-1) are available for patients with PKU.

Maple Syrup Urine Disease (MSUD)

MSUD is caused by the deficiency of the enzyme complex chain alpha ketoacid dehydrogenase that is responsible for the decarboxylation of branched chain amino acids. The name comes from the sweet odor of maple syrup in urine, sweat, and cerumen.

In MSUD, high levels of leucine lead to neurological injury. Depending on the severity of clinical presentation, symptoms can vary from vomiting to central nervous system involvement, coma, and death. Plasma concentrations of branched chain amino acids are also elevated.[98,103]

The acute treatment of MSUD symptoms includes intravenous hydration and sometimes the administration of parenteral nutrition free of branched chain amino acids. Long-term management consists of a low branched chain amino acids diet. Special nutritional preparations (such as MSUD Diet Powder and Ketonex-1) are available for MSUD patients.

Organic Acidemias and Acidurias

Examples of organic acidemias and acidurias include propionic acidemia, methylmalonic acidemia, isovaleric acidemia, multiple carboxylase deficiency, and mevalonic aciduria. Patients may present with hyperammonemia, encephalopathy, and metabolic acidosis. These symptoms result from the accumulation of toxic metabolites in the central nervous system.

Once an infant is suspected of having organic acidemia, treatment must be initiated immediately. Treatment of acute attacks consists of hydration, correction of metabolic acidosis, and removal of accumulated organic acids or ammonia through hemodialysis. Intramuscular vitamin B_{12} injections should be given in the case of vitamin B_{12}-responsive methylmalonic acidemia. Biotin should be supplemented in acidemias associated with biotin deficiency.[98-99] Special nutritional preparations are available for patients with isovaleric acidemia (such as I-Valex-1) and for propionic acidemia and methylmalonic acidemia (such as Propimex-1).

ENTERAL FEEDINGS

Enteral feedings are indicated in the pediatric patient with a functioning gastrointestinal tract when ingestion of sufficient nutrients by mouth is compromised. Even if the patient cannot tolerate full enteral feedings, small volume feedings should be attempted to preserve intestinal function.[104] Contraindications to enteral feedings include necrotizing enterocolitis (NEC), bowel obstruction, severe inflammatory bowel disease, and intestinal atresia.

Enteral Formulas

Various infant and pediatric enteral formulas are available in different formulations to address individual patients' needs. They are formulated based on age-specific nutrient requirements and the maturity of the child's gastrointestinal, liver, and kidney function. Formulas are available for premature infants, full-term infants under 1 year of age, children 1–10 years of age, children over 10 years of age, and children with inborn errors of metabolism. Preterm and term infant formulas and special formulas for children with inborn errors of metabolism are discussed earlier in this chapter.

For children 1–10 years of age, a cow's milk-based intact protein formula with a caloric density of 1 kcal/mL may be used. Some formulas contain

TABLE 6-9 Guidelines for Enteral Feeding Initiation in Premature Infants

Birth weight (g)	≤1000	>1000–<1250	1250–1500	>1500–2000	>2000–2500
Feeding Rate or Volume*	0.5 mL/hr	1 mL/hr	3 mL	4 mL	5 mL
Frequency*	continuous	continuous	q 3 hrs	q 3 hrs	q 3 hrs

* Keep feeding at this rate or volume and frequency for the first 24 hours. Advance feeding volume afterwards in the clinically stable infant by 10–20 mL/kg/day based on tolerance.

MCT to improve fat supplementation in patients with malabsorption. These formulas provide the RDA for vitamins and minerals in quantities of 1000 mL/day for children 1–6 years of age, and 1300 mL/day for children 7–10 years of age. For patients with normal gastrointestinal function, a standard formula is recommended (such as Pediasure, Kindercal, or Nutren Jr). Fiber-containing formulas (such as Pediasure with fiber) are also available and benefit patients experiencing constipation or diarrhea. For children who are intolerant to milk protein or with malabsorption, a hydrolyzed whey formula (such as Peptamen Jr or Pro-Peptide for Kids) may be provided. Amino acid-based formulas for children are also available (such as Vivonex Pediatric and Neocate One +). Table 6-5 shows examples of formulas used for children.

For adolescents, adult enteral formulas are usually used. Adult enteral feeding formulas are described in Chapter 7.

Modular components including protein, carbohydrates, and fat modules are available to supplement standard and specialized formulas as needed depending on the clinical situation and nutrient requirements. Modular protein products (such as ProMod, Casec, or Resource Instant Protein Powder) increase the protein caloric density. Modular glucose polymers (such as Polycose or Moducal) enhance the caloric density with carbohydrates. Fat products (such as Microlipid or MCT oil) may also be used for fat supplementation.

Enteral Feeding Methods and Guidelines

The enteral feeding delivery route and feeding method depend on the patient's clinical condition and tolerance. Initiation and advancement of feedings are largely based on institutional practices.

Bolus enteral feedings is the preferred method for children under 1 year of age in order to resemble nipple feeds and mimic physiologic postprandial hormonal and enzymatic release. However, continuous feeding is better tolerated and preferred in patients at risk for aspiration, in patients with a history of intolerance to enteral feeding, or following a prolonged bowel rest. Feeding begins with low volumes and slow rate to allow the gastrointestinal tract to adapt gradually. Enteral feedings are usually advanced to goal over 2–5 days with adjustments made to meet individual needs.

Table 6-9 gives guidelines for initiating enteral feedings in premature infants.

In term infants and older children, continuous feedings can be initiated at 0.5–2 mL/kg/hour and advanced in increments of 0.5–1 mL/kg/hour

> ### Parenteral Nutrition
>
> Parenteral nutrition (PN) is the intravenous administration of complete and balanced nutrition to support anabolism, maintain weight, or promote weight gain. PN is a source of macronutrients for energy (amino acids, dextrose, lipids), micronutrients (vitamins, trace minerals), fluids, and electrolytes.
>
> PN is a life-saving therapy in patients with gastrointestinal failure. PN is indicated when oral or enteral feedings are contraindicated or as a supplemental energy source when enteral feeding fails to meet nutritional needs.

every 8–12 hours as tolerated until the nutritional goal is reached. Bolus feedings are initiated at 2–5 mL/kg every 3–4 hours and advanced to goal as tolerated in increments of 2–5 mL/kg every two feedings.

In adolescents, continuous enteral feedings may be started at 25–50 mL/hr depending on tolerance, and advanced as tolerated to goal rate in increments of 20–25 mL/hr every 8–12 hours.[14]

To avoid feeding intolerance, enteral feedings may be initiated at half-strength in patients with altered gastrointestinal function and advanced slowly in critically ill and malnourished patients. The rate and strength of enteral feeding formula should not be advanced simultaneously. If feeding intolerance develops while advancing feeding, the previously tolerated concentration or volume should be used and re-advanced at a slower rate.

Before each intermittent feeding, gastric residuals should be checked to assess for tolerance. If the residual volume is greater than twice the volume previously given, feedings should be stopped. Residuals should then be rechecked in 1 hour. If residuals decrease, feeding can be restarted at the previous rate. Complications of enteral feedings and their management are described in Chapter 7.

PARENTERAL NUTRITION

Parenteral nutrition (PN) is the intravenous administration of complete and balanced nutrition to support anabolism, maintain weight, or promote weight gain. PN is a source of macronutrients for energy (amino acids, dextrose, lipids), micronutrients (vitamins, trace minerals), fluids, and electrolytes.

Indications for Parenteral Nutrition in Children

Hypermetabolism and hypercatabolism occur with severe illness and cause mobilization of the patient's energy stores. Inadequate caloric and protein intake along with increased energy expenditure place children at risk for malnutrition, growth failure, and delayed recovery.[105]

PN, a life-saving therapy in patients with gastrointestinal failure, is indicated when oral or enteral feedings are contraindicated or as a supplemental energy source when enteral feeding fails to meet nutritional needs. The decision to initiate PN should be balanced against its complications and high

Clinical Conditions Likely to Require PN in Children

❑ Congenital anomalies: severe Hirshprung's disease, gastroschisis, bowel atresia, volvolus, meconium ileus.
❑ Gastrointestinal disorders: short bowel syndrome, malabsorption, intractable diarrhea, bowel obstruction, protracted vomiting, necrotizing enterocolitis, motility disorders, inflammatory bowel disease, acute pancreatitis, enteric fistulas.
❑ Risk for aspiration pneumonia in acute illness.
❑ Severe mucositis secondary to chemotherapy.
❑ Premature infants with very low birth weight, where enteral feeding is inadequate.
❑ Premature infants with severe respiratory distress syndrome.

cost. Because bowel rest during PN causes alteration in the structural and functional integrity of the intestines,[106] early initiation of enteral nutrition is essential to stimulate gut function, prevent gut villi atrophy,[107] and reduce PN-associated hepatobiliary complications.[108] The sidebar above lists clinical conditions in children where PN may be indicated.

Parenteral Nutrition Components and Requirements

Amino Acids

The available intravenous crystalline amino acid formulas differ in their amino acid composition, concentration, and electrolyte content. All pediatric formulations contain the eight essential amino acids. The amino acids cysteine, tyrosine, glycine, and taurine are considered conditionally essential under certain circumstances. Neonatal-specific amino acid formulas are associated with greater weight gain and more positive nitrogen balance compared to standard formulas.[109]

Neonatal-specific amino acid formulas have added taurine, an amino acid that enhances bile acid conjugation, improves bile flow, and has a role in neurotransmission.[48,110] Premature infants are at risk for taurine deficiency due to increased taurine renal losses and low cystathionase activity—the rate-limiting enzyme in taurine biosynthesis from cysteine.[48,111] Also, long-term PN without taurine supplements may result in low plasma taurine concentrations.[112-133] Table 6-10 gives examples of neonatal and pediatric intravenous amino acid formulas.

Amino acids are a source of calories and nitrogen for protein synthesis, with an energy contribution of 4 kcal/g of amino acids. However, the question of whether amino acids should be included in the total energy calculation is up for debate. Two opposing positions address this question in a published discussion.[114] Including amino acids in the total energy calculation stems from the idea that a substantial amount of amino acids is oxidized to generate

TABLE 6-10 Examples of Neonatal and Pediatric Parenteral Amino Acid Formulas

	Product (Manufacturer)			
	Trophamine 10% (Braun)	Aminosyn-PF 10% (Abbott)	Aminosyn 10% (Abbott)	Travasol 10% (Clintec)
Crystalline Amino Acid Concentration	10%	10%	10%	10%
Nitrogen (g/100 mL)	1.55	1.52	1.57	1.65
Essential Amino Acids (mg/100 mL)				
Leucine	1400	1200	940	730
Isoleucine	820	760	720	600
Valine	780	673	800	580
Lysine	820	677	720	580
Methionine	340	180	400	400
Phenylalanine	480	427	440	560
Threonine	420	512	520	420
Tryptophan	200	180	160	180
Nonessential Amino Acids (mg/100 mL)				
Alanine	540	698	1280	2070
Arginine	1200	1227	980	1150
Histidine	480	312	300	480
Proline	680	812	860	680
Serine	380	495	420	500
Taurine	25	70	0	0
Tyrosine	240	44	44	40
Glycine	360	385	1280	1030
Glutamic acid	500	820	0	0
Aspartic acid	320	527	0	0
Cysteine	< 16	0	0	0
Electrolytes (mEq/L)				
Sodium	5	3.4	0	0
Potassium	0	0	5.4	0
Chloride	< 3	0	0	40
Acetate	97	46.3	148	87
pH	5–6	5.4	5.3	6
Osmolarity (mOsm/L)	875	829	1000	1000

adenosine triphosphate (ATP) and energy. The opposing point counters that amino acids avoid oxidation and are used to build lean body mass, get converted to glucose, or are lost as nitrogenous products in the urine or through the gut—and therefore should not be included as a source of calories.[114-115] Because of this controversy, institutional practices vary as to whether or not to include amino acids in calorie calculations.

Parenteral amino acids provide 10%–15% of total calories. For neonates, amino acids are started at 1 g/kg/day and advanced as tolerated to 2.5–3 g/kg/day. Amino acid requirements for infants are 2–2.5 g/kg/day and then decrease to 1.5–2 g/kg/day in older children, and to 1–1.5 g/kg/day in adolescents. Adjustments to the amino acid dose should consider the patient's clinical condition and nutritional status. For example, patients receiving dialysis or continuous renal replacement therapies (CRRT) require higher doses of amino acids to make up for losses via the dialysis membrane and filter.[116] Nondialyzed renal failure patients or patients with liver failure and hyperammonemia, on the other hand, require decreased dosages of amino acids.

Dextrose

Parenteral dextrose is a major source of calories and a source of carbon skeletons necessary for tissue accretion. It is available in the monohydrate form that provides 3.4 kcal/g of dextrose. In infants, continuous dextrose infusion is usually initiated at a rate of 4–8 mg/kg/minute and advanced daily at 2 mg/kg/minute until the nutritional goal is reached with a maximum of 10–14 mg/kg/minute.[117-118] In most children and adolescents receiving PN, dextrose is adjusted to provide 50%–60% of total calories.

Lipid Emulsions

Intravenous lipid emulsions are a source of condensed calories and essential fatty acids. Because lipid emulsions are derived from vegetable oils, they are a natural source of variable amounts of vitamin K[119] and vitamin E isomers.[120-121]

Available lipid emulsions are made of LCT. A mixture of LCT and MCT is available in Europe but is still investigational in the United States.

The caloric value of lipid emulsions varies with the concentration. The 10%, 20%, and 30% concentrations yield 1.1 kcal/mL, 2 kcal/mL, and 3 kcal/mL, respectively. The 30% lipid emulsion should be administered in total nutrient admixtures (TNA)—the admixture of amino acids, dextrose, and lipid emulsions in one solution.

Table 6-11 gives examples of intravenous lipid emulsions.

Lipid emulsions usually provide 20%–30% of total calories. In infants and children, lipid emulsions are initiated at 1 g/kg/day and advanced by 0.5–1 g/kg/day to a maximum dose of 3 g/kg/day. A lipid dose of 0.5–1 g/kg/day prevents essential fatty acid deficiency.[122]

Lipid emulsions should be used with caution in neonates with physiologic hyperbilirubinemia. The risk of kernicterus—a neonatal bilirubin-induced encephalopathy—is significantly increased when total serum bilirubin levels exceed 20 mg/dL. Fatty acids are highly protein-bound and may compete with bilirubin for albumin binding sites. This may displace bilirubin and increase the risk of kernicterus. The American Academy of Pediatrics recommends limiting the lipid emulsion dose to 0.5–1 g/kg/day when bilirubin levels exceed 10 mg/dL.[123]

TABLE 6-11 Examples of Intravenous Lipid Emulsion Formulas

Fat Source	Intralipid (Clintec) Soybean oil			Liposyn III (Abbott) Soybean oil			Liposyn II (Abbott) Soybean and Safflower oil (equal parts)	
Total fat (%)	10	20	30	10	20	30	10	20
Linoleic acid (%)	50	50	50	54.5	54.5	54.5	65.8	65.8
Linolenic acid (%)	9	9	9	8.3	83	8.3	4.2	4.2
Oleic acid (%)	26	26	26	22.4	22.4	22.4	17.7	17.7
Palmitic acid (%)	10	10	10	10.5	10.5	10.5	8.8	8.8
Stearic acid (%)	3.5	3.5	3.5	4.2	4.2	4.2	3.4	3.4
Egg phosphatides (%)*	1.2	1.2	1.2	1.2	1.2	1.2	1.2	1.2
Glycerin (%)†	2.25	2.25	1.7	2.5	2.5	1.7	2.5	2.5
Kcal/mL	1.1	2	3	1.1	2	3	1.1	2
pH	6–8.9	6–8.9	6–8.9	6–9	6–9	6–9	6–9	6–9
Osmolarity (mOsm/L)	260	260	310	284	292	293	276	258
PL:TG ratio¶	0.12	0.06	0.04	0.12	0.06	0.04	0.12	0.06

* Emulsifiers.
† To adjust tonicity.
¶ Phospholids:Triglycerides ratio.

Multivitamins

Multivitamins are essential for substrate metabolism, normal body resistance, and tissue repair. Pediatric parenteral multivitamins provide water- and fat-soluble vitamins that are added to the daily PN. The formulation is based on the RDA for oral intake in healthy children and follows the recommendations of the Nutrition Advisory Group of the American Medical Association (NAG-AMA). Guidelines for parenteral vitamin use were also provided by the American Society of Clinical Nutrition as part of a report on guidelines for parenteral nutrient requirements in infants and children receiving PN.[124]

There are no commercially available intravenous multivitamin products designed to meet the requirements of premature infants. The current formulation dosed at the RDA levels results in low concentrations of vitamin A and high concentrations of water-soluble vitamins in premature infants. Additionally, losses of vitamin A in PN by adherence to plastic and photooxidation results in inadequate vitamin A. As a result, additional vitamin A may be required, especially in LBW infants at risk for lung disease.

Due to higher metabolic demands under stressful conditions, depletion of water-soluble vitamins may occur in the absence of adequate vitamin intake. Thiamine deficiency, which causes lactic acidosis, has been reported with dextrose infusions.[125-126] Thiamine is a coenzyme for glucose metabolism that is essential for the metabolism of pyruvate and oxidation of keto acids. In case of thiamine deficiency, pyruvate cannot be oxidized by the citric acid

TABLE 6-12   Composition and Dosing of Parenteral Multivitamins

	Product (Manufacturer)	
	MVI® Pediatric* - 5 mL (NeoSan) **Infuvite Pediatric* - 5 mL¶ (Baxter)**	**Infuvite Adult - 10 mL (Baxter)†**
Water-soluble vitamins (units)		
Thiamine (mg)	1.2	6
Riboflavin (mg)	1.4	3.6
Niacin (mg)	17	40
Pantothenic acid (mg)	5	15
Pyridoxine (mg)	1	6
Cyanocobalamin (mcg)	1	5
Ascorbic acid (mg)	80	200
Biotin (mcg)	20	60
Folate (mcg)	140	600
Fat-soluble vitamins (units)		
A (IU)	2300	3300
D (IU)	400	200
E (IU)	7	10
K (mcg)	200	150

* Dosage: infants < 1 kg: 1.5 mL/day. Infants 1-3 kg: 3.25 mL/day. Infants and children > 3 kg up to 11 years of age: 5 mL/day.

† For patients ≥ 11 years of age. A daily dose of 10 mL added to PN (after mixing 5 mL of vial 1 and 5 mL of vial 2).

¶ 5 mL after mixing 4 mL of vial 1 and 1 mL of vial 2.

cycle and is converted instead to lactate by the action of lactate dehydrogenase.[127] Cases of lactic acidosis and deaths due to thiamine deficiency have been reported during periodic nationwide multivitamin shortages in the United States.[128-129]

Table 6-12 outlines the composition of parenteral multivitamins used in the pediatric population.

Trace Minerals

Trace minerals are cofactors for enzyme function in various biochemical reactions. Pediatric intravenous trace minerals provide a combination of zinc, copper, manganese, and chromium. Some formulations also contain selenium. These trace minerals are added to the daily PN unless restriction of any of the minerals is indicated. Table 6-13 shows various trace mineral requirements with PN in relation to age.[115,136]

Trace mineral formulations meet the recommendations of the AGA-AMA and the Society of Clinical Nutrition for daily intravenous supplements of trace minerals in the absence of deficiencies. Table 6-14 shows the composition of these formulations. Individual trace mineral formulations are also available and may be used at individual doses when it is necessary to supplement or restrict a specific trace mineral.

TABLE 6-13 Recommended Daily Requirements of Trace Minerals in Parenteral Nutrition

Trace Mineral	Preterm Infant mcg/kg	Term Infant mcg/kg	Children mcg/kg (maximum mcg/day)	Adolescents
Chromium	0.2	0.2	0.14–0.2 (5)	5–15 mcg
Copper	20	20	20 (300)	200–500 mcg
Manganese	1	1	1 (50)	50–150 mcg
Selenium	2	2–3	2–3 (30)	30–40 mcg
Zinc	400	300	50 (5000)	2–5 mg

Source: References 115, 136.

TABLE 6-14 Examples of Parenteral Trace Mineral Combination Products for Pediatrics (concentrations per mL)

	Trace Minerals				
	Zinc (mg) as sulfate	Copper (mg) as sulfate	Manganese (mcg) as sulfate	Chromium (mcg) as chloride	Selenium (mcg) as selenious acid
Product (Manufacturer)					
PTE-5 (APP*)	1	0.1	25	1	15
PTE-4 (APP)	1	0.1	25	1	0
Neotrace-4 (APP)	1.5	0.1	25	0.85	0
Pedtrace-4 (APP)	0.5	0.1	25	0.85	0
PedTE-PAK-4 (Solopak)	1	0.1	25	1	0
Multitrace-4 Neonatal (American Regent)	1.5	0.1	25	0.85	0
Multitrace-4 Pediatric (American Regent)	0.5	0.1	30	1	0

* APP = American Pharmaceutical Partners.

Although blood concentrations of trace minerals may not correlate with tissue stores, especially during the metabolic stress in response to injury, monitoring blood concentrations of trace minerals provides guidance under conditions when deficiency or toxicity may occur.[130] Here are a few examples:

- Zinc losses increase in patients with high stool losses and malabsorption, such as with short bowel syndrome.[131-132]
- Since excretion of copper and manganese is reduced in patients with cholestasis, restricting these minerals may be necessary to prevent their accumulation. When copper and manganese are restricted, their blood concentrations should be measured periodically to avoid deficiencies.

TABLE 6-15 Daily Fluid Requirements in Children

Weight	Daily Fluid Requirements*
Preterm infants	100–150 mL/kg[†]
1–10 kg	100 mL/kg
10–20 kg	1000 mL + 50 mL for each kg over 10 kg
> 20 kg	1500 mL + 20 mL for each kg over 20 kg

* May vary based on clinical conditions.
[†] Goal reached in 5 days.
Source: Reference 136.

- Neurotoxicity has been reported with high serum manganese concentrations in patients with cholestasis who were receiving long-term PN.[133-134]
- Fatal pancytopenia from copper deficiency was reported in a patient receiving PN after copper was restricted due to severe cholestasis.[135]

Fluids and Electrolytes

The PN solution provides a significant source of fluids and electrolytes. In the acute care setting, the PN solution should be tailored to provide the required calories—not to manage acute fluid and electrolyte losses. Instead, patients receive a separate intravenous solution to supplement fluid and electrolyte losses. In fluid-restricted patients, the PN solution is concentrated to avoid fluid overload. And for convenient administration in the home setting, daily fluid and electrolyte requirements are incorporated into the PN admixture. Table 6-15 details the guidelines for estimating maintenance fluid requirements in children.[136]

Electrolyte adjustments in PN are based on serum electrolyte concentrations. Adjustments should account for all electrolyte sources and losses, acid base status, clinical conditions, and medications that affect electrolyte balance. Table 6-16 gives the daily parenteral electrolyte requirements for pediatric and neonatal patients.[136-137]

Sodium is added to the PN solution as a chloride, acetate, or phosphate salt. Following birth, neonates develop natriuresis—the excretion of sodium in the urine—that may last up to 2 weeks. Postnatal natriuresis is more pronounced in premature infants due to kidney immaturity and reduced ability for sodium retention. In this case, sodium supplementation is necessary to promote appropriate protein synthesis and tissue development.[138] The maximum concentration of sodium in PN should be limited to 154 mEq/L, the equivalent of isotonic normal saline.

Potassium is added to the PN solution as a chloride, acetate, or phosphate salt. Potassium concentrations are usually limited to 80 mEq/L in PN solutions, with a potassium infusion rate not exceeding 0.5 mEq/kg/hour or the maximum of 10 mEq/hr in infants and children.[139] Since potassium, magnesium,

TABLE 6-16 Daily Parenteral Electrolyte Requirements*

Electrolyte	Neonates	Infants and Children	Adolescents
Sodium	2–5 mEq/kg	2–5 mEq/kg	Individualized
Potassium	2–4 mEq/kg	2–3 mEq/kg	80–180 mEq
Magnesium	0.25–1 mEq/kg	0.25–1 mEq/kg	8–24 mEq
Calcium	1–3 mEq/kg	1–2 mEq/kg	10–15 mEq
Phosphorus	0.5–2 mmol/kg	0.5–1 mmol/kg	10–40 mmol
Chloride	2–5 mEq/kg	2–5 mEq/kg	Individualized

* Adjusted based on clinical conditions.

Note: Sodium requirements in premature infants may be as high as 8 mEq/kg/day.

Source: References 136-137.

and phosphate are constituents of body cell mass, their requirements are increased during anabolism.[140]

Phosphates are dosed in millimoles because they dissociate in monobasic and dibasic forms depending on the pH of the solution.[141] When calculating the total contribution of electrolyte in solution, the amount of elemental sodium or potassium in phosphate salts should be considered. One mmol of potassium phosphate yields 1.47 mEq of potassium, while 1 mmol of sodium phosphate yields 1.33 mEq of sodium.

Infants and children require increased calcium and phosphate due to their accelerated growth. Phosphate is required intracellularly to generate high-energy phosphate bonds and form bones. Following birth, urinary phosphate excretion is high. This may result in hypophosphatemia, which is commonly observed in premature infants.[142]

The amount and ratio of calcium and phosphorus provided in PN are crucial to promoting bone mineralization. Maximizing calcium and phosphorus intake is essential to preventing metabolic bone disease.[143] Adequate bone mineral retention is achieved at a calcium-to-phosphorus ratio of 1.7 mg:1 mg or the approximate equivalent of 2.6 mEq:1 mmol.[144] Due to solubility limitations, however, it becomes difficult to maximize calcium and phosphorus in the neonatal PN solution.

Chloride is largely eliminated via the kidneys. When there is an excess of chlorides in the blood—known as hyperchloremia—due to excessive chloride salt infusion, metabolic acidosis may result.[145] When excess acetate is provided, metabolic alkalosis may result since acetate is converted in vivo to bicarbonate.[146]

The ability of premature infants to respond to acid base disturbances is reduced due to the inefficient kidney capacity for bicarbonate reabsorption and hydrogen ions excretion.[138,147] The chloride-to-acetate ratio can be adjusted in PN based on the acid base status of the patient.[148] For example, a low chloride-to-high acetate ratio of 0.5:1.5 helps with metabolic acidosis in cases of diarrhea or high fistula output. A high chloride-to-low acetate ratio of 1.5:0.5 helps with metabolic alkalosis, in cases such as secondary to excessive gastric fluid losses. In the absence of acid base disturbances, a chloride-to-acetate ratio of 1.5:1 may be used.

Carnitine Supplementation

Carnitine is a quaternary amine that facilitates the transport of long chain fatty acids across the mitochondrial membrane where they undergo oxidation.[149] Premature infants are at risk for carnitine deficiency due to their reduced carnitine biosynthetic capacity and limited carnitine reserves.[150-151] Since carnitine is not routinely added to PN solutions, children receiving PN can have low plasma carnitine concentrations[152-155] and tissue carnitine depletion.[156]

In clinical studies in neonates receiving PN,[157-160] carnitine supplementation normalized plasma carnitine concentrations, improved ketogenesis,[157-159] enhanced fat oxidation,[160] and fostered better tolerance of lipid emulsions.[158] Although blood and tissue levels of carnitine are low in premature infants, the correlation between these low levels and poor lipid tolerance in the parenterally fed infant is uncertain. Nonetheless, a trial of carnitine supplementation at a dose of 3–10 mg/kg/day added to neonatal PN is warranted in premature infants who develop unexplained hypertriglyceridemia while receiving lipid emulsions.[161-162]

Complications Associated with Parenteral Nutrition

Complications associated with PN can be classified as technical, metabolic, and infectious.

Technical Complications

Technical or catheter insertion-related complications are rare but can be serious. These complications depend on the vein approach and may include arrhythmias, blood vessel perforation, venous thrombosis, catheter malposition, pneumothorax, hydrothorax, hemothorax, chylothorax, and brachial plexus injury.[163]

Metabolic Complications

Metabolic complications that may be associated with PN include hyperglycemia, hypoglycemia, hypertriglyceridemia, acid base disturbances, electrolyte abnormalities, hepatobiliary complications, and metabolic bone disease.

Hyperglycemia

Hyperglycemia in patients receiving PN primarily results from excessive or rapid carbohydrate infusion. Other factors also predispose patients to hyperglycemia including prematurity,[164] sepsis, surgery,[165] and steroid therapy.

Premature infants have variable glucose regulation due to saturation of insulin receptors, or the immaturity of hepatic and pancreatic response.[166-167] Hyperglycemia may appear early after PN initiation, but blood glucose concentrations will likely return to normal after endogenous insulin secretion adjusts to dextrose infusion. If untreated, hyperglycemia can cause osmotic diuresis that may lead to hyperosmolar hyperglycemic nonketotic dehydration and electrolyte disturbances.[118] Also, excessive dextrose infusion and the resultant hyperglycemia can lead to hypertriglyceridemia,[168] impaired phagocytosis,[169] liver steatosis, and increased carbon dioxide production, which increases the patient's respiratory workload.[170-171]

The first way to manage hyperglycemia is to reduce the carbohydrate load if elevated. However, this reduction may compromise nutritional intake. When hyperglycemia occurs, a continuous regular insulin infusion at 0.01–0.1 unit/kg/hour may be started and titrated depending on blood glucose concentrations. Continuous intravenous insulin infusion corrects hyperglycemia and allows maximizing dextrose delivery to meet the infant's growth needs.[172]

Hypoglycemia

In patients receiving PN, hypoglycemia is usually due to the sudden reduction or cessation of dextrose infusion. Rebound hypoglycemia is caused by continued endogenous insulin secretion stimulated by high dextrose infusion, despite the reduction in dextrose infusion rate.[173] Rebound hypoglycemia can be avoided by gradually slowing down the PN infusion rate over 1–2 hours before discontinuation.[173-174] Intravenous administration of dextrose 10% or 12.5% in water after discontinuing PN also prevents rebound hypoglycemia. Premature infants are especially at risk for hypoglycemia due to the immaturity of their protective metabolic response including gluconeogenesis, ketogenesis, and hepatic glycogenolysis. To avoid any detrimental neurological effects, it is important to avoid and promptly correct hypoglycemia.[175]

Hypertriglyceridemia

Hypertriglyceridemia in patients receiving PN can result from excessive dextrose,[168] excessive lipid emulsion administration,[176] prematurity,[177] or sepsis.[178] It can also be drug-induced, such as with steroid therapy.[179] Hyperlipidemia may affect pulmonary gas diffusion[180] and pulmonary vascular resistance,[181] mainly in low birth weight infants with preexisting pulmonary and vascular disease.[182-183]

Premature infants and critically ill patients are at higher risk for hypertriglyceridemia with lipid infusion due to depressed lipoprotein lipase (LPL) activity,[184] the enzyme that metabolizes lipid particles in the blood.[185] If the hypertriglyceridemia is concomitant with uncontrolled hyperglycemia, then excess glucose is the most likely cause. In this case, the dextrose load should be reduced first. If reducing the dextrose load does not improve the hypertriglyceridemia, then the lipid dose should be decreased to 0.5–1 g/kg/day, especially when serum triglyceride concentrations are more than 200 mg/dL.[44] Then, the dextrose load should be increased back to avoid undernutrition. Also, infusing lipids over 24 hours whenever possible improves clearance.

Using the 20% lipid emulsion is recommended due to its favorable lipid profile. In one study, replacing the infusion of the 10% with the 20% lipid emulsion at equal lipid doses of 2 g/kg/day resulted in a rapid decline in serum triglyceride, cholesterol, and phospholipid concentrations.[186] The higher phospholipid-to-triglyceride ratio in the 10% compared to the 20% emulsion may result in the formation and accumulation of cholesterol, triglycerides and phospholipids in the form of an abnormal lipoprotein X.[187-188]

These Lipoprotein X particles compete with triglycerides for clearance, and are slowly cleared from the bloodstream.[189-190]

Acid Base Disturbances

Of the acid-base disorders associated with PN, metabolic acidosis may occur as a result of excessive chloride salts in the PN solution.[191-192] It can also result when cysteine hydrochloride is added to the PN solution to improve calcium and phosphate solubility.[193] Cysteine hydrochloride has been shown to increase the patient's need for acetate in order to counterbalance the hydrochloric acid load provided with cysteine.[194] On the other hand, metabolic alkalosis may occur as a result of excessive acetate salts in the PN solution.[146]

Electrolyte Abnormalities

Magnesium, phosphorus, and potassium, collectively referred to as "anabolic electrolytes," are electrolytes required in higher amounts for substrate metabolism. Without adequate supplementation of these electrolytes in the PN solution, increased anabolic requirements can cause hypokalemia, hypomagnesemia, and hypophosphatemia.[195]

Hypokalemia does not always imply body potassium depletion as intracellular shift of potassium occurs. Hypokalemia usually occurs with malabsorption syndromes, or may be due to intracellular shift with alkalemia, or as a side effect to medications (such as loop and thiazide diuretics or amphotericin B).[196]

Hypomagnesemia occurs in infants born to diabetic mothers,[197-198] in patients with diarrhea, or as a side effect of medications (such as diuretics, aminoglycosides, and amphotericin B).

Hypophosphatemia occurs with carbohydrate infusion due to intracellular shift of phosphate and increased renal phosphate excretion.[199]

Refeeding syndrome, characterized by fluid and electrolyte abnormalities, vitamin deficiencies, and possible secondary complications, may occur in malnourished patients following rapid initiation of nutrition support. This can cause severe hypophosphatemia, hypokalemia, and hypomagnesemia. To avoid the refeeding syndrome, nutrient delivery should begin at a low level and advance slowly with frequent monitoring and appropriate electrolyte supplementation.[140]

Hyperkalemia, hypermagnesemia, and hyperphosphatemia usually result from increased intake of electrolytes, decreased renal function, and hypercatabolism. The concentration of potassium, magnesium, and phosphorus in PN should be adjusted based on the serum concentrations of these electrolytes.

Hyperkalemia frequently occurs in very low birth weight infants[200] and results from reduced renal potassium elimination, excessive potassium load, extracellular redistribution in metabolic acidosis, or catabolism.[201] Hypermagnesemia occurs in neonates born to mothers who were treated with magnesium infusions for pre-eclampsia or preterm labor.[202-203]

Hypocalcemia can result from hypoalbuminemia, hypoparathyroidism, vitamin D deficiency, hyperphosphatemia, or medication-induced urinary calcium excretion (such as with loop diuretics or corticosteroids).[204] Hypercalciuria due to amino acid intake in PN can cause hypocalcemia. In one study, increasing amino acids from 1 to 2 g/kg/day increased urinary calcium excretion from 287 ± 46 mg/day to 455 ± 58 mg/day, respectively.[205] Hypocalcemia may also result from low calcium intake because of solubility limitations to calcium with phosphorus in the PN solution.[141] Serum ionized calcium represents the physiologically active form of calcium and is used to monitor calcium status in patients with hypoalbuminemia.[206]

Hepatobiliary Complications

Hepatobiliary complications associated with PN occur in a wide range of patients receiving PN.[207] The exact etiology of PN-associated liver dysfunction is unknown, but most likely results from multiple factors. Risk factors that correlate with PN-associated hepatobiliary complications include prematurity and low birth weight,[208-209] overfeeding,[210-211] extended duration of PN,[208,211-212] bowel rest,[213] sepsis,[209] bacterial translocation,[211-214] and short bowel syndrome.[215-216]

Transient elevation in liver enzymes occurs during PN,[217] but liver enzymes return to normal after PN is discontinued.[218-219] With prolonged PN therapy, severe liver complications such as cholestasis, steatosis, and cholelithiasis may occur.

Steatosis is primarily the result of excessive dextrose infusion.[220] Although steatosis is primarily reported in adults rather than in children, it often coexists with cholestasis. Cholestasis is the most common hepatobiliary complication in children receiving PN and may lead to liver failure and death.[221] PN-associated cholestasis (PNAC) may occur as early as 1 to 2 weeks after PN is initiated.[219] Patients with PNAC usually have elevated serum bilirubin concentrations with or without jaundice, depending on the severity of presentation. Other liver enzymes may also be elevated.[219,222-223] An elevation in serum conjugated bilirubin concentrations greater than or equal to 2 mg/dL is used as a marker of cholestasis.[224] Serum gamma glutamyl transferase (GGT) concentrations are also sensitivity markers for the early development of PNAC.[208,223] However, they lack specificity and can be elevated with other diseases, as well.[225]

Liver histopathological studies in patients with PN-associated hepatobiliary dysfunction show canalicular and intralobular cholestasis, periportal inflammation, bile duct proliferation, portal bridging, pigmented Kupfer cells, pseudoacinar formation, portal-portal bridging, steatosis, pericellular and portal fibrosis, and cirrhosis.[221-222]

Bowel rest during PN leads to increased intestinal permeability,[107,226] alteration in gut hormone secretion,[227] reduction in bile flow and excretion of bile salts,[228] bacterial overgrowth, bacterial and endotoxin translocation from the gut,[229-230] and impaired intestinal immunological mechanisms.

PN-associated liver dysfunction is reversible if PN is discontinued before irreversible liver damage occurs. Early initiation of enteral feedings and weaning PN seem best to prevent PNAC.

Other methods to prevent PNAC include avoiding overfeeding,[231] using a balanced caloric source,[232-233] initiating enteral feedings early,[210,223] avoiding and treating sepsis,[209,232] and administering PN cyclically.[234-236]

The pharmacological approach to PNAC is to improve bile flow, provide symptomatic relief of cholestasis and its associated symptoms, and reduce harm to the liver. The administration of ursodeoxycholic acid may improve bile flow and reduce the clinical signs and symptoms of cholestasis.[237-238] Cholecystokinin (CCK) has also been used to induce gallbladder contraction and improve bile flow. Preliminary experience with CCK shows improvement in hyperbilirubinemia and clinical signs of cholestasis, but its long-term protective effects on the liver are unknown.[239-240] Oral antibiotics, such as metronidazole or oral gentamicin, can be attempted to decrease intestinal bacterial overgrowth and reduce bacterial translocation.[241-242] Patients with short bowel syndrome and end stage liver disease should be assessed for bowel or combined liver and bowel transplantation.[221] Additional information about PN-associated liver complications in children can be found in sources outside this text.[243]

Metabolic Bone Disease

Metabolic bone disease (MBD), including osteopenia, osteomalacia, and rickets, may occur in children receiving long-term PN.[244-245] Although patients with underlying MBD may be asymptomatic, radiologic findings may reveal inadequate bone mineralization before bone pain or fractures appear. Biochemical markers usually show elevated serum alkaline phosphatase concentrations, hypercalciuria, low to normal plasma parathyroid hormone, normal 25-hydroxyvitamin D, and low 1,25 dihydroxyvitamin D plasma concentrations.[246-247]

Factors that predispose PN-dependent patients to MBD include deficiencies of calcium, phosphorus, and vitamin D,[143,248] aluminum toxicity,[249-250] and excessive vitamin D administration.[251]

Due to solubility problems, the limitation on calcium and phosphorus supplementation in PN solutions may result in decreased bone mineralization. Another contributing factor to MBD is increased urinary calcium excretion. Hypercalciuria can result from excessive calcium and inadequate phosphorus supplementation,[252] amino acid infusion,[205,253] cyclic PN infusion,[253-254] and chronic metabolic acidosis.[255]

Aluminum toxicity can also be the cause of MBD in patients receiving PN.[256] Small amounts of aluminum are present in vitamin, trace mineral, calcium and phosphate salts, and heparin solutions.[257] Premature infants and patients with renal failure are at higher risk for aluminum toxicity. Aluminum accumulation causes low bone formation[250,257] by impairing the fixation of calcium to the bones,[256] impairing parathyroid hormone (PTH) secretion, or reducing the conversion of 25-hydroxyvitamin D to the active 1,25-dihydroxyvitamin D.[258] Serum aluminum concentrations should be measured when aluminum-induced MBD is suspected.

Chronic metabolic acidosis may cause bone loss by affecting the bone buffering systems or impairing vitamin D metabolism.[255] Additionally, concomitant drug therapy such as with steroids may result in low bone density by reducing osteoblast proliferation, increasing renal calcium excretion, or inhibiting vitamin D-dependent calcium absorption.

Vitamin D may be an etiologic factor in PN-associated MBD. When vitamin D is withdrawn from PN, subsequent improvements in clinical and biochemical indices have been shown in adult patients who were receiving long-term PN and had evidence of bone demineralization. Specifically, subsidence of bone pain, fracture healing, decreased calciuria and phosphaturia,[251] positive calcium balance,[259] improvement in lumbar spine bone mineral content, and normalization of plasma PTH and 1,25 dihydroxyvitamin D concentrations were reported after vitamin D removal from PN.[260] Removal of vitamin D may be considered in selected patients who do not respond to calcium and phosphorus supplementation. However, it is impractical to eliminate vitamin D from the intravenous multivitamin combination formulation. If plasma 1,25 dihydroxyvitamin D and PTH concentrations are low and 25-hydroxyvitamin D concentrations are normal, then a trial course of vitamin D restriction may be warranted.[260]

An essential factor in preventing MBD is to maximize calcium and phosphorus intake.[261-262] To assess the effect of increased calcium and phosphorus intake on bone mineralization, a controlled, randomized, double-blind study was conducted in very-low birth weight infants who exclusively received PN for approximately 3 weeks. Infants who received the high amounts of calcium (1.7 mmol/dL) and phosphorus (2 mmol/dL) in their PN had greater retention of these minerals and higher bone mineral content compared to the group of infants who received the standard calcium (1.25 mmol/dL) and phosphorus (1.5 mmol/dL) amounts.[143]

Catheter-Related Infections

Catheter-related infections (CRI) predominantly result from skin flora migration from the catheter insertion site and are rarely due to microbial contamination of the PN solution.[263] CRI can be classified as catheter colonization, or as localized or systemic infections.[264] Microorganisms most commonly associated with CRI are coagulase-negative staphylococci, *Staphylococcus aureus*, *Escherichia coli*, *Enterobacter* spp., *Streptococcus* spp., *Serratia* spp., *Candida* spp., and *Malassezia furfur*.[265] Risk factors to CRI include long duration of catheterization,[266] the use of catheters for multiple purposes,[267,268] manipulation of the catheter hub,[269-270] long duration of PN therapy,[265,271] and prematurity.[271-272] Although multilumen catheters have been historically associated with increased infection rate,[271,273-274] some studies have shown no difference in infection risk between single and multilumen catheters.[275-276] Erythema, induration, and purulent exudates are signs of localized infections at the catheter exit.[264] Systemic infections are associated with fever and chills.[265,277]

Measures to prevent CRI include using sterile barriers during catheter placement, catheter management by trained personnel, using topical disinfectants, coating catheters with antimicrobials, regular catheter flushing, and using silver-impregnated subcutaneous cuffs for short-term catheters.[278] In infants who have anatomical and technical limitations for catheter placement, unnecessary catheter removal should be avoided if possible. Specific guidelines for managing CRI can be found in sources outside this text.[279-280]

Hematological Complications with Lipid Emulsions

Studies on the possible effects of lipid emulsions on platelet function and coagulation have yielded mixed results. Although some reports have shown no effects of lipid emulsions on platelet count,[281-282] others have linked thrombocytopenia to lipid infusion in children and neonates.[283-284] Although the effect on platelets may be clinically insignificant,[285] keep in mind that lipid emulsions may be a contributing factor for an unexplained change in platelet function.[283]

MONITORING PARAMETERS IN PEDIATRIC PATIENTS RECEIVING PARENTERAL NUTRITION

The frequency of monitoring parameters for PN therapy depends on the patient's clinical condition and nutritional status. More frequent monitoring of the laboratory and nutritional data is required in critically ill patients or patients with multiple medical problems.

When interpreting nutritional markers it is necessary to consider the sensitivity, specificity, and predictive value of each biochemical marker. For example, during the acute phase response that coincides with stress (such as surgery, trauma, burns, sepsis), the liver reprioritizes its synthetic function by suppressing the synthesis of the negative acute phase proteins including albumin, prealbumin, retinol-binding protein, and transferrin.[286-287] In these cases, serum concentrations of these visceral proteins may decrease in the absence of malnutrition. Table 6-17 gives guidelines for laboratory monitoring of PN therapy.

PHARMACEUTICAL ISSUES WITH PARENTERAL NUTRITION

Calcium Phosphate Solubility

Neonates have increased calcium and phosphorus requirements due to accelerated growth. However, the calcium and phosphorus requirements for optimal bone mineralization in neonates are higher than can be delivered in PN solutions. This is because calcium phosphate precipitates in-solution.[288] If precipitates are formed, they can lodge in the pulmonary capillaries during PN infusion, causing serious complications. In one report, calcium-phosphate precipitates in the infused TNA led to fatal microvascular pulmonary emboli. The precipitates were not seen because of the opaque color of the TNA due to the white lipid emulsion.[289] Using appropriate filters can prevent precipitates from reaching the blood.

Several approaches should be taken to avoid calcium phosphate precipitation. Specifically:

TABLE 6-17 Laboratory Monitoring Parameters for Acute Care Pediatric Patients Receiving Parenteral Nutrition*

Variable	Initial	Daily (Unstable)	2–3 Times/Week (Stable)	Weekly (Stable)	As Indicated
Na, K, Cl, CO_2	X	X	X		
BUN, Creatinine	X	X	X		
Glucose	X	X	X		
Liver enzymes[†¶]	X			X	
Ca, Mg, P	X	X		X	
Total Proteins, Albumin	X			X	
Triglycerides				X	
Blood indices	X				X
Vitamins					X
Trace minerals					X
Ammonia					X
Microbial blood cultures					X

* Frequency of monitoring varies with clinical conditions. In long-term PN patients, the frequency of laboratory monitoring ranges from once a week to once a month.

[†] GGT (gamma glutamyl transpeptidase) is useful to confirm the hepatobiliary origin of elevated alkaline phosphatase levels in case of PN-associated liver dysfunction.

[¶] AST (aspartate transaminase), ALT (alanine transaminase), alkaline phosphatase, total and conjugated bilirubin.

- Solubility curves for specific amino acid products should be used as a guide for the amount of calcium and phosphorus that can be safely mixed in PN solutions.[290]
- Calcium gluconate in PN should be used over calcium chloride because of its slower dissociation in solution.
- An acidic pH is more favorable for calcium and phosphate solubility because it reduces the dibasic phosphates in solution that may bind the divalent calcium. For example, adding cysteine hydrochloride at a dose of 40 mg per g of amino acids to lower the pH of PN solution allows higher calcium and phosphate amounts in PN.[291-292] However, cysteine hydrochloride may destabilize the lipid emulsion due to its low pH and should be infused separately.
- Calcium and phosphorus should not be added sequentially during the mixing process. Typically, phosphorus is added first and calcium last.
- The solution should be agitated periodically after each additive and visually inspected for any precipitates.[293]

Medication Compatibility with Parenteral Nutrition Solutions

The following guidelines should be used when adding medications to PN solutions:

- Heparin, histamine-2 receptor blockers, and regular insulin are compatible with PN.
- Iron dextran is incompatible with lipid emulsions and should not be added to the TNA.[294]
- Intravenous histamine-2 receptor blockers including ranitidine, famotidine and cimetidine may be added to PN solutions, usually for stress ulcer prophylaxis.
- Regular insulin may be added to control hyperglycemia. However, since insulin therapy is difficult to regulate in infants, intravenous insulin for these patients should be administered in a separate intravenous infusion and not in the PN solution to allow safe titration of the insulin dose.
- The addition of heparin to PN solutions at doses of 0.5–1 unit/mL[295-296] maintains the patency of the venous catheter,[297-298] minimizes the risk of phlebitis,[296,298] and improves the clearance of lipid emulsions by enhancing the LPL activity.[185]
- Heparin should be removed from the PN of patients in whom heparin is contraindicated, such as those with bleeding or thrombocytopenia.

Delivery Modalities and Administration of PN

PN can be administered via a peripheral or central venous catheter depending on the vascular access route, solution osmolarity, and expected duration of therapy. Peripheral PN (PPN) is intended for a short period of time, usually not exceeding 5 to 7 days.

Peripheral vein infusion of hyperosmolar solutions carries the risk of vein irritation and tissue damage. The risk of developing phlebitis is greater when PPN solution osmolarity exceeds 600–900 mOsm/L.[299] The maximum dextrose concentration in peripherally infused solutions for infants and children is 12.5%. Preferably, PPN should be infused with lipid emulsions to minimize the chances of phlebitis. Lipid emulsions are isotonic solutions, and their coadministration with PN prolongs the viability of peripheral intravenous catheters and lowers the final solution osmolarity.[300] Table 6-18 outlines the guidelines for estimating PN solution osmolarities.[301]

Because of the life-threatening potential of calcium phosphate precipitates in PN solutions, the Food and Drug Administration has issued a safety alert recommending the use of in-line filters during PN infusion. An in-line 0.22-micron filter should be used for nonlipid containing PN solutions, while a 1.2-micron filter should be used for lipid containing TNA. Because lipid particles measure about 0.5 micron in diameter, they should be co-infused with PN beyond the 0.22-micron filter.[293,302]

PN administration should be initiated as a continuous infusion over 24 hours with the caloric goal gradually achieved over 3 days. PN infusion can be gradually tapered if necessary to an infusion cycle over 10–14 hours, depending on tolerance. Infants may not tolerate such short cycles due to the risk of hypoglycemia. Cyclic PN infusion is especially desirable in the home care setting in order to provide infusion-free time to the patient.

TABLE 6-18 Guidelines for Estimating Osmolarity of Parenteral Nutrition Solution

PN Component	Approximate Osmolarity
Amino acids	100 mOsm/%
Dextrose	50 mOsm/%
Sodium salts	2 mOsm/mEq
Potassium salts	2 mOsm/mEq
Calcium gluconate	1.4 mOsm/mEq
Magnesium sulfate	1 mOsm/mEq

Source: Reference 301.

Table 6-11 details the osmolarities of lipid emulsions.

REFERENCES

1. Klotz KA, Wessel JJ, Hennies GA. Goals of pediatric nutrition support and nutrition assessment. In: Merritt RJ, ed. *The A.S.P.E.N. Nutrition Support Practice Manual.* 1st ed. Silver Spring, MD: American Society for Parenteral and Enteral Nutrition; 1998:1-14.

2. American Academy of Pediatrics, Committee on Nutrition. Assessment of Nutritional Status. In: Kleinman RE, ed. *Pediatric Nutrition Handbook.* 4th ed. Elk Grove Village, IL: American Academy of Pediatrics; 1998:165-84.

3. Zemel BS, Riley EM, Stallings VA. Evaluation of methodology for nutritional assessment in children: anthropometry, body composition, and energy expenditure. *Ann Rev Nutr.* 1997;17:211-35.

4. Fomon SJ, Haschke F, Ziegler EE, et al. Body composition of reference children from birth to age 10 years. *Am J Clin Nutr.* 1982;35:1169-75.

5. Corrales KM, Utter SL. Failure to thrive. In: Samour PQ, Helm KK, Lang CE, eds. *Handbook of Pediatric Nutrition.* 2nd ed. Gaithersburg, MD: Aspen Publishers, Inc; 1999:395-412.

6. Klawitter BM. Nutrition assessment of infants and children. In: Williams CP, ed. *Pediatric Manual of Clinical Dietetics.* 1st ed. Chicago: American Dietetic Association; 1998:19-34.

7. United States Department of Health and Human Services. Centers for Disease Control and Prevention. National Center for Health Statistics. CDC growth charts: United States. Available at: http://www.cdc.gov/growthcharts. Accessed April 27, 2001.

8. Baer MT, Harris AB. Pediatric nutrition assessment: identifying children at risk. *J Am Diet Assoc.* 1997; 97(10)(suppl 2):S107-15.

9. Mascarenhas MR, Zemel B, Stallings VA. Nutritional assessment in pediatrics. *Nutrition.* 1998;14:105-15.

10. Wallach J. *Interpretation of Diagnostic Tests.* 7th ed. Philadelphia: Lippincott, Williams & Wilkins; 2000:3-31.

11. Shronts EP, Fish JA, Pesce-Hammond K. Nutrition Assessment. In: Merritt RJ, ed. *The A.S.P.E.N. Nutrition Support Practice Manual.* 1st ed. Silver Spring, MD: American Society for Parenteral and Enteral Nutrition; 1998:1-17.

12. Teasley-Strausburg KM, Anderson JD. Assessment of nutrition status and nutrition requirements. In: DiPiro JT, Talbert RL, Yee GC, et al., eds. *Pharmacotherapy: A Pathophysiologic Approach.* 4th ed. Stamford, CT: Appleton & Lange; 1999:2221-36.

13. Loughery CM, Duggan C. Laboratory assessment of nutritional status. In: Hendricks KM, Duggan C, Walker WA, eds. *Manual of Pediatric Nutrition.* 3rd ed. Hamilton, Ontario: BC Decker Inc; 2000:66-76.

14. Morgan SL, Weinsier RL, eds. *Fundamentals of Clinical Nutrition.* 2nd ed. St. Louis, MO: Mosby-Year Book, Inc; 1998:174-87.

15. Food and Nutrition Board. *Recommended Dietary Allowances.* 10th ed. Washington, DC: National Academy Press; 1989.

16. Fomon SJ, Filer LJ. Milks and formulas. In: Fomon SJ, ed. *Infant Nutrition.* 2nd ed. Philadelphia: WB Saunders Company; 1974:359-407.

17. Lau C, Hurst N. Oral feeding in infants. *Curr Probl Pediatr.* 1999;29:105-24.

18. American Academy of Pediatrics, Committee on Nutrition. Encouraging Breastfeeding. *Pediatrics.* 1980;65:657-8.

19. American Academy of Pediatrics. Breastfeeding and the use of human milk. *Pediatrics.* 1997;100:1035-9.
20. Akers SM, Groh-Wargo SL. Normal nutrition during infancy. In: Samour PQ, Helm KK, Lang CE, eds. *Handbook of Pediatric Nutrition.* 2nd ed. Gaithersburg, MD: Aspen Publishers Inc; 1999:65-97.
21. Lteif AN, Schwenk WF. Breast milk: revisited. *Mayo Clin Proc.* 1998;73:760-3.
22. Nutrition Committee of the Canadian Paediatric Society and the Committee on Nutrition of the American Academy of Pediatrics. Breastfeeding: a commentary in celebration of the International Year of the Child: 1979. *Pediatrics.*1978;65:591-601.
23. American Academy of Pediatrics, Committee on Nutrition. Nutrition and Oral Health. In: Kleinman RE, ed. *Pediatric Nutrition Handbook.* 4th ed. Elk Grove Village, IL: American Academy of Pediatrics; 1998:523-9.
24. American Academy of Pediatrics, Committee on Nutrition. Breastfeeding. In: Kleinman RE, ed. *Pediatric Nutrition Handbook.* 4th ed. Elk Grove Village, IL: American Academy of Pediatrics; 1998:3-20.
25. Haller CA, Simpser E. Breastfeeding: 1999 perspective. *Curr Opin Pediatr.* 1999;11:379-83.
26. American Academy of Pediatrics, Committee on Nutrition. Iron fortification of infant formulas. *Pediatrics.* 1999;104:119-23.
27. American Academy of Pediatrics, Committee on Nutrition. Commentary on breast-feeding and infant formulas, including proposed standards for formulas. *Pediatrics.* 1976; 57:278-85.
28. American Academy of Pediatrics, Committee on Nutrition. Recommended nutrient levels of infant formulas (per 100 kcal). In: Kleinman RE, ed. *Pediatric Nutrition Handbook.* 4th ed. Elk Grove Village, IL: American Academy of Pediatrics; 1998:653-4.
29. Hall RT, Carroll RE. Infant feeding. *Pediatr Rev.* 2000;21:191-9.
30. American Academy of Pediatrics, Committee on Nutrition. Soy protein-based formulas: recommendations for use in infant feeding. *Pediatrics.* 1998;101:148-53.
31. Maldonado J, Gil A, Narbona E, et al. Special formulas in infant nutrition: a review. *Early Hum Dev.* 1998;53(suppl):S23-32.
32. Burks AW, Casteel HB, Fiedorek SC, et al. Prospective oral food challenge study of two soybean protein isolates in patients with possible milk or soy protein enterocolitis. *Pediatr Allergy Immunol.* 1994;5:40-5.
33. American Academy of Pediatrics, Committee on Nutrition. Formula Feeding of Term Infants. In: Kleinman RE, ed. *Pediatric Nutrition Handbook.* 4th ed. Elk Grove Village, IL: American Academy of Pediatrics; 1998:29-42.
34. Halken S, Host A. How hypoallergenic are hypoallergenic cow's milk-based formulas? *Allergy.* 1997;52:1175-83.
35. Redel CA, Shulman RJ. Controversies in the composition of infant formulas. *Pediatr Clin North Am.* 1994;41:909-24.
36. Anderson DM. Nutrition for premature infants. In: Samour PQ, Helm KK, Lang CE, eds. *Handbook of Pediatric Nutrition.* 2nd ed. Gaithersburg, MD: Aspen Publishers Inc; 1999:43-63.
37. Battaglia FC, Lubchenco LO. A practical classification of newborn infants by weight and gestational age. *J Pediatr.* 1967;71:159-63.
38. American Academy of Pediatrics, Committee on Nutrition. Nutritional needs of preterm infants. In: Kleinman RE, ed. *Pediatric Nutrition Handbook.* 4th ed. Elk Grove Village, IL: American Academy of Pediatrics; 1998:55-87.
39. Greene HL, Smidt LJ. Water-soluble vitamins: C, B_1, B_2, B_6, niacin, pantothenic acid, and biotin. In: Tsang RC, Lucas A, Uauy R, et al., eds. *Nutritional Needs of the Preterm Infant: Scientific Basis and Practical Guidelines.* Pawling, NY: Williams & Wilkins; 1993:121-33.
40. Hansen JW. Appendix: Consensus recommendations, nutritional needs of the stable/growing infants. In: Tsang RC, Lucas A, Uauy R, et al., eds. *Nutritional Needs of the Preterm Infant: Scientific Basis and Practical Guidelines.* Pawling, NY: Williams & Wilkins; 1993:287-95.
41. Ehrenkranz RA. Iron, folic acid, and vitamin B_{12}. In: Tsang RC, Lucas A, Uauy R, et al., eds. *Nutritional Needs of the Preterm Infant: Scientific Basis and Practical Guidelines.* Pawling, NY: Williams & Wilkins; 1993:177-94.
42. Heird WC. Nutritional requirements during infancy. In: Shils ME, Olson JA, Shike M, et al., eds. *Modern Nutrition in Health and Disease.* 9th ed. Baltimore: Lippincott, Williams & Wilkins; 1999:839-55.
43. Lucas A. Enteral nutrition. In: Tsang RC, Lucas A, Uauy R, et al., eds. *Nutritional Needs of the Preterm Infant: Scientific Basis and Practical Guidelines.* Pawling, NY: Lippincott Williams & Wilkins; 1993:209-23.
44. Thureen PJ, Hay WW. Intravenous nutrition and postnatal growth of the micropremie. *Clin Perinatol.* 2000;27:197-234.
45. American Academy of Pediatrics, Committee on Nutrition. Nutritional needs of low-birth-weight infants. *Pediatrics.* 1977;60:519-30.
46. Ziegler EE. Protein in premature feeding. *Nutrition.* 1994;10:69-71.

47. Bayes R, Campoy C, Molina-Font JA. Some current controversies on nutritional requirements of full-term and pre-term newborn infants. *Early Hum Dev.* 1998;53(suppl):S3-13.
48. Chesney RW, Helms RA, Christensen M, et al. The role of taurine in infant nutrition. *Adv Exp Med Biol.* 1998;442:463-76.
49. Cicco R, Holzman IR, Brown DR, et al. Glucose polymer tolerance in premature infants. *Pediatrics.* 1981;67:498-501.
50. Siimes MA, Jarvenpaa AL. Prevention of anemia and iron deficiency in very low-birth-weight infants. *J Pediatr.* 1982;101:277-80.
51. Stekel A, Olivares M, Pizarro F, et al. Absorption of fortification iron from milk formulas in infants. *Am J Clin Nutr.* 1986;43:917-22.
52. Dallman PR, Yip R. Changing characteristics of childhood anemia. *J Pediatr.* 1989;114:161-4.
53. Koo WW, Tsang RC. Calcium, magnesium, phosphorus, and vitamin D. In: Tsang RC, Lucas A, Uauy R, et al., eds. *Nutritional Needs of the Preterm Infant: Scientific Basis and Practical Guidelines.* Pawling, NY: Williams & Wilkins; 1993:135-55.
54. Koo WW, MacLaughlin K, Saba M. Nutrition support for the preterm infant. In: Merritt RJ, ed. *The A.S.P.E.N. Nutrition Support Practice Manual.* 1st ed. Silver Spring, MD: American Society for Parenteral and Enteral Nutrition; 1998:1-16.
55. American Academy of Pediatrics, Vitamin K Ad Hoc Task Force. Controversies concerning vitamin K and the newborn. *Pediatrics.* 1993;91:1001-3.
56. Greer FR. Vitamin metabolism and requirements in the micropremie. *Clin Perinatol.* 2000;27:95-118.
57. American Academy of Pediatrics, Committee on Nutrition. The use of whole cow's milk in infancy. *Pediatrics.* 1992;89:1105-9.
58. Underwood BA, Hofvander Y. Appropriate timing for complementary feeding of the breast-fed infant: a review. *Acta Paediatr Scand.* 1982;294(suppl):1-32.
59. American Academy of Pediatrics, Committee on Nutrition. Supplemental foods for infants. In: Kleinman RE, ed. *Pediatric Nutrition Handbook.* 4th ed. Elk Grove Village, IL: American Academy of Pediatrics; 1998:43-53.
60. American Academy of Pediatrics, Committee on Nutrition. Feeding From Age 1 Year to Adolescence. In: Kleinman RE, ed. *Pediatric Nutrition Handbook.* 4th ed. Elk Grove Village, IL: American Academy of Pediatrics; 1998:125-39.
61. Bock SA. Prospective appraisal of complaints of adverse reactions to foods in children during the first 3 years of life. *Pediatrics.* 1987;79:683-8.
62. Host A, Koletzko B, Dreborg S, et al. Dietary products used in infants for treatment and prevention of food allergy: joint statement of the European Society for Paediatric Allergology and Clinical Immunology (ESPACI) Committee on hypoallergenic formulas and the European Society for Paediatric Gastroenterology, Hepatology and Nutrition (ESPGHAN) Committee on Nutrition. *Arch Dis Child.* 1999;81:80-4.
63. Bruijnzeel-Koomen C, Ortolani C, Aas K, et al. Adverse reactions to food: European Academy of Allergology and Clinical Immunology Subcommittee. *Allergy.* 1995;50:623-35.
64. Chandra RK. Food hypersensitivity and allergic disease: a selective review. *Am J Clin Nutr.* 1997;66:526S-9S.
65. Sampson HA. Diagnosis and management of food allergies. In: Shils ME, Olson JA, Shike M, et al., eds. *Modern Nutrition in Health and Disease.* 9th ed. Baltimore: Lippincott, Williams & Wilkins; 1999:1503-11.
66. Sampson HA, Mendelson L, Rosen JP. Fatal and near-fatal anaphylactic reactions to foods in children and adolescents. *N Engl J Med.* 1992;327:380-4.
67. Watson WT. Food allergy in children. *Clin Rev Allergy Immunol.* 1995;13:347-59.
68. James JM, Burks AW. Food hypersensitivity in children. *Curr Opin Pediatr.* 1994;6:661-7.
69. Christie L. Food hypersensitivities. In: Samour PQ, Helm KK, Lang CE, eds. *Handbook of Pediatric Nutrition.* 2nd ed. Gaithersburg, MD: Aspen Publishers Inc; 1999:149-72.
70. American Academy of Pediatrics. Hypoallergenic infant formulas. *Pediatrics.* 2000;106:346-9.
71. Burks AW, Stanley JS. Food allergy. *Curr Opin Pediatr.* 1998;10:588-93.
72. Host A, Jacobsen HP, Halken S, et al. The natural history of cow's milk protein allergy/intolerance. *Eur J Clin Nutr.* 1995;49(suppl 1):S13-8.
73. Saarinen KM, Juntunen-Backman K, Jarvenpaa AL, et al. Supplementary feeding in maternity hospitals and the risk of cow's milk allergy: a prospective study of 6209 infants. *J Allergy Clin Immunol.* 1999;104:457-61.
74. Bernstein M, Day JH, Welsh A. Double-blind food challenge in the diagnosis of food sensitivity in the adult. *J Allergy Clin Immunol.* 1982;70:205-13.
75. Bock SA, Sampson HA, Atkins FM, et al. Double-blind, placebo-controlled food challenge (DBPCFC) as an office procedure: a manual. *J Allergy Clin Immunol.* 1988;82:986-97.

76. Bock SA, Atkins FM. Patterns of food hypersensitivity during sixteen years of double-blind, placebo-controlled food challenges. *J Pediatr.* 1990;117:561-7.

77. Bock SA. In vivo diagnosis: skin testing and oral challenge procedures. In: Metcalfe DD, Sampson HA, Simon RA, eds. *Food Allergy: Adverse Reactions to Foods and Food Additives.* 2nd ed. Cambridge, MA: Blackwell Scientific Publications; 1997:151-66.

78. Sampson HA, Albergo R. Comparison of results of skin tests, RAST, and double-blind placebo-controlled food challenges in children with atopic dermatitis. *J Allergy Clin Immunol.* 1984;74:26-33.

79. Bock SA, Buckley J, Holst A, et al. Proper use of skin test with food extracts in diagnosis of hypersensitivity to food in children. *Clinical Allergy.* 1977;7:375-83.

80. Zeiger RS, Heller S. The development and prediction of atopy in high-risk children: follow-up at age seven years in a prospective randomized study of combined maternal and infant food allergen avoidance. *J Allergy Clin Immunol.* 1995;95:1179-90.

81. Businco L, Dreborg S, Einarsson R, et al. Hydrolysed cow's milk formulae, allergenicity and use in treatment and prevention: an European Society of Pediatric Allergy and Clinical Immunology (ESPACI) position paper. *Pediatr Allergy Immunol.* 1993;4:101-11.

82. Businco L, Bruno G, Giampietro PG. Prevention and management of food allergy. *Acta Paediatr Suppl.* 1999;430:104-9.

83. Vanderhoof JA, Murray ND, Kaufman SS, et al. Intolerance to protein hydrolysate infant formulas: an underrecognized cause of gastrointestinal symptoms in infants. *J Pediatr.* 1997;131:741-4.

84. De Boissieu D, Matarazzo P, Dupont C. Allergy to extensively hydrolyzed cow milk proteins in infants: identification and treatment with an amino acid-based formula. *J Pediatr.* 1997;131:744-7.

85. Zeiger RS, Sampson HA, Bock SA, et al. Soy allergy in infants and children with IgE-associated cow's milk allergy. *J Pediatr.* 1999;134:614-22.

86. Saarinen UM, Kajosaari M. Breastfeeding as prophylaxis against atopic disease: prospective follow-up study until 17 years old. *Lancet.* 1995;346:1065-9.

87. Chandra RK. Five-year follow-up of high-risk infants with family history of allergy who were exclusively breast-fed or fed partial whey hydrolysate, soy, and conventional milk formulas. *J Pediatr Gastroenterol Nutr.* 1997;24:442-6.

88. Fälth-Magnuson K, Kjellman N-IM. Allergy prevention by maternal elimination diet during late pregnancy: a 5-year follow-up of a randomized study. *J Allergy Clin Immunol.* 1992;89:709-13.

89. Järvinen KM, Mäkinen-Kiljunen S, Suomalainen H. Cow's milk challenge through human milk evokes immune responses in infants with cow's milk allergy. *J Pediatr.* 1999;135:506-12.

90. Sigurs N, Hattevig G, Kjellman B. Maternal avoidance of eggs, cow's milk, and fish during lactation: effect on allergic manifestations, skin-prick tests, and specific IgE antibodies in children at age 4 years. *Pediatrics.* 1992;89:735-9.

91. Sampson HA, Metcalfe DD. Food allergies. *JAMA.* 1992;268:2840-4.

92. Zeiger RS. Dietary aspects of food allergy prevention in infants and children. *J Pediatr Gastroenterol Nutr.* 2000;30(suppl 1):S77-86.

93. Wood RA. Prospects for the prevention of allergy in children. *Curr Opin Pediatr.* 1996;8:601-5.

94. Halken S, Jacobsen HP, Host A, et al. The effect of hypo-allergenic formulas in infants at risk of allergic disease. *Eur J Clin Nutr.* 1995;49(suppl 1):S77-83.

95. Bock SA, Sampson HA. Food allergy in infancy. *Pediatr Clin North Am.* 1994;4:1047-67.

96. Elsas LJ, Acosta PB. Nutritional support of inherited metabolic disease. In: Shils ME, Olson JA, Shike M, et al., eds. *Modern Nutrition in Health and Disease.* 9th ed. Baltimore: Lippincott, Williams & Wilkins; 1999:1003-56.

97. Acosta PB. Nutrition support of inborn errors of metabolism. In: Samour PQ, Helm KK, Lang CE, eds. *Handbook of Pediatric Nutrition.* 2nd ed. Gaithersburg, MD: Aspen Publishers Inc; 1999:243-92.

98. Rezvani I. Metabolic disease. In: Behrman RE, Kleigman RM, Jenson HB, eds. *Nelson Textbook of Pediatrics.* 16th ed. Philadelphia: WB Saunders Company; 2000:344-67.

99. Burton BK. Inborn errors of metabolism in infancy: a guide to diagnosis. *Pediatrics.* 1998;102:E69.

100. Leonard JV, Morris AAM. Inborn errors of metabolism around time of birth. *Lancet.* 2000;356:583-7.

101. Kirby RB. Maternal phenylketonuria: a new cause for concern. *J Obstet Gynecol Neonatal Nurs.* 1999;28:227-34.

102. Start K. Treating phenylketonuria by a phenylalanine-free diet. *Professional Care of Mother & Child.* 1998;8:109-10.

103. Chuang DT. Maple syrup urine disease: it has come a long way. *J Pediatr.* 1998;132: S17-23.

104. American Society for Parenteral and Enteral Nutrition. Guidelines for the use of parenteral and enteral nutrition in adult and pediatric patients. *J Parenter Enteral Nutr.* 1993;17(suppl 4):1SA-52SA.

105. Nordenstrom J, Pesson E. Energy supply during total parenteral nutrition-how much and what source? *Acta Anaesthesiol Scand.* 1985;29:95-9.

106. Utili R, Abernathy CO, Zimmerman HJ. Endotoxin effects on the liver. *Life Sci*. 1977;20:553-68.
107. Williamson RCN, Chir M. Intestinal adaptation: structural, functional and cytokinetic changes. *N Engl J Med*. 1978;298:1393-402.
108. Wilmore DW, Smith RJ, O'Dwyer ST, et al. The gut: a central organ after surgical stress. *Surgery*. 1988;104:917-23.
109. Thornton L, Griffin E. Evaluation of a taurine containing amino acid solution in parenteral nutrition. *Arch Dis Child*. 1991;66:21-5.
110. Okamoto E, Rassin DK, Zucker CL, et al. Role of taurine in feeding the low-birth-weight infant. *J Pediatr*. 1984;104:936-40.
111. Zelikovic I, Chesney RW, Friedman AL, et al. Taurine depletion in very low birth weight infants receiving total parenteral nutrition: role of renal immaturity. *J Pediatr*. 1990;116:301-6.
112. Vinton NE, Laidlaw SA, Ament ME, et al. Taurine concentrations in plasma, blood cells, and urine of children undergoing long-term total parenteral nutrition. *Pediatr Res*. 1987;21:399-403.
113. Forchielli ML, Gura KM, Sandler R, et al. Aminosyn PF or Trophamine: which provides more protection from cholestasis associated with total parenteral nutrition? *J Pediatr Gastroenterol Nutr*. 1995;21:374-82.
114. Miles JM, Klein JA. Should protein be included in calorie calculations for a TPN prescription: point-counterpoint. *Nutr Clin Pract*. 1996;11:204-6.
115. Shils ME, Brown R. Parenteral Nutrition. In: Shils ME, Olson JA, Shike M, et al., eds. *Modern Nutrition in Health and Disease*. 9th ed. Baltimore: Lippincott, Williams & Wilkins; 1999:1657-88.
116. Maxvold NJ, Smoyer WE, Custer JR, et al. Amino acid loss and nitrogen balance in critically ill children with acute renal failure: a prospective comparison between classic hemofiltration and hemofiltration with dialysis. *Crit Care Med*. 2000;28:1161-5.
117. Farrag HM, Nawrath LM, Healey JE, et al. Persistent glucose production and greater peripheral sensitivity to insulin in the neonate vs the adult. *Am J Physiol*. 1997;272:E86-93.
118. Stonestreet BS, Rubin L, Pollak A, et al. Renal functions of low birth infants with hyperglycemia and glucosuria produced by glucose infusions. *Pediatrics*. 1980;66:561-7.
119. Lennon C, Davidson KW, Sadowski JA, et al. The vitamin K content of intravenous lipid emulsions. *J Parenter Enteral Nutr*. 1993;17:142-4.
120. Steephen AC, Traber MG, Ito Y, et al. Vitamin E status of patients receiving long-term parenteral Nutrition: is vitamin E supplementation adequate? *J Parenter Enteral Nutr*. 1991;15:647-52.
121. Gutcher GR, Lax AA, Farrell PM. Tocopherol isomers in intravenous lipid emulsions and resultant plasma concentrations. *J Parenter Enteral Nutr*. 1984;8:269-73.
122. Hay WW Jr, Lucas A, Heird WC, et al. Workshop summary: nutrition of the extremely low birth weight infant. *Pediatrics*. 1999;104:1360-8.
123. American Academy of Pediatrics, Committee on Nutrition. Use of intravenous fat emulsions in pediatric patients. *Pediatrics*. 1981;68:738-43.
124. Greene HL, Hambidge KM, Schanler R, et al. Guidelines for the use of vitamins, trace elements, calcium, magnesium, and phosphorus in infants and children receiving total parenteral nutrition: report of the subcommittee on pediatric parenteral nutrient requirements from the committee on clinical practice issues of the American Society for Clinical Nutrition. *Am J Clin Nutr*. 1988;48:1324-42.
125. Kitamura K, Takahashi T, Tanaka H, et al. Two cases of thiamine deficiency-induced lactic acidosis during total parenteral nutrition. *Tohoku J Exp Med*. 1993;171:129-33.
126. Barrett TG, Forsyth JM, Nathavitharana KA, et al. Potentially lethal thiamine deficiency complicating parenteral nutrition in children. *Lancet*. 1993;341:901-2.
127. Romanski SA, McMahon M, Molly M. Metabolic acidosis and thiamine deficiency. *Mayo Clin Proc*. 1999;74:259-63.
128. Centers for Disease Control and Prevention. Deaths associated with thiamine-deficient total parenteral nutrition. *MMWR Morb Mortal Wkly Rep*. 1989;38:43-6.
129. Centers for Disease Control and Prevention. Lactic acidosis traced to thiamine deficiency related to nationwide shortage of multivitamins for total parenteral nutrition. *MMWR Morb Mortal Wkly Rep*.1997;46:523-8.
130. Shenkin A. Trace elements and inflammatory response: implications for nutritional support. *Nutrition*. 1995;11:100-5.
131. McClain CJ. Zinc metabolism in malabsorption syndromes. *J Am Coll Nutr*. 1985;4:49-64.
132. Ladefoged K. Intestinal and renal loss of infused minerals in patients with severe short bowel syndrome. *Am J Clin Nutr*. 1982;36:59-67.
133. Fitzgerald K, Mikalunas V, Rubin H, et al. Hypermanganesemia in patients receiving total parenteral nutrition. *J Parenter Enteral Nutr*. 1999;23:333-6.
134. Taylor S, Manara AR. Manganese toxicity in a patient with cholestasis receiving total parenteral nutrition. *Anaesthesia*. 1994;49:1013.

135. Spiegel JE, Willenbucher RF. Rapid development of severe copper deficiency in a patient with Crohn's disease receiving parenteral nutrition. *J Parenter Enteral Nutr.* 1999;23:169-72.

136. American Society for Parenteral and Enteral Nutrition National Advisory Group on Standards and Practice Guidelines for Parenteral Nutrition. Safe Practices of Parenteral Nutrition Formulations. *J Parenter Enteral Nutr.* 1998;22:49-66.

137. Baugh N, Recupero MA, Kerner JA. Nutritional requirements for pediatric patients. In: Merritt RJ, ed. *The A.S.PE.N. Nutrition Support Practice Manual.* 1st ed. Silver Spring, MD: American Society for Parenteral and Enteral Nutrition; 1998: 1-13.

138. Chevalier RL. Developmental renal physiology of the low birth weight pre-term newborn. *J Urol.* 1996;156(suppl 2):714-9.

139. Taketomo CK, Hodding JH, Kraus DM. *Pediatric Dosage Handbook.* 8th ed. Hudson, OH: Lexi-Comp Inc; 2001:816-8.

140. Brooks MJ, Melnik G. The refeeding syndrome: an approach to understanding its complication and prevention. *Pharmacotherapy.* 1995;15:713-26.

141. Dunham B, Marcuard S, Khazanie PG, et al. The solubility of calcium and phosphorus in neonatal total parenteral nutrition solutions. *J Parenter Enteral Nutr.* 1991;15:608-11.

142. Karlen J, Aperia A, Zetterstorm R. Renal excretion of calcium and phosphate in preterm and term infants. *J Pediatr.* 1985;106:814-9.

143. Prestridge LL, Schanler RJ, Shulman R, et al. Effect of parenteral calcium and phosphorus on mineral retention and bone mineral content in very low birth weight infants. *J Pediatr.* 1993;122:761-8.

144. Pelegano JF, Rowe JC, Carey DE, et al. Effect of calcium/phosphorus ratio on mineral retention in parenterally fed premature infants. *J Pediatr Gastroenterol Nutr.* 1991;12:351-5.

145. Scheingraber S, Rehm M, Sehmisch C, et al. Rapid saline infusion produces hyperchloremic acidosis in patients undergoing gynecologic surgery. *Anesthesiology.* 1999;90:1265-70.

146. Eliahou HE, Feng PH, Weinberg U, et al. Acetate and bicarbonate in the correction of uraemic acidosis. *Br Med J.* 1970;4:399-401.

147. Kalhoff H, Wiese B, Kunz C, et al. Increased renal net acid excretion in prematures below 1,600 g body weight compared with prematures and small-for-date newborns above 2,100 g on alimentation with commercial preterm formula. *Biol Neonate.* 1994;66:10-5.

148. Kushner RF. Total parenteral nutrition-associated metabolic acidosis. *J Parenter Enteral Nutr.* 1986;10:306-10.

149. Boehm KA, Helms RA, Christensen ML, et al. Carnitine: a review for the pharmacy clinician. *Hosp Pharm.* 1993;28:843-50.

150. Borum PR, Bennett SG. Carnitine as an essential nutrient. *J Am Coll Nutr.* 1986;5:177-82.

151. Schmidt-Sommerfeld E, Penn D. Carnitine and parenteral nutrition of the neonate. *Biol Neonate.* 1990;58(suppl 1):81-8.

152. Dahlstrom KA, Ament ME, Moukarzel AA, et al. Low blood and plasma carnitine levels in children receiving long-term parenteral nutrition. *J Pediatr Gastroenterol Nutr.* 1990;11:375-9.

153. Penn D, Schmidt-Sommerfeld E, Wolf H. Carnitine deficiency in premature infants receiving total parenteral nutrition. *Early Hum Dev.* 1980;4:23-34.

154. Schiff D, Chan G, Secombe D, et al. Plasma carnitine levels during intravenous feeding of the neonate. *J Pediatr.* 1979;95:1043-6.

155. Moukarzel AA, Dahlstrom KA, Buchman AL, et al. Carnitine status of children receiving long-term total parenteral nutrition: a longitudinal prospective study. *J Pediatr.* 1992;120:759-62.

156. Penn D, Schmidt-Sommerfeld E, Pascu F. Decreased tissue carnitine concentrations in newborn infants receiving total parenteral nutrition. *J Pediatr.* 1981;98:976-8.

157. Helms RA, Mauer EC, Hay WW Jr, et al. Effect of intravenous L-carnitine on growth parameters and fat metabolism during parenteral nutrition in neonates. *J Parenter Enteral Nutr.* 1990;14:448-53.

158. Bonner CM, DeBrie KL, Hug G, et al. Effects of parenteral L-carnitine supplementation on fat metabolism and nutrition in premature infants. *J Pediatr.* 1995;126:287-92.

159. Schmidt-Sommerfeld E, Penn D, Wolf H. Carnitine deficiency in premature infants receiving total parenteral nutrition: effect of L-carnitine supplementation. *J Pediatr.* 1983;102:931-5.

160. Larsson LE, Olegard R, Ljung ML, et al. Parenteral nutrition in preterm neonates with and without carnitine supplementation. *Acta Anaesthesiol Scand.* 1990;34:501-5.

161. Borum PR. Is L-carnitine stable in parenteral nutrition solutions prepared for preterm neonates? *Neonatal Intensive Care.* 1993;6:30-2.

162. Tibboel D, Delemarre FMC, Przyrembel H, et al. Carnitine deficiency in surgical neonates receiving total parenteral nutrition. *J Pediatr Surg.* 1990;25:418-21.

163. Perdue M. Intravenous complications. In: Terry J, Baranowski L, Lonsway RA, eds. *Intravenous Therapy Clinical Principles and Practice.* Philadelphia: WB Saunders Company; 1995:419-46.

164. Dweck HS, Cassady G. Glucose intolerance in infants of very low birth weight. Incidence of hyperglycemia in infants of birth weights 1,100 grams or less. *Pediatrics*. 1974;53:189-95.
165. Campbell IT. Limitations of nutrient intake. The effect of stressors: trauma, sepsis and multiple organ failure. *Eur J Clin Nutr*. 1999;53(suppl 1):S143-7.
166. Pollak A, Cowett RM, Schwartz R, et al. Glucose disposal in low-birth-weight infants during steady-state hyperglycemia: effects of exogenous insulin administration. *Pediatrics*. 1978;61:546-9.
167. Farrag HM, Cowett RM. Glucose homeostasis in the micropremie. *Clin Perinatol*. 2000;27:1-22.
168. Aarsland A, Chinkes D, Wolfe RR. Hepatic and whole-body fat synthesis in humans during carbohydrate overfeeding. *Am J Clin Nutr*. 1997;65:1774-82.
169. Alexiewicz JM, Kumar D, Smogorzewski M, et al. Polymorphonuclear leukocytes in non-insulin-dependent diabetes mellitus: abnormalities in metabolism and function. *Ann Intern Med*. 1995;123:919-24.
170. Forsyth JS, Murdock N, Crighton A. Low birthweight infants and total parenteral nutrition immediately after birth. Part III. Randomized study of energy substrate utilisation, nitrogen balance, and carbon dioxide production. *Arch Dis Child*. 1995;73:F13-6.
171. Liposky JM, Nelson LD. Ventilatory response to high caloric loads in critically ill patients. *Crit Care Med*. 1994;22:796-802.
172. Ditzenberger GR, Collins SD, Binder N. Continuous insulin intravenous infusion therapy for VLBW infants. *J Perinat Neonat Nurs*. 1999;13:70-82.
173. Dudrick SJ, Macfadyen BV Jr, Van Buren CT, et al. Parenteral hyperalimentation: metabolic problems and solutions. *Ann Surg*. 1972;176:259-64.
174. Ladefoged K, Jarnum S. Metabolic complications to total parenteral nutrition. *Acta Anaesthesiol Scand*. 1985;29:89-94.
175. Cornblath M, Hawdon JM, Williams AF, et al. Controversies regarding the definition of neonatal hypoglycemia: suggested operational thresholds. *Pediatrics*. 2000;105:1141-5.
176. Andrew F, Chan G, Schiff D. Lipid metabolism in the neonate. I. The effects of Intralipid infusion on plasma triglyceride and free fatty acid concentrations in the neonate. *J Pediatr*. 1976;88:273-8.
177. Shennan AT, Bryan MH, Angel A. The effect of gestational age on Intralipid tolerance in newborn infants. *J Pediatr*. 1977;91:134-7.
178. Park W, Paust H, Schroder H. Lipid infusion in premature infants suffering from sepsis. *J Parenter Enteral Nutr*. 1984;8:290-2.
179. Bagdade JD, Porte D, Bierman EL. Steroid-induced lipemia: a complication of high-dosage corticosteroid therapy. *Arch Intern Med*. 1970;125:129-34.
180. Periera GR, Fox WW, Stanley CA, et al. Decreased oxygenation and hyperlipemia during intravenous fat infusions in premature infants. *Pediatrics*. 1980;66:26-30.
181. Prasertsom W, Phillipos EZ, Van Aerde JE, et al. Pulmonary vascular resistance during lipid infusion in neonates. *Arch Dis Child*. 1996;74:F95-8.
182. Greene HL, Hazlett D, Demaree R. Relationship between Intralipid-induced hyperlipemia and pulmonary function. *Am J Clin Nutr*. 1976;29:127-35.
183. Brans YW, Dutton EB, Andrew DS, et al. Fat emulsion tolerance in very low birth weight neonates: effect on diffusion of oxygen in the lungs and blood pH. *Pediatrics*. 1986;78:79-84.
184. Dhanireddy R, Hamosh M, Sivasubramanian KN, et al. Postheparin lipolytic activity and Intralipid clearance in very low-birth-weight infants. *J Pediatr*. 1981;98:617-22.
185. Zaidan H, Dhanireddy R, Hamosh M, et al. Lipid clearing in premature infants during continuous heparin infusion: role of circulating lipase. *Pediatr Res*. 1985;19:23-5.
186. Haumont D, Richelle M, Deckelbaum RJ, et al. Effect of liposomal content of lipid emulsions on plasma lipid concentrations in low birth weight infants receiving parenteral nutrition. *J Pediatr*. 1992;121:759-63.
187. Tashiro T, Mashima Y, Yamamori H, et al. Intravenous Intralipid 10% vs. 20%, hyperlipidemia, and increase in lipoprotein X in humans. *Nutrition*. 1992;8:155-60.
188. Haumont D, Deckelbaum RJ, Richelle M, et al. Plasma lipid and plasma lipoprotein concentrations in low birth weight infants given parenteral nutrition with twenty or ten percent lipid emulsion. *J Pediatr*. 1989;115:787-93.
189. Carpentier YA. Intravascular metabolism of fat emulsions. *Clin Nutr*. 1989;8:115-25.
190. Griffin E, Breckenridge WC, Kuksis MH, et al. Appearance and characterization of lipoprotein X during continuous Intralipid infusion in the neonate. *J Clin Invest*. 1979;64:1703-12.
191. Richards CE, Drayton M, Jenkins H, et al. Effect of different chloride infusion rates on plasma base excess during neonatal parenteral nutrition. *Acta Paediatr*. 1993;82:678-82.
192. Groh-Wargo S, Ciaccia A, Moore J. Neonatal metabolic acidosis: effect of chloride from normal saline flushes. *J Parenter Enteral Nutr*. 1988;12:159-61.

193. Heird WC, Hay W, Helms RA, et al. Pediatric parenteral amino acid mixture in low birth weight infants. *Pediatrics*. 1988;81:41-50.
194. Laine L, Shulman RJ, Pitre D, et al. Cysteine usage increases the need for acetate in neonates who receive total parenteral nutrition. *Am J Clin Nutr*. 1991;54:565-7.
195. Nesbakken R, Reinlie S. Magnesium and phosphorus: the electrolytes of energy metabolism. *Acta Anaesthesiol Scand*. 1985;29:60-4.
196. Weiner ID, Wingo CS. Hypokalemia-consequences, causes, and correction. *J Am Soc Nephrol*. 1997;8:1179-88.
197. Ahsan SK, al-Swoyan S, Hanif M, et al. Hypomagnesemia and clinical implications in children and neonates. *Indian J Med Sci*. 1998;52:541-7.
198. Weintrob N, Karp M, Hod M. Short- and long-range complications in offspring of diabetic mothers. *J Diabetes Complications*. 1996;10:294-301.
199. Rasmussen A. Carbohydrate induced hypophosphatemia. *Acta Anaesthesiol Scand*. 1985;29:68-70.
200. Shaffer SG, Kilbride HW, Hayen LK, et al. Hyperkalemia in very low birth weight infants. *J Pediatr*. 1992;121:275-9.
201. Fukuda Y, Kojima T, Ono A, et al. Factors causing hyperkalemia in premature infants. *Am J Perinatol*. 1989;6:76-9.
202. McGuinness GA, Weinstein MM, Cruikshank DP, et al. Effects of magnesium sulfate treatment on perinatal calcium metabolism. II. *Obstet Gynecol*. 1980;56:595-600.
203. Donovan EF, Tsang RC, Steichen JJ, et al. Neonatal hypermagnesemia: effect on parathyroid hormone and calcium homeostasis. *J Pediatr*. 1980;96:305-10.
204. Schultz NJ, Chitwood-Dagner KK. Body electrolyte homeostasis. In: Dipiro JT, Talbert RL, Yee GC, et al., eds. *Pharmacotherapy: A Pathophysiologic Approach*. Stamford, CT: Appleton & Lange; 1997: 1105-37.
205. Bengoa JM, Sitrin MD, Wood RJ, et al. Amino acid-induced hypercalciuria in patients on total parenteral nutrition. *Am J Clin Nutr*. 1983;38:264-9.
206. Ladenson JH, Lewis JW, Boyd JC. Failure of total calcium corrected for protein, albumin, and pH to correctly assess free calcium status. *J Clin Endocrinol Metab*. 1978;46:986-93.
207. Kelly DA. Liver complications of pediatric parenteral nutrition: epidemiology. *Nutrition*. 1998;14:153-7.
208. Beale E, Nelson R, Bucciarelli R, et al. Intrahepatic cholestasis associated with parenteral nutrition in premature infants. *Pediatrics* 1979;64:342-7.
209. Beath SV, Davies P, Papadopoulou A, et al. Parenteral nutrition-related cholestasis in postsurgical neonates: multivariate analysis of risk factors. *J Pediatr Surg*. 1996;31:604-6.
210. Lucas A, Bloom R, Aynsley-Green A. Metabolic and endocrine consequences of depriving preterm infants of enteral nutrition. *Acta Pediatr Scand*. 1983;72:245-9.
211. Colomb V, Goulet O, Rambaud C, et al. Long-term parenteral nutrition in children: liver and gallbladder disease. *Transplant Proc*. 1992;24:1054-5.
212. Suita S, Masumoto K, Yamanouchi T, et al. Complications in neonates with short bowel syndrome and long-term parenteral nutrition. *J Parenter Enteral Nutr*. 1999;23 (suppl 5):S106-9.
213. Drongowski RA, Coran AG. An analysis of factors contributing to the development of total parenteral nutrition-induced cholestasis. *J Parenter Enteral Nutr*. 1989;13:586-9.
214. Pierro A, van Saene HKF, Donnell SC, et al. Microbial translocation in neonates and infants receiving long-term parenteral nutrition. *Arch Surg*. 1996;131:176-9.
215. Cavicchi M, Beau P, Crenn P, et al. Prevalence of liver disease and contributing factors in patients receiving home parenteral nutrition for permanent intestinal failure. *Ann Intern Med*. 2000;132:525-32.
216. Ito Y, Shils ME. Liver dysfunction associated with long-term total parenteral nutrition in patients with massive bowel resection. *J Parenter Enteral Nutr*. 1991;15:271-6.
217. Nanji AA, Anderson FH. Sensitivity and specificity of liver function tests in the detection of parenteral nutrition-associated cholestasis. *J Parenter Enteral Nutr*. 1985;9:307-8.
218. Rodgers BM, Hollenbeck JI, Donnelly WH, et al. Intrahepatic cholestasis with parenteral alimentation. *Am J Surg*. 1976;131:149-55.
219. Sheldon GF, Petersen SR, Snaders R. Hepatic dysfunction during hyperalimentation. *Arch Surg*. 1978;113:504-8.
220. Postuma R, Trevenen CL. Liver disease in infants receiving total parenteral nutrition. *Pediatrics*. 1979;63:110-5.
221. Beath SV, Needham SJ, Kelly DA, et al. Clinical features and prognosis of children assessed for isolated small bowel or combined small bowel and liver transplantation. *J Pediatr Surg*. 1997;32:459-61.
222. Hodes JE, Grosfeld JL, Weber TR, et al. Hepatic failure in infants on total parenteral nutrition (TPN): clinical and histopathologic observations. *J Pediatr Surg*. 1982;17:463-8.
223. Benjamin DR. Hepatobiliary dysfunction in infants and children associated with long-term total parenteral nutrition: a clinico-pathologic study. *Am J Clin Pathol*. 1981;76:276-83.

224. Vileisis RA, Inwood RJ, Hunt CE. Laboratory monitoring of parenteral nutrition-associated hepatic dysfunction in infants. *J Parenter Enteral Nutr.* 1981;5:67-9.

225. Goldberg DM, Martin JF. Role of gamma–glutamyl transpeptidase activity in the diagnosis of hepatobiliary disease. *Digestion.* 1975;12:232-46.

226. Deitch EA, Winterton J, Li M, et al. The gut as a portal of entry for bacteremia. Role of protein malnutrition. *Ann Surg.* 1987;205:681-92.

227. Aynsley-Green A. Plasma hormone concentrations during enteral and parenteral nutrition in the human newborn. *J Pediatr Gastroenterol Nutr.* 1983;2(suppl 1):S108-12.

228. Rager R, Finegold MJ. Cholestasis in immature newborn infants: is parenteral alimentation responsible? *J Pediatr.* 1975;86:264-9.

229. Alverdy JC, Aoys E, Moss GS. Total parenteral nutrition promotes bacterial translocation from the gut. *Surgery.* 1988;104:185-90.

230. Go LL, Healy PJ, Watkins SC, et al. The effect of endotoxin on intestinal mucosal permeability to bacteria in vitro. *Arch Surg.* 1995; 130:53-8.

231. Messing B, Colombel JF, Heresbach D, et al. Chronic cholestasis and macronutrient excess in patients treated with prolonged parenteral nutrition. *Nutrition.* 1992;8:30-6.

232. Buchmiller CE, Kleiman-Wexler RL, Ephgrave KS, et al. Liver dysfunction and energy source: results of a randomized clinical trial. *J Parenter Enteral Nutr.* 1993;17:301-6.

233. Meguid MM, Akahoshi MP, Jeffers S, et al. Amelioration of metabolic complications of conventional total parenteral nutrition. *Arch Surg.* 1984;119:1294-8.

234. Collier S, Crough J, Hendricks K, et al. Use of parenteral nutrition in infants less than 6 months of age. *Nutr Clin Pract.* 1994;9:65-8.

235. Maini B, Blackburn GL, Bistrian BR, et al. Cyclic hyperalimentation: an optimal technique for preservation of visceral proteins. *J Surg Res.* 1976;20:515-25.

236. Ternullo SR, Burckart GJ. Experience with cyclic hyperalimentation in infants [abstract]. *J Parenter Enteral Nutr.* 1979;3:516.

237. Spagnuolo MI, Iorio R, Vegnente A, et al. Ursodeoxycholic acid for the treatment of cholestasis in children on long-term total parenteral nutrition: a pilot study. *Gastroenterology.*1996;111:716-9.

238. Narkewicz MR, Smith D, Gregory C, et al. Effect of ursodeoxycholic acid therapy on hepatic function in children with intrahepatic cholestatic liver disease. *J Pediatr Gastroenterol Nutr.* 1998;26:49-55.

239. Rintala RJ, Lindahl H, Pohjavuori M. Total parenteral nutrition-associated cholestasis in surgical neonates may be reversed by intravenous cholecystokinin: a preliminary report. *J Pediatr Surg.* 1995;30:827-30.

240. Teitelbaum DH, Han-Markey T, Schumacher RE. Treatment of parenteral nutrition associated cholestasis with cholecystokinin-octapeptide. *J Pediatr Surg.* 1995;30:1082

241. Vanderhoof JA, Langnas AN, Pinch LW, et al. Short bowel syndrome. *J Pediatr Gastroenterol Nutr.* 1992;14:359-70.

242. Booth IW, Lander AD. Short bowel syndrome. *Baillieres Clin Gastroenterol.* 1998;12:739-73.

243. Btaiche IF, Khalidi N. Parenteral nutrition-associated liver complications in children. *Pharmacotherapy.* 2002;22:188-211.

244. The TS, Kollee LA, Boon JM, et al. Rickets in a preterm infant during intravenous alimentation. *Acta Pediatr Scand.* 1983;72:769-71.

245. Kien CL, Browning C, Jona J, et al. Rickets in premature infants receiving parenteral nutrition: a case report and review of the literature. *J Parenter Enteral Nutr.* 1982;6:152-6.

246. Shike M, Shils ME, Heller A, et al. Bone disease in prolonged parenteral nutrition: osteopenia without mineralization defect. *Am J Clin Nutr.* 1986;44:89-98.

247. de Vernejoul MC, Messing B, Modrowski D, et al. Multifactorial low remodeling bone disease during cyclic total parenteral nutrition. *J Clin Endocrinol Metab.* 1985;60:109.

248. Leape LL, Valaes T. Rickets in low birth weight infants receiving total parenteral nutrition. *J Pediatr Surg.* 11:665-74.

249. Koo WW, Kaplan LA, Horn J, et al. Aluminum on parenteral nutrition solution-sources and possible alternatives. *J Parenter Enteral Nutr.* 1986;10:591-5.

250. Ott SM, Maloney NA, Klein GL, et al. Aluminum is associated with low bone formation in patients receiving chronic parenteral nutrition. *Ann Intern Med.* 1983;98:910-4.

251. Shike M, Sturtridge WC, Tam CS, et al. A possible role for vitamin D in the genesis of parenteral nutrition-induced metabolic bone disease. *Ann Intern Med.* 1981;95:560-8.

252. Larchet M, Garabedian M, Bourdeau A, et al. Calcium metabolism in children during long-term total parenteral nutrition: the influence of calcium, phosphorus, and vitamin D intakes. *J Pediatr Gastroenterol Nutr.* 1991;13:367-75.

253. Lipkin EW, Ott SM, Chesnut CH III. Mineral loss in the parenteral nutrition patient. *Am J Clin Nutr.* 1988;47:515-23.

254. Wood RJ, Bengoa JM, Sitrin MD, et al. Calciuric effect of cyclic versus continuous total parenteral nutrition. *Am J Clin Nutr.* 1985;41:614-9.

255. Cunningham J, Fraher LJ, Clemens TL, et al. Chronic acidosis with metabolic bone disease. *Am J Med.* 1982;73:199-204.

256. Vargas JH, Klein GL, Ament ME, et al. Metabolic bone disease of total parenteral nutrition: course after changing from casein to amino acids in parenteral solutions with reduced aluminum content. *Am J Clin Nutr.* 1988;48:1070-8.

257. Koo WW, Kaplan LA, Bendon R, et al. Response to aluminum in parenteral nutrition during infancy. *J Pediatr.* 1986;109:883-7.

258. Klein GL. Metabolic bone disease of total parenteral nutrition. *Nutrition.* 1998;14:149-52.

259. Shike M, Harrison JE, Sturtridge WC, et al. Metabolic bone disease in patients receiving long-term total parenteral nutrition. *Ann Intern Med.* 1980;92:343-50.

260. Verhage AH, Cheong WK, Allard JP, et al. Increase in lumbar spine bone mineral content in patients on long-term parenteral nutrition without vitamin D supplementation. *J Parenter Enteral Nutr.* 1995;19:431-6.

261. Sloan GM, White DE, Brennan MF. Calcium and phosphorus metabolism during total parenteral nutrition. *Ann Surg.* 1983;197:1-6.

262. Wood RJ, Sitrin MD, Cusson GJ, et al. Reduction of total parenteral nutrition-induced urinary calcium loss by increasing the phosphorus in the total parenteral nutrition prescription. *J Parenter Enteral Nutr.* 1986;10:188-90.

263. Lewis WJ, Sherertz RJ. Microbial interactions with catheter material. *Nutrition.* 1997;13(suppl):5S-9S.

264. Mermel LA. Defining intravascular catheter-related infections: a plea for uniformity. *Nutrition.* 1997;13(suppl): 2S-4S.

265. Widmer AF. Management of catheter-related bacteremia and fungemia in patients on total parenteral nutrition. *Nutrition.* 1997;13(suppl):18S-25S.

266. Maki DG, Goldman DA, Rhame FS. Infection control in intravenous therapy. *Ann Intern Med.* 1973;79:867-87.

267. Snydman DR, Murray SA, Kornfeld SJ, et al. Total parenteral nutrition-related infections. Prospective epidemiologic study using semiquantitative methods. *Am J Med.* 1982;73:695-9.

268. Nahata MC, King DR, Powell DA, et al. Management of catheter-related infections in pediatric patients. *J Parenter Enteral Nutr.* 1988;12:58-9.

269. Sitges-Serra A, Puig P, Linares J, et al. Hub colonization as the initial step in an outbreak of catheter-related sepsis due to coagulase negative staphylococci during parenteral nutrition. *J Parenter Enteral Nutr.* 1984;8:668-72.

270. Linares J, Sitges-Serra A, Garau J, et al. Pathogenesis of catheter sepsis: a prospective study with quantitative and semiquantitative cultures of catheter hub and segments. *J Clin Microbiol.* 1985;21:357-60.

271. Yeung C, May J, Hughes R. Infection rate for single lumen vs triple lumen subclavian catheters. *Infect Control Hosp Epidemiol.* 1988;9:154-8.

272. Beganovic N, Verloove-Vanhorick SP, Brand R, et al. Total parenteral nutrition and sepsis. *Arch Dis Child.* 1988;63:66-7.

273. Pemberton LB, Lyman B, Lander V, et al. Sepsis from triple- vs single-lumen catheters during total parenteral nutrition in surgical or critically ill patients. *Arch Surg.* 1986;121:591-4.

274. McCarthy MC, Shives JK, Robison RJ, et al. Prospective evaluation of single and triple lumen catheters in total parenteral nutrition. *J Parenter Enteral Nutr.* 1987;11:259-62.

275. Shulman RJ, Smith EO, Rahman S, et al. Single- vs double-lumen central venous catheters in pediatric oncology patients. *Am J Dis Child.* 1988;142:893-5.

276. Ma TY, Yoshinaka R, Banaag A, et al. Total parenteral nutrition via multilumen catheters does not increase the risk of catheter-related sepsis: a randomized prospective study. *Clin Infect Dis.* 1998;27:500-3.

277. Garrison RN, Wilson MA. Intravenous and central catheter infections. *Surgical Clinics of North America.* 1994;74:557-70.

278. Darouiche RO, Raad II. Prevention of catheter-related infections: the skin. *Nutrition.* 1997;13(suppl):26S-9S.

279. Raad II, Sabbagh MF. Optimal duration of therapy for catheter-related Staphylococcus aureus bacteremia: a study of 55 cases and review. *Clin Infect Dis.* 1992;14:75-82.

280. Mermel LA, Farr BM, Sherertz RJ, et al. Guidelines for the management of intravascular catheter-related infections. *Clin Infect Dis.* 2001;32:1249-72.

281. Panter-Brick M, Wagget J, Dale G. Intralipid and thrombocytopenia [letter]. *Lancet.* 1975;1:857-8.

282. Cohen IT, Dahms B, Hays DM. Peripheral total parenteral nutrition employing a lipid emulsion (Intralipid): complications encountered in pediatric patients. *J Pediatr Surg.* 1977;12:837-45.

283. Goulet O, Girot R, Maier-Redelsperger M, et al. Hematologic disorders following prolonged use of intravenous fat emulsions in children. *J Parenter Enteral Nutr.* 1986;10:284-8.

284. Lipson AH, Pritchard J, Thomas G. Thrombocytopenia after intralipid infusion in a neonate [letter]. *Lancet.* 1974;2:1462-3.

285. Stahl GE, Spear ML, Hamosh M. Intravenous administration of lipid emulsions to premature infants. *Clin Perinatol.* 1986;13:133-62.

286. Gabay C, Kushner I. Mechanisms of disease: acute-phase proteins and other systemic responses to inflammation. *N Engl J Med.* 1999;340:448-54.

287. Winkler MF, Gerrior SA, Pomp A, et al. Use of retinol-binding protein and prealbumin as indicators of the response to nutrition therapy. *J Am Diet Assoc.* 1989;89:684-7.

288. Mirtallo JM. The complexity of mixing calcium and phosphate. *Am J Hosp Pharm.* 1994;51:1535-6.

289. Hill SE, Heldman LS, Goo ED, et al. Fatal microvascular pulmonary emboli from precipitation of a total nutrient admixture solution. *J Parenter Enteral Nutr.* 1996;20:81-7.

290. Lenz GT, Mikrut BA. Calcium and phosphate solubility in neonatal parenteral nutrient solutions containing Aminosyn-PF or Trophamine. *Am J Hosp Pharm.* 1988;45:2367-71.

291. MacKay MW, Fitzgerald KA, Jackson D. The solubility of calcium and phosphate in two specialty amino acid solutions. *J Parenter Enteral Nutr.* 1996;20:63-6.

292. Fitzgerald KA, MacKay MW. Calcium and phosphate solubility in neonatal parenteral nutrient solutions containing TrophAmine. *Am J Hosp Pharm.* 1986;43:88-93.

293. Driscoll DF, Newton DW, Bistrian BR. Precipitation of calcium phosphate from parenteral nutrient fluids. *Am J Hosp Pharm.* 1994;51:2834-6.

294. Vaughan LM, Small C, Plunkett V. Incompatibility of iron dextran and a total nutrient admixture. *Am J Hosp Pharm.* 1990;47:1745-6.

295. Moclair AE, Bates I. The efficacy of heparin in maintaining peripheral infusions in neonates. *Eur J Pediatr.* 1995;154:567-70.

296. Wright A, Hecker J, McDonald G. Effects of low dose heparin on failure of intravenous infusions in children. *Heart Lung.* 1995;24:79-82.

297. Treas LS, Latinis-Bridges B. Efficacy of heparin in peripheral venous infusion in neonates. *J Obstet Gynecol Neonatal Nurs.* 1992;21:214-9.

298. Alpan G, Eyal F, Springer C, et al. Heparinization of alimentation solutions administered through peripheral veins in premature infants: a controlled study. *Pediatrics.* 1984;74:375-8.

299. Isaacs JW, Millikan WJ, Stackhouse J, et al. Parenteral nutrition of adults with 900-milliosmolar solution via peripheral veins. *Am J Clin Nutr.* 1977;30:552-9.

300. Matsusue S, Nishimura S, Koizumi S, et al. Preventive effect of simultaneously infused lipid emulsion against thrombophlebitis during postoperative peripheral parenteral nutrition. *Surg Today.* 1995;25:667 71.

301. Strausburg KM. Parenteral nutrition admixture. In: Merritt RJ, ed. *The A.S.P.E.N. Nutrition Support Practice Manual.* 1st ed. Silver Spring, MD: American Society for Parenteral and Enteral Nutrition; 1998:1-12.

302. US Food and Drug Administration. Safety alert: hazards of precipitation associated with parenteral nutrition. *Am J Hosp Pharm.* 1994;51:1427-8.

CHAPTER 7

BASICS OF ENTERAL AND PARENTERAL NUTRITION

Carol J. Rollins

When food consumption is restricted for a significant time, energy stores become depleted and body proteins are lost. Consequences of the ensuing malnutrition include decreased wound healing, increased infections, impaired immunity, increased morbidity, and a rise in mortality. When patients will not, should not, or cannot eat, malnutrition is inevitable unless nutrition can be provided another way.

Specialized nutrition support offers two important options. Enteral nutrition (EN) bypasses the upper gastrointestinal (GI) tract by placing a feeding tube into the stomach or small bowel. Parenteral nutrition (PN) bypasses the entire GI tract to provide nutrients intravenously.

Man has attempted to provide specialized nutrition support since ancient times, but efforts were limited by sparse knowledge of internal anatomy, physiology, bacteriology, and nutrition. By the late 1800s, however, successful gastrostomy placement had been performed, and in 1913 goats were successfully fed with intravenous (IV) protein hydrolysate for over 2 weeks.[1]

Knowledge of nutrition expanded rapidly during the early 20th century. By 1950 most of the vitamins had been discovered, the essential amino acids had been identified, protein hydrolysate and crystalline amino acids had been infused into humans, and hypertonic glucose had been infused through a polyethylene catheter located in the superior vena cava. The hallmark study for PN came in the mid-1960s when Dr. Stanley Dudrick showed that normal growth and development could be achieved in beagle puppies fed intravenously through a central line; then he sustained a newborn infant for 22 months with intravenous feeding.[1] Advances in both EN and PN since that time have made specialized nutrition support routinely available.

Growing interest in specialized nutrition support during the 1970s, and the realization that these therapies could be both life-sustaining and life-threatening, led to formation of the American Society for Parenteral and Enteral Nutrition (ASPEN) in 1975. ASPEN is interdisciplinary, composed of

Types of Specialized Nutrition Support
❏ Enteral nutrition (EN): feeding that bypasses the upper gastrointestinal tract by placing a tube into the stomach or small bowel.
❏ Parenteral nutrition (PN): feeding that bypasses the entire gastrointestinal tract to provide nutrients intravenously.

pharmacy, medicine, nursing, dietetics, and nutrition professionals "dedicated to assuring that every patient receives optimal nutrition care."[2] ASPEN's stated mission is "to serve as a preeminent, interdisciplinary, research-based, patient-centered clinical nutrition society throughout the world."[2] To help accomplish this mission, ASPEN has developed guidelines and standards of practice, and participating professions have developed certification processes. Certified nutrition support physicians (CNSP), nurses (CNSN), and dietitians (CNSD) must pass a basic profession-specific certification examination in the specialty practice area of EN and PN therapy, which is developed through the National Board of Nutrition Support Certification. Pharmacists can be designated a board-certified nutrition support pharmacist (BCNSP) through the Board of Pharmaceutical Specialties (see sidebar).

This chapter first provides basic information to help you decide on patients' nutritional goals and assess whether specialized nutrition support is appropriate. It also covers principles of EN and PN therapy. Although evidence-based practice is always desirable, studies related to nutrition support are often small and nutrition is rarely the primary problem in the population being studied. Disease-state effects frequently overshadow nutrition support decisions. Even so, it is critical to realize that mismanaging nutrition support can significantly harm patients and even cause death.

NUTRITION SCREENING

It's best to use an organized approach to pinpoint patients who require nutritional intervention. Nutrition screening that employs parameters associated with nutrition-related complications helps you rapidly identify both patients at risk of malnutrition and those already malnourished. The screening criteria you use should have documented efficacy.

The Nutrition Screening Initiative, a joint project of the American Academy of Family Physicians, the American Dietetic Association, and the National Council on the Aging, has developed several tools for nutrition screening.[3] One of these tools uses the acronym DETERMINE as a mnemonic device for remembering the risk factors for malnutrition (see sidebar below).

Hospital and home care organizations accredited by the Joint Commission on Accreditation of Healthcare Organizations (JCAHO) are expected to have a nutrition screening process in place and a procedure, based on screening results, for referring patients to a qualified health professional for nutrition assessment. Because JCAHO requires screening for all patients admitted to

Nutrition Support Pharmacy

Since 1988 the specialty of *nutrition support pharmacy* has been recognized by the Board of Pharmaceutical Specialties in Washington, D.C. These specialists promote, maintain, and restore proper nutrition for patients in all settings, including hospitals and home care. To become board certified, which is voluntary, pharmacists must have a specified level of experience and training and are required to pass a rigorous exam. Currently there are more than 400 board-certified nutrition support pharmacists. Their required knowledge and abilities include:

❑ Interviewing the patient, obtaining a medical, nutritional, medication, psychosocial, and socioeconomic history, and reviewing the history to assess nutritional status.

❑ Estimating or measuring daily requirements for energy, protein, vitamins, minerals, and fluids.

❑ Understanding the components of a nutritionally adequate diet as well as the processes of normal ingestion, digestion, absorption, metabolism, and excretion of nutrients.

❑ Understanding the effects of diseases, clinical conditions, altered metabolism, and medical or surgical therapies on nutritional status.

❑ Understanding the effects of nutritional status on diseases.

❑ Identifying, monitoring, and managing interactions between drugs and nutrients.

❑ Being familiar with diseases and clinical conditions that affect ingestion, digestion, absorption, metabolism, and excretion of nutrients.

❑ Identifying potentially malnourished patients.

❑ Understanding all aspects of enteral and parenteral feeding.

❑ Developing therapeutic plans and communicating them to patients and caregivers.

More information on board certification can be found on the Internet at http://www.bpsweb.org.

accredited health care organizations, the process must be carried out efficiently by personnel who are readily available. Periodic rescreening is also required. JCAHO does not specify the criteria to be included in nutrition screening, the time period for rescreening, or the profession that qualified health providers must be part of to accept referrals for nutrition assessment. The sidebar on page 216 lists parameters commonly used for nutrition screening. Screening instruments often include one or two criteria from each category, but information corresponding to all the criteria may not be available for all patients.

ASPEN suggests the following timing for nutrition screening: within 24 hours for acute care, on admission or within 24 hours for long-term care, and on the initial nursing visit for home care.[2]

Nutritional Health Checklist

The "Determine Your Nutritional Health" checklist developed by the American Academy of Family Physicians, the American Dietetic Association, and the National Council on the Aging, is a nutrition screening tool that uses the mnemonic device below as a reminder of malnutrition risk factors. It is available on the Web at http://www.aafp.org/nsi.

Disease
Eating poorly
Tooth loss/mouth pain
Economic hardship
Reduced social contact
Multiple medicines
Involuntary weight loss/gain
Needs assistance in self care
Elderly years above 80

Nutrition Screening Parameters

Presence of one or more of the following indicates that a patient is at nutritional risk and should undergo nutrition assessment.

Anthropometric Parameters

1. Low body weight
   —Current weight under 80% of ideal body weight (IBW)
   —Current weight under 85% of usual body weight (UBW)
2. Unplanned weight loss
   —10 pounds (4.5 kg) or more in 6 months or less
   —Over 1% of usual weight per week for 1 or more weeks
   —Over 5% of usual weight in 1 month
   —Over 10% of usual weight in 6 months
3. Body mass index (BMI)
   —Under 18.5
   —30 or greater

Laboratory Parameters

1. Serum albumin 3.2 g/dL or less
2. Total lymphocyte count (TLC) under 1500 mm^3
3. Total iron binding capacity (TIBC) over 400 mcg/dL

Diagnosis

1. Altered gastrointestinal (GI) function
   —delayed gastric emptying or gastroparesis
   —diarrhea (500 ml or more for > 3 days)
   —vomiting > 5 days
2. Altered tissue repair
   —decubitus or pressure ulcer
   —nonhealing wounds
3. Cachexia
4. Cancer
5. Depression or dementia (forgets to eat)
6. Diabetes mellitus
7. Dialysis
8. End stage organ failure (cardiac, hepatic, pulmonary, renal)
9. Gastrointestinal disease
   —inflammatory bowel disease
   —active Crohn's disease or ulcerative colitis
   —graft versus host disease of liver/GI tract
   —short bowel syndrome
10. Major GI surgery within past year
11. Major trauma/surgery within the past 60 days
12. Mesenteric ischemia
13. Organ transplant
    —solid organ: heart, kidney, liver, lung, pancreas
    —hematopoietic: bone marrow, peripheral blood stem cells, umbilical cord blood

Reduced Nutritional Intake

1. Less than 50% of estimated requirements for > 5 days
2. 50% to 80% of estimated requirements for 2 to 4 weeks

Source: References 3, 6–9, 13, 24–26, 31–36, 73.

NUTRITION ASSESSMENT

Once a patient is identified as "at risk" by the nutrition screening process, further evaluation is appropriate to assess the patient's current nutritional status, risk of developing protein-energy malnutrition, and risk of specific nutrient deficiencies. The patient's response to nutritional intervention must also be monitored and his or her risk of complications from malnutrition must be quantified.[4] Nutrition assessment should include five major components, as listed in the following sidebar.

Key Components of Nutrition Assessment

1. History.
2. Body measurements or anthropometrics.
3. Physical examination.
4. Biochemical evaluation.
5. Functional evaluation.

Although the depth of information may vary from case to case, it should correlate with the degree of risk for malnutrition (higher risk, more in depth evaluation) and the complexity of the patient presentation. When objective data are unreliable or not available, subjective data provide valuable information in the assessment process.

History

Medical, dietary, social, and medication histories all provide useful data in assessing nutritional status. An interdisciplinary approach is highly valuable in obtaining a complete history. Each health care professional should be able to gather a basic history, but it's useful—especially when patients' cases are complex—to have the various disciplines handle specific segments of the history (i.e., physicians/medical history, dietitians/nutrition history, pharmacists/medication history, and nurses/social and family history).

Information in the medical history that may be pertinent to nutritional status includes:

- History of present illness.
- Type and duration of other illnesses.
- Surgical history.
- Addictive habits (tobacco, alcohol, illicit drugs).
- Psychological evaluation.
- Contributing family history.

Dietary history provides information on the quantity and quality of intake relative to population requirements, such as percent of Dietary Reference Intakes (DRIs) for selected nutrients.[5] It also covers:

- Usual meal patterns.
- Dietary restrictions.
- Food allergies and aversions.
- Use of dietary supplements.
- Changes in food intake, appetite, satiety, taste acuity, and bowel function (constipation, diarrhea, steatorrhea).
- Gastrointestinal disturbances (nausea, vomiting, dyspepsia), which may be listed here as well as in the medical history.

Social history may provide clues to the patient's ability to buy and prepare appropriate foods, uncover problems related to social isolation, and identify other factors that contribute to nutritional risk. The type and quantity of medications a patient receives can influence income available for food, appetite, weight loss or gain, drug-nutrient interactions, nutrient requirements, and nutrient tolerance (e.g., hyperglycemia with glucocorticoids).

Body Measurements or Anthropometrics

Anthropometric measurements use quantitative techniques to assess the size and proportions of the body. By applying the data derived from anthropometric measurements you can estimate body composition and the body's lean and fat masses. Anthropometric criteria used in nutrition assessment are more specific for the degree of malnutrition than the criteria used for screening. Height and weight, the most common anthropometric measurements, are inexpensive, easy to obtain for most patients, require minimal personnel training, and are generally reliable. Weight, or derivations of height and weight, is considered one of the best parameters for determining nutritional status in many situations.[6] The sidebar on page 220 lists equations used in calculating common parameters, including percent of ideal body weight (IBW), percent of usual body weight (UBW), body mass index (BMI), and percent weight loss. Typical classifications used for degree of malnutrition are:

- Mild malnutrition with weight at 80% to 90% IBW or 85% to 95% UBW.
- Moderate malnutrition with weight at 70% to 79% IBW or 75% to 84% UBW.
- Severe malnutrition when weight is below 70% IBW or 75% UBW.

BMI is strongly correlated with certain obesity-related comorbid conditions, such as type 2 diabetes mellitus, and has a relatively strong correlation with total body fat. Using BMI in nutrition assessment requires caution, however, since patients can be mistakenly classified as malnourished due to large individual variations in the correlation. There is no universally accepted interpretation of BMI for nutrition assessment. A BMI of 14 to 15 kg/m^2 is associated with significant morbidity, and malnutrition is generally considered to be present when the BMI is 18.5 kg/m^2 or under.[7] One suggested scheme for determining the degree of malnutrition is the following[8]:

- Mild malnutrition with BMI 17 to 18.5.
- Moderate malnutrition with BMI 16 to 17.
- Severe malnutrition with BMI under 16.

Other anthropometric measurements include subscapular skinfold thickness (SSF), triceps skinfold thickness (TSF), mid-arm circumference (MAC), and mid-arm muscle circumference (MAMC). Skinfold thickness serves as

Calculations and Equations

Ideal Body Weight (IBW)
    Males: 50 kg + 2.3 kg per inch (2.54 cm) over 5 feet (152 cm) or
                 106 lb (48 kg) + 6 lb (2.7 kg) per inch over 5 feet (152 cm)
    Females: 45.5 kg + 2.3 kg per inch (2.54 cm) over 5 feet (152 cm) or
                 100 lb + 5 lb per inch (2.54 cm) over 5 feet (152 cm)

Percent of IBW
    (current weight ÷ IBW) x 100

Percent of Usual Body Weight (UBW)
    (current weight ÷ UBW) x 100

Percent Weight Change
    [(UBW - current weight) ÷ UBW] x 100

Body Mass Index (BMI)
    (weight in kg) ÷ (height in meters)^2 or
    (weight in kg x 1540) ÷ (height in inches)^2 or
    (weight in lb x 700) ÷ (height in inches)^2

Total Lymphocyte Count (TLC)
    (% lymphocytes ÷ 100) x white blood cell count/mm^3

Nitrogen Balance
    nitrogen intake − nitrogen loss = nitrogen balance, using
    nitrogen intake = protein intake as grams per 24 hours ÷ 6.25
    nitrogen loss = 24 hour urine urea nitrogen loss + 4 g insensible losses or
        24 hour total urine nitrogen loss + 2 g insensible losses

Source: References 6–9, 13, 14, 73.

an indirect measure of subcutaneous fat, while MAC and MAMC indirectly evaluate skeletal muscle mass. These measurements require inexpensive equipment (skinfold caliper, tape measure), but training and consistent practice are necessary to avoid measurement errors. Interpreting SSF, TSF, MAC, and MAMC can be difficult because hydration status influences the measurements. Usefulness in hospitalized patients is limited since reference values were developed in nonhospitalized populations, and measurements change slowly. These measurements are best suited to monitoring when used with serial evaluations obtained periodically over a long time.

For instance, TSF and MAMC could be obtained on each visit for a patient scheduled to receive eight cycles of monthly chemotherapy in an oncology clinic. To improve accuracy, the same clinician should do the measurements every month. The measurements should be obtained before IV fluids and chemotherapy are started on each visit to avoid fluctuations due to fluid status.

Several direct measures of body composition exist, but the majority are applicable only in the research setting. Underwater weighing (hydrodensitometry) is the "gold standard" to determine fat and fat-free mass using a two-compartment model. Isotope dilution and neutron activation ascertain lean body mass or body cell mass; whole body conductivity determines fat-free mass; and infrared interactance measures subcutaneous fat thickness. Large imaging equipment used for other medical purposes, including ultrasound, magnetic resonance imaging (MRI), computed tomography (CT), and dual energy x-ray absorptiometry (DEXA), can provide body composition information as well.[9]

These advanced technologies have limited application to body composition analysis in the clinical setting for several reasons, including that some are not approved by the Food and Drug Administration (FDA) for this purpose in the United States. Furthermore, CT and DEXA expose the patient to ionizing radiation and MRI cannot provide images of all body compartments that relate to body composition. Determining body composition from MRI, CT, or DEXA imaging obtained for other purposes is rare because it requires expensive computer software that is generally not included with the equipment. Even if the software were readily available, ethical and legal restrictions could prevent use of imaging data without obtaining informed consent specifically for body composition analysis.

Bioelectrical impedance analysis (BIA) is a relatively inexpensive, rapid, and noninvasive method of evaluating body composition, including fat-free mass and total body water.[10] In 1994, a National Institutes of Health (NIH) Technology Assessment concluded that BIA provides a reliable estimate of total body water under most circumstances, but that fat-free mass and percent body fat predicted from the data have variable validity.[11] For healthy people and those with certain chronic diseases not associated with abnormal water distribution, such as diabetes mellitus, BIA was judged to be a useful technique for body composition analysis. It was not deemed useful for monitoring short-term changes, however, such as those from dietary intervention. At the time of its assessment, NIH noted the lack of well-defined methods and instrument standards for BIA.[11] Although BIA is now used routinely in some clinical settings, the results' validity may be questioned because of the lack of reference standards and because hydration status, obesity, fever, and electrolyte abnormalities can alter the results.

Physical Examination

In conjunction with the patient history, the nutrition-oriented physical examination allows a comprehensive nutrition plan to be developed. Using a systems approach, you should identify any signs and symptoms of malnutrition that are present and note problems that place the patient at continued nutritional risk, such as poor dentition. Although not everyone warrants an exhaustive physical examination, a general overview and history-directed examination is appropriate for each patient. If, for example, a patient's history appears to be

Key Terms and Abbreviations in Chapter 7

Miscellaneous terms related to feeding and diet:

Central venous access device (CVAD)
Dietary Reference Intakes (DRIs)
Internal jugular (IJ) catheters
Nonprotein calorie to nitrogen ratio (NPC:N)
Peripheral parenteral nutrition (PPN)
Peripherally inserted central catheter (PICC)
Recommended dietary allowance (RDA)
Respiratory quotient (RQ)
Total nutrient admixture (TNA)

Body size and measurement:

Actual body weight (ABW)
Adjusted dosing weight (ADW)
Body mass index (BMI)
Ideal body weight (IBW)
Mid-arm circumference (MAC)
Mid-arm muscle circumference (MAMC)
Subscapular skinfold thickness (SSF)
Triceps skinfold thickness (TSF)
Usual body weight (UBW)

Medical tests and procedures:

Bioelectrical impedance analysis (BIA)
Blood urea nitrogen (BUN) measurements
Bone marrow transplant (BMT)
Computed tomography (CT)
Creatinine-height index (CHI)
Delayed hypersensitivity testing (DHT)
Dual energy x-ray absorptiometry (DEXA)
Magnetic resonance imaging (MRI)
Retinol-binding protein (RBP)
Total lymphocyte count (TLC)
Total urine nitrogen (TUN)
Urine urea nitrogen (UUN)

Eicosanoids:

Leukotriene B_4 (LTB_4)
Prostaglandin E_2 (PGE_2)
Thromboxane A_2 (TXA_2)

Nutritional assessments:

Mini Nutritional Assessment (MNA)
Nutrition Risk Index (NRI)

Patient-generated subjective global assessment (PG-SGA)
Prognostic Inflammatory and Nutrition Index (PINI)
Prognostic Nutrition Index (PNI)
Subjective global assessment (SGA)

Medical conditions:

Acute renal failure (ARF)
Chronic obstructive pulmonary disease (COPD)
Chronic renal failure (CRF)

Energy and metabolic rate:

Basal energy expenditure (BEE)
Basal metabolic rate (BMR)
Resting energy expenditure (REE)
Resting metabolic rate (RMR)
Total energy expenditure (TEE)

Types and placement of tubes:

Jejunal tube placed through a PEG (JET-PEG)
Nasoduodenal (ND)
Nasogastric (NG)
Nasojejunal (NJ)
Percutaneous endoscopic gastrostomy (PEG)
Percutaneous endoscopic jejunostomy (PEJ)

Components of nutrients:

Aromatic amino acids (AAAs)
Branched-chain amino acid (BCAA)
Docosahexaenoic acid (DHA)
Essential amino acid (EAA)
Eicosapentaenoic acid (EPA)
Fatty acid (FA)
Fructooligosaccharides (FOS)
Long chain fatty acid (LCFA)
Medium chain fatty acid (MCFA)
Medium chain triglyceride (MCT)
Monounsaturated fatty acid (MUFA)
Polyunsaturated fatty acid (PUFA)
Short chain fatty acid (SCFA)

Plastics used in PN delivery:

Diethylhexylphthalate (DEHP)
Ethylene vinyl acetate (EVA)
Polyvinyl chloride (PVC)

consistent with fat malabsorption, the nutrition-oriented physical examination should focus on signs and symptoms associated with potential deficiencies of vitamins A, D, E, and K.

Through this general overview, you gain an appreciation of the patient's weight for height, muscle wasting, and loss of subcutaneous fat. Observing the musculoskeletal system yields helpful information: for example, the temporalis muscles provide a subjective assessment of muscle wasting not easily camouflaged by edema, and the hands provide an initial impression of subcutaneous fat stores. You should also review anthropometric data and vital signs. To complete the examination, look for alterations that could be nutrition-related in the skin, hair, nails, face, eyes, lips, mouth, teeth, gums, neck, thorax, cardiac system, gastrointestinal system, urinary tract, musculoskeletal system, and nervous system. Few classic vitamin deficiencies are seen today in clinical practice in the United States, but subclinical deficiencies may be present in many patients at risk nutritionally. For more information on nutritional deficiencies see Chapter 1, and you can look at other references for excellent comprehensive reviews of the nutrition-focused physical examination.[12,13]

Biochemical Evaluation

Biochemical parameters included in a complete nutrition assessment allow clinicians to evaluate somatic protein status, immune function, nutritional anemias, nitrogen balance, and visceral protein status.

Creatinine-height index (CHI) and urinary 3-methylhistidine can be used to estimate skeletal muscle (somatic protein) or lean tissue mass, but they are rarely used in clinical practice and have largely been replaced by more direct methods of body composition analysis. Total lymphocyte count (TLC), which evaluates B-cell and T-cell function, and delayed hypersensitivity testing (DHT), which evaluates cell-mediated immunity, lack specificity for malnutrition, severely limiting their application to clinical nutrition assessment. Both, however, should be considered secondary parameters for nutrition assessment. A reduced TLC and anergy on DHT suggests immunosuppression, which is associated with malnutrition. TLC can generally be obtained in hospitalized patients because only a white blood count with a differential is needed to calculate it (see the Calculations and Equations sidebar on page 220). For DHT, intradermal administration of three to six antigens is typically required, with induration evaluated 24 to 48 hours later.

Several issues too complex to discuss here surround the selection and interpretation of tests used to evaluate nutritional anemias resulting from deficiencies of iron, folic acid, vitamin B_{12}, or copper. Most likely, biochemical parameters for evaluating nutritional anemias will be ordered as the result of the initial nutrition assessment, rather than being available beforehand. Tests must be interpreted correctly to avoid adding nutrients when they are not necessary. For example, many patients have low serum iron who are not iron deficient. Administering iron to a sick patient who is not iron deficient could increase the risk of infection and mortality.

Nitrogen Balance

The biochemical parameters for nutrition assessment most likely to be encountered in the clinical setting are nitrogen balance (N-balance) and visceral protein status. Nitrogen balance—nitrogen intake minus nitrogen losses from urine and other sources (see sidebar on page 220)—is an indicator of physiological stress and protein requirements. Nitrogen intake is generally calculated from protein intake, assuming that protein has a 16% nitrogen content. Thus the number of grams of nitrogen is equal to grams of protein divided by 6.25. Altering the "natural" amino acid content of protein by adding individual amino acids may invalidate this assumption; so the nitrogen content of modified amino acid products should be checked before doing the conversion. Urinary losses are measured as urine urea nitrogen (UUN) or as total urine nitrogen (TUN).

Negative N-balance occurs when losses are greater than intake, which indicates catabolism, or protein breakdown. Initially the protein is lost from skeletal muscle, but if the negative N-balance is prolonged, losses come from visceral organs (heart, liver, lung, kidneys) and from functional proteins, such as enzymes and transport proteins. Urinary nitrogen loss increases with physiological stress associated with certain illnesses and injuries (e.g., closed head injury, long bone fractures, severe infection). N-balance becomes significantly negative unless there is a concomitant increase in nitrogen (protein) intake. The more negative the N-balance, the quicker protein malnutrition will occur—and the sooner nutritional intervention is needed. Positive N-balance is associated with anabolism, or tissue repair and protein synthesis.

Urinary nitrogen loss is not routinely evaluated in most health care facilities because it requires patients' urine to be carefully collected for 24 hours without contamination by stool or blood. Only selected patients at high nutritional risk are likely to be evaluated routinely for urinary nitrogen loss, such as those in the intensive care unit (ICU) or those requiring specialized nutrition support.

Some nutrition support clinicians use N-balance as a weekly monitoring parameter for patients receiving specialized nutrition support, either enteral or parenteral. Others choose not to use it routinely because of its limitations: problems with accurate 24-hour urine collection, inability to reliably account for unmeasured nitrogen losses, poor correlation between UUN and TUN in hospitalized patients, and failure of UUN or TUN to reflect catabolism in patients with altered urine output (i.e., renal failure, renal insufficiency, diuretic induced urine output).

Accuracy is an issue for nearly all evaluations based on timed urine collection. Accurate collections are more likely in patients with a urinary catheter in place who are cared for by well-trained personnel, such as in the ICU setting, but much less likely in general medical or surgical units. Nevertheless, problems can occur with timed urine collection in any setting.

Unmeasured nitrogen losses are accounted for in the N-balance calculation by adding 4 g "insensible" loss to the measured UUN or 2 g "insensible" loss to the measured TUN. These values reflect normal unmeasured daily nitrogen losses from feces, skin, and miscellaneous sources in healthy non-stressed adults. The difference in grams of insensible loss between UUN and TUN is based on the assumption that UUN normally represents 80% to 90% of TUN.[14] In stressed patients, however, this assumption does not hold true—instead, UUN represents a highly variable percent of TUN. Measuring ammonia plus UUN may provide a more reliable estimate of TUN than using UUN alone.[15] Of course, measuring TUN itself provides the most accurate assessment of urinary nitrogen loss because no assumptions are necessary regarding UUN to TUN ratios, but TUN measurement is not widely available in clinical practice.

Determining N-balance, difficult even under the best of conditions, is further complicated when nitrogen losses result from disrupted tissue (not included in normal "insensible" losses), such as wounds, burns, and sloughed tissue following chemotherapy or radiation as well as losses from high-output enterocutaneous fistulas and excessive stool output. Nitrogen lost through such routes can exceed losses in the urine, and are typically very difficult to measure or estimate accurately. As a result, the utility of N-balance for assessing nutrition or monitoring medical nutrition therapy is highly questionable when there are significant nonurinary nitrogen losses.

Adaptations of the N-balance calculation, referred to as urea kinetics or urea appearance,[16] are available for use in patients with reduced urinary nitrogen clearance, including renal failure or insufficiency. The concept is simple—account for the accumulation of urea in the body in addition to losses in the urine—but its application is time consuming and complex. Patient weights and blood urea nitrogen (BUN) must be measured when 24-hour urine collection starts and again when it is complete. Urine collection, weight recording, and BUN measures must be coordinated with dialysis times unless nitrogen loss in the dialysate is measured, and you must make assumptions related to urea distribution and total body water. Although urea kinetics poses potential problems, these calculations can provide valuable information for assessing protein requirements in renally compromised patients.

Visceral Proteins

Visceral proteins are the most commonly used biochemical parameters for nutrition assessment and monitoring in the clinical setting, especially albumin, transferrin, and transthyretin (prealbumin, or thyroxin-binding pre-albumin) and occasionally retinol-binding protein (RBP). The name prealbumin, a synonym for transthyretin, reflects that this protein moves ahead of albumin during paper electrophoresis; it is not a precursor to albumin, as some might think.[17] Table 7-1 summarizes information on these visceral proteins.

The long half-life of albumin limits its usefulness for short-term monitoring of nutrition support.[18-20] RBP's extremely short half-life results in rapid serum concentration changes in response to both nutrition and nutrition independent factors—changes that may occur too rapidly to allow a good correlation between nutrition therapy and serum concentration of RBP. Thus transthyretin is often preferred as a parameter for nutrition assessment and monitoring.

The large total body pool of albumin renders it susceptible to concentration and dilution effects from dehydration and overhydration, respectively. Fluid status influences the serum concentration of all visceral proteins, but the effect decreases as the total body pool decreases. RBP is the least affected by fluid status, followed by transthyretin, transferrin, and albumin.[20,21]

From the clinical standpoint, considerably greater fluid imbalance is necessary to significantly alter RBP, serum transthyretin, or transferrin concentrations as compared to serum albumin, although transferrin will be more readily affected than the other two proteins.

Factors affecting synthesis, distribution, or degradation of visceral proteins will influence serum concentrations. Because synthesis of visceral proteins occurs in the liver, hepatic insufficiency or failure decreases production—and consequently, serum concentrations—of these proteins. To assess the nutrition of patients with hepatic insufficiency or failure, subjective parameters are usually better because concentrations of visceral proteins do not correlate with nutritional status or respond to adequate provision of calories and protein.

Physiological stress, such as inflammation and infection, alters protein production in the liver and diverts synthetic capacity so that acute-phase reactants, such as C-reactive protein, haptoglobin, fibronectin, and ceruloplasmin, are produced.[22] Consequently, synthesis of the visceral proteins declines and serum concentrations fall regardless of the patient's nutritional status. Serum albumin drops an average of 0.5 g/dL in roughly two-thirds to three-quarters of patients who undergo surgery.[22] Compounding the effects of stress on protein synthesis are changes in the distribution of visceral proteins that occur during acute catabolic states, such as surgery and trauma. During these states, microvascular permeability increases and albumin distribution shifts from the vascular to the interstitial space.[23] Although the drop in other visceral protein concentrations is partially mitigated by their smaller total body pools, all decline somewhat. In contrast to albumin, short half-life proteins—transferrin, transthyretin, RBP—recover rapidly and are better for monitoring patients' response to specialized nutrition support. Transferrin can be monitored weekly and transthyretin twice weekly (i.e., every 3 to 4 days) to detect changes in protein status.

Because visceral proteins serve as carriers of substances in the plasma, changes in the amount of the substance are associated with increases or decreases in the carrier protein's serum concentration. Transferrin, a carrier for iron, provides a regulatory mechanism for iron absorption. With iron deficiency, the transferrin concentration increases to allow increased iron absorption and transport. Transthyretin, a secondary carrier for thyroxin, forms complexes with RBP, thereby carrying retinol. Hyperthyroidism, a condition characterized by excessive free thyroxin, is associated with decreased transthyretin concentrations. On the other hand, corticosteroid therapy is associated with increased transthyretin, which may be related to

TABLE 7-1 Visceral Proteins Used in Nutrition Assessment and Monitoring

	Albumin	Transferrin	Transthyretin	RBP[a]
Half-Life	20 days	8 to 10 days	2 to 3 days	12 hours
Total Body Pool	3 to 5 g/kg	Under 100 mg/kg	10 mg/kg	2 mg/kg
Normal Serum Levels	3.5 to 5 g/dL	200 to 400 mg/dL	15 to 40 mg/dL	2.8 to 7.6 mg/dL
Mild Malnutrition	2.8 to 3.4 g/dL[b]	150 to 199 mg/dL	10 to 14 mg/dL	2.7 to 2.9 mg/dL
Moderate Malnutrition	2.1 to 2.7 g/dL[c]	100 to 149 mg/dL	5 to 9 mg/dL[h]	2.4 to 2.6 mg/dL
Severe Malnutrition	Under 2.1 g/dL[d]	Under 100 mg/dL	Under 5 mg/dL[h]	Under 2.4 mg/dL
Nutrition-Independent Increases	Exogenous albumin administration Dehydration	Iron-deficiency Chronic blood loss Acute hepatitis Dehydration	Renal failure Corticosteroid therapy Dehydration	Renal disease Dehydration
Nutrition-Independent Decreases	Liver disease Acute catabolic states[e] Stress[f] Protein loss Overhydration	Liver disease Acute catabolic states[e] Stress[f] Protein loss Overhydration Iron excess	Liver disease Acute catabolic states[e] Stress[f] Protein loss Overhydration Hyperthyroidism Dialysis Zinc deficiency	Liver disease Acute catabolic states[e] Stress[f] Protein loss Overhydration Hyperthyroidism Cystic fibrosis Vitamin A deficiency
Appropriateness for Screening	Excellent	Poor - expensive; not readily available	Poor - expensive; not readily available	Very poor - changes too rapidly; expensive; not readily available
Appropriateness for Assessment	Acceptable for initial assessment	Acceptable to good - may not be reliable during antibiotic therapy; not reliable in patients with iron deficiency. Not as well studied as transthyretin.	Good - not reliable to determine degree of malnutrition in patients in renal failure.	Marginally acceptable to acceptable - changes may be too rapid with nutrition-independent factors.

Appropriateness for Monitoring Response to Nutrition Therapy	Poor - responds too slowly; too sensitive to fluid, acute catabolic states for use in most hospitalized patients. Acceptable for long-term stable patients (HPN, HEN)[g]	Good for moderate duration therapy - can evaluate weekly. May not be reliable during antibiotic therapy. Not as well studied as transthyretin.	Excellent for short and moderate duration therapy - can evaluate every 3–4 days. Trends can be monitored in patients in renal failure.	Marginally acceptable for short and moderate duration therapy - can evaluate every 1–2 days. May change too quickly with non-nutrition factors for good correlation to nutrition.

a. Retinol-binding protein.
b. Serum albumin 3.2 g/dL or less with 10% to 15% weight loss has been suggested to define mild marasmus-hypoalbuminemia (see Table 7-2).
c. Serum albumin 3.2 g/dL or less with over 15% weight loss has been suggested to define moderate marasmus-hypoalbuminemia (see Table 7-2).
d. Serum albumin under 2.5 g/dL with 10% weight loss or less has been suggested to define kwashiorkor (see Table 7-2).
e. Acute catabolic states include trauma, surgery, and protein-wasting conditions.
f. Stress includes conditions resulting in an inflammatory response, such as infection. Cachexia represents an outcome from a chronic inflammatory response.
g. Home parenteral nutrition (HPN), home enteral nutrition (HEN).
h. When the laboratory uses 7 mg/dL as the lower limit of sensitivity, consider 7 to 10 mg/dL as moderate malnutrition and under 7 mg/dL as severe malnutrition.

Source: References 6,17–21, 28.

vitamin A mobilization. Transthyretin forms complexes with RBP, which increases during vitamin A mobilization and decreases with vitamin A deficiency when there is less vitamin A to transport.

Serum albumin, an inexpensive laboratory test that is often included in routine chemistry panels, such as the comprehensive metabolic panel, serves well as a nutrition screening parameter.[24-26] Hypoalbuminemia correlates with several negative prognostic indicators: prolonged hospital stays, poor clinical outcomes, and increased morbidity and mortality.

During initial nutrition assessments, serum albumin is used with anthropometric measurements to define the type of malnutrition. Kwashiorkor is primarily a protein malnutrition in which serum albumin is severely depleted but weight loss is minimal. Nutritional marasmus is primarily an energy malnutrition with severe weight loss or extremely low weight relative to IBW, but with limited reduction of serum albumin. Table 7-2 lists the malnutrition terms included in the *International Classification of Diseases, ninth edition, Clinical Modification* (ICD-9-CM), and the corresponding code numbers, along with proposed serum albumin and anthropometric parameters for applying each term to adults.[27] The table also provides the protein-energy malnutrition (PEM) terminology commonly used in practice and the corresponding ICD-9-CM definition. Using the proper ICD-9-CM codes for malnutrition is critical when billing Medicare and other insurance carriers to ensure that payment covers the cost of care. Numerous studies have shown that malnutrition increases the cost of care because of associated complications.[24]

When visceral proteins degrade, their serum concentrations are affected. During the acute-phase response to injury, albumin degradation accelerates, its serum concentration decreases, and the amino acid pool for synthesizing acute-phase proteins increases. During renal failure, transthyretin and RBP concentrations increase independent of nutrition. Increased serum RBP is attributed to altered glomerular filtration and reduced metabolism by the kidneys.[17,28] Higher serum transthyretin may be secondary to the rise in RBP, since transthyretin forms complexes with RBP.[28]

Given the many factors that influence visceral protein concentrations independent of nutritional status, laboratory results alone are often of minimal value. You must evaluate them in light of the patient's current status and history to determine if they are useful in assessing nutritional status. For monitoring the response to specialized nutrition support, trends in serum protein concentrations are often useful. For instance, trends in transthyretin can be used to monitor patients in renal failure. The absolute number on the laboratory report, however, does not correspond to the degree of malnutrition.

For patients with liver failure, you can expect little or no response in visceral protein concentrations despite adequate nutrition support. Therefore, both single readings and trends in visceral protein concentrations are of little value in assessing nutritional status of patients with severe hepatic impairment, and you must select other methods.

TABLE 7-2 Classification of Adult Protein-Energy Malnutrition

ICD-9-CM Term	ICD-9-CM Code	Clinical Description	Serum Albumin	Weight Loss	% IBW
Kwashiorkor	260	Severe Protein Malnutrition	Under 2.5 g/dL	10% or less	
Nutritional Marasmus	261	Severe Energy Malnutrition	2.5 g/dL or above	Over 20%	Under 80%
Nutritional Marasmus	261	Severe Energy Malnutrition	2.5 g/dL or above		Under 70%
Other Severe PEM[a]	262	Severe PEM	Under 2.5 g/dL	Over 10%	
Moderate Marasmus-Hypoalbuminemia	263.0	Moderate PEM	3.2 g/dL or less	Over 15%	
Mild Marasmus-Hypoalbuminemia	263.0	Mild PEM	3.2 g/dL or less	10% to 15%	
Other PEM; Anticipate Prolonged LOS[b]	263.8[c]				
Septic or stressed; not depleted		Moderate Protein Malnutrition	3.2 g/dL or less	Under 5%	
Moderate weight loss; major surgery planned		Moderate Energy Malnutrition	Over 3.2 g/dL	Over 10%	
Mild weight loss; moderate depletion		Moderate Protein with Mild Energy Malnutrition	3.2 g/dL or less	Over 5%	
Inability to eat for 7 days or more[d]		At risk of PEM			

a. PEM = Protein-energy malnutrition.

b. LOS = Length of stay.

c. The last four descriptions are proposed to be included for ICD-9-CM Code 263.8 (Other PEM).

d. Actual or predicted time

Source: References 6–8, 17, 27.

Functional Evaluation

The body's ability to function normally depends on adequate nutrition. Calories are necessary for energy-requiring activity; protein must be provided to maintain muscle mass and muscle strength; calcium, phosphorus, and magnesium are necessary for accretion of bone mass; and specific vitamins serve as cofactors for biochemical processes in the body. Assessing nutrient-dependent functions can often yield important information about nutritional status. For instance, measuring whole blood or erythrocyte transketolase activity provides an assessment of thiamin activity that is more useful than serum thiamin concentrations. Activity of specific enzymes, rather than serum concentrations, is sometimes used to evaluate vitamin status. Other functional status assessments may rely more on subjective data, such as the patient's ability to walk a selected distance.

Strength, a functional assessment of muscle, can reflect nutritional status in patients who do not have neuromuscular disease. Hand grip strength, for example, appears to reflect nutritional status and to serve as a prognostic indicator in surgical patients.[29] Dynamometers, which are relatively inexpensive and can be operated with minimal training, have been used to measure hand grip and forearm muscle strength.[30]

Subjective Global Assessment

Subjective global assessment (SGA) combines segments of patients' medical and dietary histories with portions of the physical examination to determine nutritional status based on physiologic status, not physical appearance alone. The SGA technique was initially used to prospectively predict the need for preoperative nutrition support in GI surgery patients.[31-33] Later, a patient-generated subjective global assessment (PG-SGA) was developed for use in oncology clinics.[34] Neither version of the SGA is population specific; both have been used in a variety of patient populations and are effective alternatives to the more commonly used objective assessment tools—weight for height and visceral protein concentrations. Use of SGA or PG-SGA is particularly beneficial when objective measurements are poor indicators of nutritional status, as with end-stage liver disease. In patients with end-stage liver disease, weight fluctuates significantly based on the amount of edema or ascites present and visceral protein concentrations reflect poor hepatic synthetic capability. Because neither is a reliable indicator of nutritional status in these patients, SGA is a better assessment tool.[35]

The SGA and PG-SGA are essentially the same except that the patient completes much of history in the PG-SGA and its wording is more patient-friendly. The clinician completes the entire SGA survey. They include these history components:

- Weight change evaluated on the basis of amount lost or gained in the past 6 months, rate of change, and pattern of change.
- Alteration in dietary intake, which subjectively compares current to normal intake (change or no change), and notes the duration of

Stages of Malnutrition

❑ Stage A: well nourished. Patients with improved weight (nonfluid weight gain), normalization of dietary intake, adequately managed GI symptoms, or improved functional status fit in this category, although they may remain nutritionally at risk.

❑ Stage B: moderate or suspected malnutrition. Characteristics of this group include potentially significant weight loss within a few weeks, lack of desirable weight gain, clear reduction in dietary intake, or mild subcutaneous fat or muscle loss.

❑ Stage C: significant weight loss or obvious malnutrition. Patients in this group are severely malnourished.

a change as well as whether the patient is on a special or restrictive diet (i.e., hypocaloric liquids, full liquids). No food diary or other records are required.

- GI symptoms, such as presence of nausea, vomiting, diarrhea, and anorexia lasting more than 2 weeks.
- Functional capacity, such as whether the patient is able to complete normal daily tasks at work or is ambulatory or bedridden, and the duration of functional limitations.
- Primary diagnosis, including its relationship to metabolic demand (normal, low, moderate, or high demand).
- Physical characteristics, which are scored on a four point scale (normal, mild, moderate, severe). Characteristics that are evaluated include loss of subcutaneous fat in the chest and triceps, muscle wasting in quadriceps and deltoids, edema in the ankles and sacral area, and ascites.

After the history and physical data are gathered for SGA, the patient is categorized by stages of malnutrition described in the sidebar above.

Mini Nutritional Assessment

The Mini Nutritional Assessment (MNA), developed for the geriatric population but not age-specific, scores objective and subjective data in four areas.[36] The scores from each section are totaled to determine the malnutrition indicator score.

- Anthropometric assessment, including BMI, MAC, calf circumference, and weight loss over the preceding 3 months. (Maximum of 8 points.)
- General assessment, including functional evaluations of mobility and neuropsychological problems—parameters that distinguish the MNA from most other nutrition assessment tools and add to its value in the geriatric population. Other key questions for geriatric

patients involve independent living, number of prescription drugs, presence of pressure sores or skin ulcers (no staging of the ulcer is required). (Maximum of 9 points.)

■ Dietary assessment, involving six questions about the number of meals eaten per day, selective markers of protein intake (daily servings of dairy products, legumes, eggs, meat, fish, poultry), consumption of fruits and vegetables, changes in food intake, fluid intake, and mode of feeding. (Maximum of 11 points.)

■ Self-assessment, which asks whether patients view themselves as having nutrition problems and how they think their health compares to others of the same age. (Maximum of 4 points.)

A total score of 24 or more is classified as well-nourished; 17 to 23.5 means the person is at risk of malnutrition; and 17 or less means the person is malnourished.

Prognostic Indicators

Nutrition assessment parameters are rarely used alone because multiple parameters can better identify patients needing intervention. Some specific equations have been developed that combine parameters to identify patients at risk of nutrition-related complications.

The Prognostic Nutrition Index (PNI) uses serum albumin, triceps skin fold thickness, transferrin, and DHT to predict the patient's risk of operative morbidity and mortality based on nutrition status.[13]

The Prognostic Inflammatory and Nutrition Index (PINI) combines markers of inflammatory response (alpha-1 acid glycoprotein and C-reactive protein) with nutritional markers (serum albumin and transthyretin) to predict the risk of infectious complications and death.[13]

The Nutrition Risk Index (NRI) stratifies operative morbidity and mortality in the Veteran's Affairs Cooperative Group study of preoperative nutrition support.[37] The NRI combines serum albumin and the ratio of current weight to usual weight. The concept of the NRI is similar to the classifications of malnutrition shown in Table 7-2. NRI is the most practical prognostic index for routine nutrition assessments because all the information needed for most patients is readily available, it is inexpensive, and it requires minimal personnel training.

NUTRIENT REQUIREMENTS

Dietary guidelines and nutrient standards for healthy people provide the template for nutrient requirements during EN and PN therapy. Specialized nutrition support per se does not alter nutrient requirements, but the disease or condition that necessitates its use can have a large impact. In addition, differences in bioavailability based on the route of administration may call for adjustments in nutrient amounts. For instance, delivering 1 mg/day of iron to the body requires administering 1 mg elemental iron intravenously or 10 mg via the GI tract, since normally only about 10% of the iron ingested is absorbed, or about 20% when a person is iron deficient. General guidelines for nutrient requirements during EN and PN therapy are discussed later in this chapter, including limited information on renal and liver dysfunction.

Degree of metabolic stress, disease states, nutritional status, organ function, drug-nutrient interactions, expected duration of therapy, and other factors can also influence requirements. The results of your nutrition assessment should guide you in determining specific nutrient requirements for individual patients.

It is best to use lean body mass to establish nutrient requirements because it represents the metabolically active component of the body. Unfortunately, lean body mass is not typically available in clinical practice and you must choose a weight that best represents metabolically active tissue for calculating nutrient goals. Actual body weight (ABW) is considered appropriate when actual weight is 120% or less of IBW.[38] However, some clinicians prefer to use ABW only when weight is at IBW or below.

In many hospitalized patients receiving nutrition support, ABW reflects fluid retention, edema, or ascites. Therefore, using IBW in this setting may prevent overfeeding patients who weigh up to 120% of IBW. At weights above 120% of IBW, an adjusted dosing weight (ADW) is recommended.[38] Since IBW is actually represented as a range of $\pm$ 10% from the calculated IBW value, some clinicians use ADW above 130% IBW.[13,39]

Guidelines and equations for determining an ADW in obese patients[40] recognize that not all excess weight (that above IBW) is adipose tissue—some is metabolically active lean tissue. But the percent of excess weight added to IBW to obtain the ADW is different in various equations. Studies of overfeeding have reported from 20% to 50% gain in fat-free mass, but there is little evidence indicating the percentage of excess weight metabolically active in critically ill patients. This means that no particular ADW equation is superior to another.[41,42] Most clinicians estimate that lean mass makes up 25% to 40% of excess weight in these patients. Unfortunately, there are no equations for determining ADW based on BMI, which—if available—would allow you to adjust for the degree of obesity.

Protein Requirements

Protein is required for preventing or slowing catabolism of body protein, repairing damaged tissue, and maintaining normal tissue. The goal of protein provision in specialized nutrition support depends on patients' protein status and degree of metabolic stress. In highly catabolic patients, the initial goal is to reduce catabolism of body proteins. Anabolism (or repletion) is not a realistic goal during the stress response, but is in order when patients are depleted. Stable patients on longer-term specialized nutrition support simply need to maintain their protein status. Tools for gauging catabolism and depletion include nutrition assessment, visceral proteins, nitrogen balance, and subjective global assessment.

Requirements for protein are influenced by such factors as the patient's disease states, degree of metabolic stress, extent of tissue repair required (i.e., magnitude of tissue damage from burns, trauma, surgery, chemotherapy, or radiation), organ function, and caloric needs. In healthy adults, the minimum protein intake necessary to maintain and repair tissue is approximately 0.5 to 0.7 g/kg/day.[43,44] To assure that requirements for nearly all healthy adults are met, the recommended dietary allowance (RDA) is set just above the minimum, at 0.8 g/kg/day.[43] Healthy geriatric patients appear to require slightly more protein than younger adults, with 1 to 1.25 g/kg/day suggested.[45] When fat-free mass is used for the calculations, however, protein needs may actually decline with increased age.[46] The ASPEN National Advisory Group on Standards and Practice Guidelines for PN suggests that 0.8 to 1 g/kg/day is a standard protein range for maintenance.[38] For catabolic patients, 1.2 to 2 g/kg/day is considered the standard range. This assumes normal organ function and does not account for excessive losses beyond the catabolic state. Losses from fistula output, protein-losing enteropathy, extensive open wounds, or other unusual sources must be added to the standard range. For most hospitalized patients, however, protein provided at 1 to 1.5 g/kg/day is probably adequate.[47]

There is some question as to whether protein synthesis is promoted by intake above 1.5 g/kg/day, at least in severely septic patients.[48] Higher protein intake may simply serve as a caloric source. Results of the nutrition assessment should be used to guide decisions on protein provision to individual patients. Table 7-3 summarizes protein recommendations for patients with normal organ function, as well as those with renal and hepatic insufficiency.

Organ function, specifically renal and hepatic function, can alter protein tolerance. The goals of protein provision—reduced catabolism, anabolism, or maintenance—depend on the patient's protein status and remain the same for patients with or without organ dysfunction. With organ dysfunction, you may need to make concessions in reaching these goals, especially in the rate at which goals can be achieved. When protein intake is restricted because of organ dysfunction, the patient must receive enough calories to avoid oxidation of protein as an energy source. Recommendations for protein intake in patients with renal dysfunction are affected by the patient's catabolic state, severity and duration of renal dysfunction, type and duration of renal replacement therapy (dialysis), if any, and other disease states. When patients have hypercatabolism or high urinary protein losses, as occurs in nephrotic syndrome, protein requirements increase.

Patients developing acute renal failure (ARF) are generally hypermetabolic and hypercatabolic. Hypercatabolic renal failure patients receiving dialysis may benefit from protein provided at 1.5 to 1.8 g/kg/day, although it may be necessary to initiate support with 1.2 to 1.5 g/kg/day.[49] Similar protein provision may be necessary in less catabolic, protein-depleted patients receiving dialysis because they need more than the amount lost in

TABLE 7-3 Protein Requirements and Recommendations

Description	Protein (g/kg/day)	Examples/Comments
Minimum requirement	0.5 to 0.7	Healthy adults based on nitrogen balance studies
RDA	0.8	Healthy adults, includes factors for protein efficiency
Maintenance	0.8 to 1	Nonstressed, otherwise healthy adults requiring long-term EN or PN therapy, generally at home
Geriatric	1 to 1.25	Healthy older persons; Less if lean body mass used
Minimal catabolism or Protein repletion	1 to 1.2	Hospitalized adults; Elective surgery without complications; Evidence of protein depletion but nonstressed
Moderate catabolism	1.2 to 1.5	Surgery with minor complications or wound infection
Highly catabolic state	1.5 to 2	Closed head injury; Pelvic fracture; Sepsis; Peritonitis
ARF or CRF without dialysis, noncatabolic[a]	0.6 to 0.8 usual, up to 1	Controversial since MDRD[b] study showed little benefit of protein restriction in most CRF patients
Hemodialysis	1 to 1.2	ARF or CRF[a] 3 times weekly
Peritoneal dialysis	1.2 to 1.5	Highest requirement with peritonitis
Continuous renal replacement therapy	1 to 1.2	Usual for stable, not hypercatabolic, patients receiving CVVHD or CVVH[c]; Rate, dialysate affect protein loss
ARF or CRF with dialysis, hypercatabolic[a]	1.5 to 1.8 usual, up to 2.5	Above 2 g/kg/day may be needed with CVVHD, CVVH[c] in hypercatabolic ARF or CRF patients
Cirrhosis, uncomplicated	1 to 1.2 initially, up to 1.5	No encephalopathy; Increase to positive N-balance or 1.5 as tolerated
Cirrhosis, complicated	1 to 1.2 initially, up to 1.8	No encephalopathy; Increase, as tolerated, to positive N-balance or 1.5 if cholestasis or 1.8 when malnourished
Hepatitis, uncomplicated acute or chronic	1 to 1.2 initially, up to 1.5	No ascites, no encephalopathy; Increase to positive N-balance or 1.5 as tolerated, especially if PEM present
Liver disease with encephalopathy (cirrhosis or fulminant hepatitis)	0.5 to 1.2	Grade 1 to 2 encephalopathy; Below 1 only short-term
	0.5 to 0.6	Grade 3 to 4 encephalopathy
	0.6 to 0.8	Chronic encephalopathy; Increase to 1 if possible

a. ARF = Acute renal failure; CRF = Chronic renal failure.
b. MDRD = Modified diet in renal disease study.[50]
c. CVVHD = Continuous veno-venous hemodialysis; CVVH = Continuous veno-venous hemofiltration.

Source: References 43–50, 52–54.

renal replacement therapy to accomplish repletion. The amount of protein lost varies considerably based on the type of dialysis, membrane characteristics of the dialysis method, flow rate, and duration of therapy. Patients receiving peritoneal dialysis tend to require more protein than those on hemodialysis, especially when peritonitis is present. Stable, nondialyzed patients with renal failure have the least losses.

The prevailing practice is routine protein restriction at 0.6 to 0.8 g/kg/day in noncatabolic patients with chronic renal failure (CRF) not receiving dialysis. Results from the Modification of Diet in Renal Disease (MDRD) study, in which protein restriction was shown to benefit only patients with advanced CRF,[50] has prompted questions about this practice, but the results cannot necessarily be applied to the overall CRF population.

Liver disease alters amino acid metabolism and suppresses protein synthesis.[51] Adequate protein provision, however, is essential to prevent catabolism of body protein in stressed patients and to provide amino acids for the acute-phase response to stress. Hepatic repair and regeneration also require adequate protein provision, as does reversal of protein depletion. The key in liver dysfunction is to provide enough protein without inducing hepatic encephalopathy. Protein should be initiated cautiously and adjusted frequently based on tolerance in patients with liver dysfunction. In general, most of these patients do not require severe protein restriction.

It may be appropriate to withhold protein over the short term in patients with acute decompensated liver disease.[52] As soon as possible, usually within 24 to 48 hours—when the overall condition improves and encephalopathy clears—you should provide protein cautiously, starting with about 0.5 to 0.6 g/kg/day and increasing as tolerated to achieve positive N-balance.

In patients with cirrhosis, restricting protein for a short time to 0.5 to 0.6 g/kg/day may be appropriate during episodes of decompensation manifested by hepatic encephalopathy, but protein should be increased to at least 1 g/kg/day as soon as possible. Cirrhotic patients appear to require at least this level of protein intake to attenuate muscle wasting and promote positive N-balance.[53]

In patients with alcoholic hepatitis, failure to achieve positive N-balance is associated with poor survival rates.[54] When applying the guidelines for patients with liver dysfunction included in Table 7-3, you should titrate from the lower to the upper amount of protein based on tolerance (lack of encephalopathic symptoms).

Energy Requirements

Because the body requires energy to function, it will consume itself if an adequate supply of exogenous energy is not provided. In healthy adults, the greatest share of energy is expended to maintain critical body functions (respiration, circulation, muscle tone, and core temperature) and vital organs. The rate at which a person uses energy while at complete physical and mental rest, the basal metabolic rate (BMR), should be measured soon after awakening and 12 to 16 hours after taking food. Resting metabolic rate (RMR) is also taken at complete rest, but is not usually done soon after awakening and may include residual effects from the previous meal. RMR, the measure used in clinical practice, is about 10% higher than true BMR and approximates 1 kcal/kg/hour in adults and 65% to 70% of total daily energy requirements.[17,55] Considerable variation can exist, however, due to differences in lean body mass and other variables.

Other ways that healthy adults expend energy include digestion of food and physical activity. When people are ill they use additional energy to handle inflammation, the stress response, thermal regulation, and tissue repair. To replenish fat stores and muscle mass, nutritionally depleted adult patients require additional energy above the resting amount. Fat synthesis is estimated to require 12 kcal/g of fat, while fat-free mass requires about 1.7 kcal/g.[42,56]

Of the many ways to measure or estimate caloric requirements, direct calorimetry is the "gold standard," but it is not practical in any setting except metabolic research units. The subject must stay alone in the direct calorimetry chamber—a large, sophisticated machine that measures heat exchange—for anywhere from several hours to days. Indirect calorimetry, which measures gas exchange rather than heat exchange, is the most accurate way to determine caloric needs in most people. Various indirect calorimetry machines are available—ranging from metabolic rooms to portable metabolic carts that are suitable for the clinical setting. They use oxygen consumption and carbon dioxide production to calculate caloric requirements indirectly. They lack precision when the oxygen concentration of inspired air is above 60%, as sometimes occurs with mechanical ventilation,[57] and they must be calibrated properly. Another potential cause of error is air leakage through chest tubes or around an endotracheal or tracheostomy tube. Still, in the clinical setting it is usually simpler to obtain indirect calorimetry on mechanically ventilated patients because the oxygen content of air coming from an oxygen tank can be determined easily. For spontaneous breathing persons, a nose clamp and mouth piece or a hood system must be used.

When indirect calorimetry is not available, caloric requirements can be estimated using an equation derived through linear regression analysis that relates various factors to BMR or RMR. Seven of more than a dozen equations available are listed in Table 7-4; all except the Ireton-Jones and Swinamer equations are for healthy adults.[39,55,58,59] Some equations list BMR or basal energy expenditure (BEE) as their unit of measure, but all are essentially calculations of RMR or resting energy expenditure (REE), so there is no 10% adjustment between BEE and REE. These predictive equations calculate total calories.

Studies have shown a 5% to 15% overestimation of BEE in healthy subjects using the Harris-Benedict equations,[60] the most recognized and widely used of the predictive equations.[61] Published in 1919, Harris-Benedict uses ABW in obese patients, as do most other equations for predicting caloric requirements. New equations continue to use ABW instead of fat-free mass because these two body measurements correlate strongly enough to make them the

TABLE 7-4 Equations for Estimating Resting Energy Expenditure (REE)

Name	Equations for Men	Equations for Women
Harris-Benedict	$66 + 13.75(W) + 5(H) - 6.8(A)$	$655 + 9.5(W) + 1.9(H) - 4.7(A)$
Owen	$879 + 10.2(W)$	$795 + 7.18(W)$
Mifflin	$9.99(W) + 6.25(H) - 4.92(A) + 5$	$9.99(W) + 6.25(H) - 4.92(A) - 161$
James	18-30 yr: $692 + 15.1(W)$ 30-60 yr: $873 + 11.6(W)$ Over 60 yr: $588 + 11.7(W)$	18-30 yr: $487 + 14.8(W)$ 30-60 yr: $845 + 8.17(W)$ Over 60 yr: $658 + 9.01(W)$

World Health Organization (WHO)	18-30 yr:
	  $[64.4(W) - 113(H/100) + 3000] \div 4.184$
	30-60 yr:
	  $[19.2(W) + 66.9(H/100) + 3769] \div 4.184$
		18-30 yr:
		  $[55.6(W) + 139.7(H/100) + 146] \div 4.184$
		30-60 yr:
		  $[36.4(W) - 104.6(H/100) + 3619] \div 4.184$

Ireton-Jones*	Spontaneously breathing:
	  $629 - 11(A) + 25(W) -609(O)$
	Ventilated:
	  $1784 - 11(A) + 5(W) + 244 + 239(T) + 804(B)$
		Spontaneously breathing:
		  $629 - 11(A) + 25(W) - 609(O)$
		Ventilated:
		  $1784 - 11(A) + 5(W) + 239(T) + 804(B)$

Swinamer*	$941(BSA) - 6.3(A) + 104(Tmax) + 24(RR) + 804(V_T) - 4243$	$941(BSA) - 6.3(A) + 104(Tmax) + 24(RR) + 804(V_T) - 4243$

A   = age in years
B   = burn
BSA = body surface area
H   = height in cm
O   = 1 if obese; zero if not obese
RR   = respiratory rate
T   = trauma
Tmax = maximum temperature in past 24 hours, degrees Celsius
V_T = tidal volume
W   = weight in kg

* These equations measure energy expenditure, including stress and activity, not REE.

Source: References 39, 55, 58–64.

same in predicting RMR—and ABW is more readily available.[62-64] The World Health Organization (WHO) equations were developed using results of over 11,000 measurements and appear to be the best predictors of RMR in healthy normal-weight persons.[55] Most equations overpredict caloric requirements with obese subjects, but those based on body surface area appear to perform better than those based on weight, height, and age.[58]

To obtain total energy expenditure (TEE) or estimated caloric requirements, you can adjust RMR calculations by adding nonresting energy expenditures. Adding both an activity factor of 1.2 to 1.3 times RMR plus a stress factor of 1.1 to 2 times RMR has been recommended for hospitalized patients.[17]

The stress factor is based on the premise that caloric requirements increase proportionally to the severity of stress; thus, lower factors are for mild stress, while the highest are for severe stress, such as major sepsis, multiple trauma, and severe burns.[17,65] Many studies, however, have indicated that increases in caloric requirements are not commensurate with severity of stress.[66-68] Because advances in critical care medicine over the past two decades have decreased the amount of energy that patients expend, previously used stress factors may no longer be accurate. For example, better control of ambient temperature and improved wound care and skin grafting appear to have decreased the hypermetabolism associated with burns.[69,70] Adding both an activity and a stress factor to the BEE obtained from the Harris-Benedict equations will generally cause caloric requirements to be overestimated, as will applying the stress factors proposed by Long alone.[65] Even critically ill patients, such as those with multiple trauma or sepsis, require energy in the range of 100% to 120% of the BEE calculated from the Harris-Benedict equations.[47] Severely marasmic patients tend to be hypometabolic, with an RMR that is below predicted values, at least until tissue repletion begins.

Overestimating caloric needs using activity and stress factors is a potential problem that may contribute to substrate intolerance and complications. As advances are made in patient care it is important to evaluate their effects on energy consumption. Equations that include factors for temperature, minute ventilation, ventilatory status, and cardiac output, are dynamic and may self-adjust for the impact of changes in care. These equations and those that contain factors for trauma, burns, or other stress conditions are estimating caloric expenditure, not REE, and should not have activity or stress factors added to the calculated number. For example, the Ireton-Jones equations already include ventilatory status, trauma, burns, and obesity factors, and should not have activity or stress factors added to the calculated number.[39] The Swinamer equation, developed using data from critically ill patients requiring mechanical ventilation, accounts for changes associated with ventilatory status.[59] Swinamer, Ireton-Jones, and similar equations may be better suited to hospitalized patients than are those derived by adding stress factors to RMR calculated from equations developed in healthy subjects.

The other method of determining caloric requirements is kcal/kg/day estimation. The ASPEN National Advisory Group on Standards and Practice

Guidelines for PN suggests total calories of 25 to 30 kcal/kg/day as the standard range for adults with normal organ function.[38] Although it is "not the intent of the document to provide guidelines on the nutrient requirements in various disease states and conditions," this range suggests that estimations derived from adding activity and stress factors to RMR must be viewed cautiously. If RMR is 1 kcal/kg/hour (24 kcal/kg/day), the range of 25 to 30 kcal/kg/day is only 1 to 1.25 times RMR.[17] Using the kcal/kg/day method, mildly catabolic patients are expected to need about 25 kcal/kg/day; moderately catabolic, 25 to 27 kcal/kg/day; and hypercatabolic and hypermetabolic patients, 28 kcal/kg/day or more. Elderly patients probably require about 5 kcal/kg/day less than their younger counterparts. Total caloric intake of about 35 kcal/kg/day is typically recommended for patients with restricted protein intake, such as those with renal or hepatic dysfunction.[71,72] If these patients do not receive enough calories they risk protein malnutrition because their bodies use the limited protein as a caloric source.

For patients requiring specialized nutrition support in the home, Medicare recognizes 20 to 35 kcal/kg/day as the standard; below 20 kcal/kg/day or above 35 kcal/kg/day the prescribing physician must provide additional documentation to justify the caloric prescription.[73] Rarely should patients be provided more than 35 kcal/kg/day for a significant period without clear justification, such as findings from indirect calorimetry. Evidence of malabsorption and need for significant body mass repletion may also justify high-calorie enteral feedings. Parenteral calorie requirements, however, should not be affected by malabsorption.

Caloric Sources

Nonprotein calories come from fats and carbohydrates, the latter being the primary source of energy in most diets and in the majority of EN and PN formulations. Glucose, the primary oxidative fuel of the body, is required in the amount of 2 mg/kg/minute (2.88 g/kg/day) for adenosine triphosphate (ATP) to be produced in the brain, medulla of the kidneys, leukocytes, and erythrocytes.[57,74] The body needs at least 50 g of carbohydrate daily to prevent ketosis, although 100 g may better suppress gluconeogenesis and, consequently, reduce protein catabolism.[17]

The normal diet contains about 125 to 150 g of carbohydrate per 1000 calories, or 50% to 60% of *total* calories as carbohydrate. Enteral formulas range from about 25% to 85% of *total* calories as carbohydrate, although most formulas contain 40% to 60%. The standard distribution for *nonprotein* calories in PN therapy is 70% to 85% carbohydrate.[38] The highest dextrose dose recommended is not more than 5.75 g/kg/day (4 mg/kg/minute) for critically ill, and 7 g/kg/day (5 mg/kg/minute) for most other patients, as this represents the maximum oxidation rate for glucose.[38,75] Up to 10 g/kg/day (7 mg/kg/minute) may be acceptable in stable patients.[75]

Dietary fibers are polysaccharides and lignin, which resist digestion in the human GI tract. Short chain fatty acids—produced when colonic flora ferment soluble fibers—can be absorbed and metabolized, but they contribute little to caloric intake.

Fatty acids become the body's primary fuel source after available carbohydrates (glucose and glycogen) have been utilized. Fatty acids also serve essential functions as precursors to prostaglandins, leukotrienes, and thromboxanes, as well as structural components of phospholipids in cell membranes and insulators along nerve conduction pathways. Linoleic, linolenic, and arachidonic acids are considered physiologically essential, but only the first two must be present in the diet since linoleic acid serves as a precursor to arachidonic acid.[17]

To meet the body's need for essential fatty acids, patients should receive at least 1% to 2% of the total caloric requirement as linoleic acid (3 to 6 g daily). Some references recommend at least 2% to 4% of total caloric intake as linoleic and alpha-linolenic acid to prevent essential fatty acid deficiency.[17,57] Up to 30% of total calories as fat is generally recognized as satisfactory for healthy people, although lower fat intake may have health benefits, such as reduced risk of cardiovascular disease and obesity, for some people.[17]

The recommended split is one-third of fat intake as polyunsaturated fatty acids, one-third as monounsaturated fatty acids, and one-third as other fatty acids, including omega-3 fatty acids, medium chain fatty acids, and saturated fats. The percentage of calories supplied as carbohydrate and fat during specialized nutrition support may differ from recommendations for a healthy diet due to complex issues related to substrate oxidation during metabolic stress, immune-modulation, and substrate tolerance. Formulas used in EN therapy frequently manipulate fatty acid content to achieve specific goals, as discussed under specialized EN formulas.

During PN therapy, the amount of fat can be altered, but the fatty acid content of all commercially available parenteral lipid emulsions is essentially the same. The recommendation for intravenous fats is 15% to 30% of *nonprotein* calories as fat, not to exceed 2.5 g/kg/day.[38] Others have suggested a maximum of 1 g/kg/day for either critically ill or stable patients.[75] The generally recognized upper limit for calories from intravenous fat is 60% of *total* calories.[76] Caloric requirements and substrate composition should be reassessed frequently based on the patient's substrate tolerance, response to nutrition support, and attainment of nutritional goals.

Fluid Requirements

Water is required for digestion, absorption, transport, and nutrient utilization. It is also essential for eliminating waste products and toxins. Among the many methods available for calculating fluid requirements is caloric intake—estimated as 1 mL fluid per kcal.[43] For healthy people weighing 80% to 120% of IBW, average maintenance fluid requirements are as follows.[77]

- Active young adults 16 to 30 years of age: 40 mL/kg/day.
- Adults 20 to 55 years of age: 35 mL/kg/day.
- Older adults 55 to 75 years of age: 30 mL/kg/day.
- Adults 75 years and older: 25 mL/kg/day.

To estimate maintenance fluid, use a baseline of 1500 mL for the first 20 kg body weight. Then, above that weight, add the following:

- For pediatric patients, 25 mL/kg.
- For adults up to 50 years of age, 20 mL/kg.
- For adults over age 50, 15 mL/kg.

Depending on caloric density, 70% to 85% of an enteral formula's volume is free water. The standard fluid volume for adult PN is 20 to 40 mL/kg/day.[38] Both dehydration and overhydration can be issues in patients receiving specialized nutrition support. Fever, diarrhea, surgical drains, and open wounds or burns contribute to excess fluid loss in many patients. On the other hand, multiple IV medications often contribute excess fluid in hospitalized patients. In critically ill patients, organ dysfunction may further complicate the picture by contributing to altered fluid distribution. It is important to evaluate fluid status frequently in patients receiving specialized nutrition support by monitoring daily weight and intake/output. Blood pressure, skin turgor, and thirst may be other useful parameters.

Micronutrient Requirements

Micronutrients include electrolytes, vitamins, minerals, and trace minerals. The Food and Nutrition Board of the National Academy of Sciences has established Dietary Reference Intakes (DRIs) for 14 vitamins and 12 other elements,[78-81] as discussed in Chapter 1 of this book. These new DRIs provide the best reference point for patients receiving specialized nutrition support. Table 7-5 gives the dosage range for adult men and women in the new DRIs (shown under the enteral column). For specific disease states and preexisting deficiencies, you should make the same adjustments as with oral feeding.

Bypassing the stomach and duodenum could, at least theoretically, affect absorption of nutrients such as vitamin B_{12} and iron. There are no studies comparing bioavailability of specific nutrients by site of delivery, however, so no alterations in nutrients can be recommended based on gastric versus duodenal versus jejunal administration. As of this writing ASPEN has not released guidelines for micronutrients, but if they do the ASPEN guidelines would be the best ones to use because they would be specific for enteral or parenteral nutrition.

Micronutrients provided by the parenteral route should follow the American Medical Association Nutrition Advisory Group (AMA-NAG) guidelines for parenteral multivitamin preparations (listed in the parenteral column in Table 7-5).[82] Because these guidelines were published over 25 years ago, they do not reflect more recent vitamin-related knowledge, nor do they incorporate the DRIs, which give more consideration to optimal nutrition than do their predecessors, the RDAs.[43,78-81] Studies have generally confirmed that the AMA-NAG quantities prevent vitamin deficiencies in patients requiring PN therapy.[83-85] Even so, the Food and Drug Administration (FDA) has amended the conditions for marketing effective adult parenteral multivitamin products

TABLE 7-5 Daily Micronutrient Requirements

Micronutrient	Enteral: DRIs[a]		Parenteral
	Men	**Women**	
Electrolytes			
Sodium	22 mmol[b]	22 mmol[b]	1–2 mEq/kg + losses[c]
Potassium	51 mmol[b]	51 mmol[b]	1–2 mEq/kg[c]
Calcium	1000–1200 mg	1000–1200 mg	10–15 mEq[c]
Magnesium	420 mg	320 mg	10 mEq
Phosphorus	700 mg	700 mg	30 mmol
Vitamins			
Thiamine	1.2 mg	1.1 mg	3 mg (6 mg)[d]
Riboflavin	1.3 mg	1.1 mg	3.6 mg
Niacin	16 mg	14 mg	40 mg
Folic Acid	400 mcg	400 mcg	400 mcg (600 mcg)[d]
Pantothenic Acid	5 mg	5 mg	15 mg
Vitamin B$_6$	1.3–1.7 mg	1.3–1.5 mg	4 mg (6 mg)[d]
Cyanocobalamin	2.4 mcg	2.4 mcg	5 mcg
Biotin	30 mcg	30 mcg	60 mcg
Ascorbic Acid	90 mg	75 mg	100 mg (200 mg)[d]
Vitamin A	900 mcg	700 mcg	1000 mcg = 3300 IU
Vitamin D	5–15 mcg	5–15 mcg	5 mcg = 200 IU
Vitamin E	15 mg	15 mg	10 mg = 10 IU
Vitamin K	120 mcg	90 mcg	Zero (150 mcg)[d]
Choline	550 mg	425 mg	
Trace Elements			
Chromium	30–35 mcg	20–25 mcg	10–15 mcg
Copper	900 mcg	900 mcg	0.3–0.5 mg
Manganese	2.3 mg	1.8 mg	60–100 mcg
Selenium	55 mcg	55 mcg	20–60 mcg
Zinc	11 mg	8 mg	2.5–5 mg
Iodine	150 mcg	150 mcg	
Iron	8 mg	8–18 mg	
Fluoride	4 mg	3 mg	
Molybdenum	45 mcg	45 mcg	

a. DRIs = Dietary reference intakes.
b. Estimated minimum requirement for healthy adults.
c. Standard intake.[38]
d. New Food and Drug Administration requirement (effective 2003) is in parentheses.[86]

Source: References 38, 78-81, 86.

by increasing the content of thiamin, pyridoxine, folic acid, and ascorbic acid and adding vitamin K.[86] (These changes appear in parentheses under the parenteral column in Table 7-5.) Patients on PN who have not received the appropriate vitamin supplementation have developed serious complications, and some have died.[87-89]

It can be a complex process to translate DRIs for oral intake of nutrients (and especially minerals), which are set for normal absorption, into requirements for parenteral intake, which requires no absorption.[78-81] Most minerals are only partially absorbed from the GI tract and they often bind with other food components. For example, only about one-third of oral calcium and magnesium is absorbed, and many factors affect their absorption. Therefore the equivalent parenteral dosage should be about one-third the enteral dosage for calcium and magnesium.

To illustrate the relationship between AMA-NAG standards and RDAs, if you use the 1989 RDA of 800 mg/day for calcium (parenteral recommendations for calcium have not been updated to reflect the new RDIs), about 266 mg (13 mEq) of calcium would be absorbed.[43,79] This does indeed correspond with the AMA-NAG parenteral standard intake of 10 to 15 mEq/day.[38]

Most vitamins are well absorbed, in contrast to minerals, so it isn't necessary to adjust for absorption between enteral and parenteral recommendations. Vitamins in solution are subject to stability issues, however, and as a result the dosing recommendations for vitamin A and most water-soluble vitamins tend to be higher for parenteral than for enteral administration. Oxidation, hydrolysis, photodegradation, adsorption to the container, and precipitation are problems that affect vitamin delivery and dosage during PN therapy.[90-92] (For more information on this issue, see the PN section that starts on page 277.)

INDICATIONS FOR SPECIALIZED NUTRITION SUPPORT

When patients do not receive the proper nutrients by mouth to maintain health, specialized nutrition support should be considered within 5–10 days. Malnourished patients need intervention in the first few days of this window, whereas the later few days relate to well-nourished patients—unless they have sustained severe trauma or burns, in which case earlier nutrition support is called for. Figure 7-1 outlines the steps in determining appropriate routes for nutrition intervention.

Patients who receive EN must have some degree of digestive and absorptive capacity, but otherwise, there are few contraindications to EN therapy. By selecting the proper formulas and manipulating the EN regimen appropriately, you can use EN therapy even with patients who have decreased GI functional capacity.[4,93] GI tract obstruction is an absolute contraindication unless the obstruction can be bypassed. Nasopharyngeal or esophageal obstruction and severe stricture can be bypassed by surgical placement of a feeding ostomy (gastrostomy or jejunostomy). You must compare the risk of this more invasive tube placement with the risk of PN therapy and consider the expected duration of therapy, potential complications, and costs. A proximal colostomy or end-ileostomy may allow an otherwise obstructed colon to be bypassed, making EN a viable option when aggressive therapy is warranted.

Advanced directives, ethical and moral reasons involving prolongation of life, or family wishes may preclude EN therapy or nutritional intervention

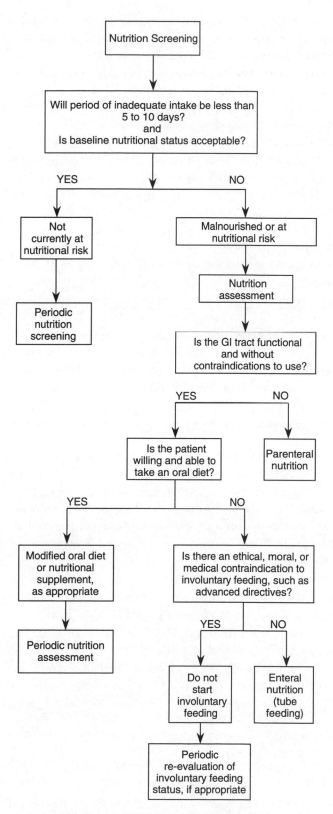

FIGURE 7-1 Nutrition Intervention Algorithm

in some patients. Other potential contraindications include diffuse peritonitis, severe acute necrotizing pancreatitis, intractable vomiting, diarrhea so severe that fluid and electrolyte management are difficult, and high-output enterocutaneous fistulas that prevent feeding distal or proximal to the fistulas. Once such problems have been dealt with, however, EN should be the route of choice for patients who will not, should not, or cannot maintain their nutritional health through normal eating. When EN therapy is contraindicated or cannot alone meet the patient's nutritional goals, PN therapy is appropriate. If necessary, EN and PN therapy can be used concomitantly.

Unless there is a contraindication, EN is the route of choice for people who cannot eat by the oral route because it helps preserve the GI barrier, while PN allows it to deteriorate and predisposes patients to infection and septic morbidity.[94-98] EN is generally considered safer, more physiologic, and more cost-effective than PN therapy and is now used instead of PN in many patients once thought to require bowel rest.[4,93]

For example, pancreatitis patients are not usually on bowel rest long enough to require specialized nutrition support, but if necessary a feeding tube can be placed beyond the Ligament of Treitz (i.e., jejunal feeding). In a trial comparing EN and PN in patients with pancreatitis, the two feeding methods resulted in the same clinical outcome even though fewer EN patients reached caloric goals.[99] In another trial, EN reduced the incidence of infection and possibly preserved the GI barrier and immune function better than PN.[100] Similar outcomes have also been seen in trials comparing EN and PN in patients with inflammatory bowel disease, except that EN was associated with fewer adverse events.[4]

Postoperative EN is now commonly started within hours after surgery in patients expected to remain without adequate nutrition for more than a week.[101] Early postoperative nutrition has not been found to benefit well-nourished patients able to eat within 5 to 7 days, but malnourished patients undergoing major surgery and those with severe trauma may benefit. Severely malnourished patients may even benefit from preoperative nutrition support, but in better nourished patients the benefits may not outweigh the risks.[37,101] Unfortunately, preoperative PN has not been compared to EN therapy in severely malnourished patients who have a functioning GI tract. It is considered safe and effective to initiate EN soon after patients are admitted to intensive care and burn units.[102-105] To determine the appropriateness of EN or PN therapy for specific patients you can refer to comprehensive literature reviews that assess data on when and how to feed.[4,93,106]

ENTERAL NUTRITION

Feeding Tube Placement

It goes without saying that for EN therapy to be an option, it must be possible to place a feeding tube. You must consider both the site of feeding (either the stomach or small bowel) and the method of tube placement. The enteral nutrition algorithm in Figure 7-2 reflects these considerations.

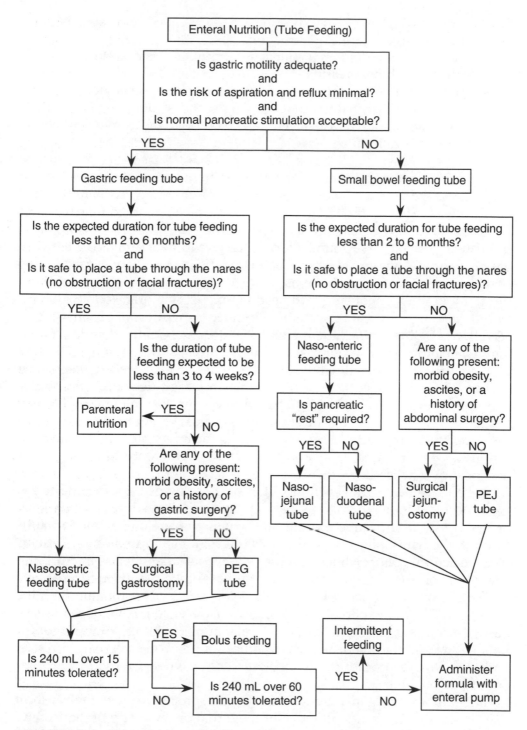

FIGURE 7-2   Enteral Nutrition Algorithm

The stomach is the site of choice because gastric feedings are more physiologic, tubes are easier to place, and more options exist for the feeding regimen. Post-pyloric (small bowel) feeding is generally reserved for:

- Patients who have gastric dysfunction, such as gastroparesis, gastric atony, or gastric outlet obstruction.
- Those for whom minimal pancreatic stimulation is desired, such as patients with pancreatitis.
- Patients at risk of aspiration, including those on mechanical ventilation and those with poor gag, cough, and swallowing reflexes, neurological injury, or delayed gastric emptying (a common problem in critically ill patients).[107]

Post-pyloric tube placement may also facilitate early postoperative feeding because the stomach tends to regain function more slowly than the small bowel after surgery. Although post-pyloric feeding is the standard of practice for patients at risk of aspiration, most studies (including a review of 45 published papers) have found little difference in aspiration risk between gastric and post-pyloric feeding.[108] Failure to distinguish between aspiration of oropharyngeal secretions versus gastric content often contributes to indeterminate results. In patients with head injury, post-pyloric feeding may fail to reduce complications because of continued aspiration of oropharyngeal secretions.[109] Different feeding methods, inadequately defined patient populations, heterogeneous groups, small sample sizes, and poor data collection also contribute to the difficulty of determining which feeding site better reduces aspiration risk. Even when studies are well designed and clearly distinguish oropharyngeal secretions from feeding formula, however, they fail to show a difference in aspiration between gastric and post-pyloric feeding. One study that radio-tagged the feeding formula noted an overall aspiration risk of 8.6% in 35 patients, but found no difference between gastric and post-pyloric feeding.[110]

Tube placements are generally either nasal or by ostomy, depending on the expected duration of therapy. Nasal tubes are indicated for patients likely to require short-term tube feedings and when passage of a small-bore tube through the nares, pharynx, and esophagus is not contraindicated. Patients with structural abnormalities in these regions, facial and sinus fractures, or severe sinusitis may not be candidates for nasal tube placement. In patients with facial or sinus fractures, it may be possible to place a tube through the mouth (oral tube). Experienced nurses can use bedside techniques to place nasogastric (NG), nasoduodenal (ND), and nasojejunal (NJ) tubes in most patients. Nasal placement of feeding tubes—a relatively noninvasive, safe, and inexpensive procedure—is most successful when handled by experienced personnel.

Patients are not generally sedated for the procedure, although a local anesthetic may be used at the back of the throat or on the tip of the feeding tube. Placing post-pyloric tubes is more challenging than placing gastric tubes. Fluoroscopic guidance may be necessary for ND or NJ tube placement in some patients. Nasal tubes (small bore, of soft material) can often be used safely for months if patients receive meticulous care and if tube placement is alternated between nostrils. Long-term nasal tube placement can, however, erode the nasal septum.

Up to 60% of patients may experience ulceration or mucosal bruising of the esophagus and hypopharynx from tube placement, but clinically evident injury is rare.[111,112] If small-bore tubes are inadvertently inserted in the lungs, significant harm can result if the pleura are perforated or the tube's misplacement is not recognized before feeding formula is infused. The actual incidence of pulmonary placement is probably no more than 4%, although widely varying estimates can be found in the literature.[113,114] The problem is most likely to occur in neurologically compromised patients without a functional cough reflex. Infusing enteral formula into the lungs or pleural space can result in pleuritis, pneumonitis, empyema, bacterial superinfection, or sepsis.[113]

Auscultating to detect air insufflation, assessing pH of fluids drawn through the tube, and determining whether gastric fluid is being aspirated are ways to assess tube location. Tube placement should be confirmed radiographically when other methods of evaluating tube location yield unclear results, as is often the case with mechanically ventilated, heavily sedated, and neurologically compromised patients. All methods, however, including radiographs, can be misinterpreted.[113]

Feeding ostomies (enterostomies) are reserved for patients requiring longer-term feedings. Enterostomies (i.e., gastrostomies and jejunostomies) can be placed by either percutaneous endoscopy or surgery. Although there is no definitive time period for "longer-term" feedings, a minimum of 4 weeks is typically necessary to justify a feeding enterostomy in any patient. An expected duration of at least 6 months justifies an enterostomy for nearly all patients.[115] If tube feeding is expected to last between a few weeks and 6 months, multiple factors will influence whether nasal tube placement or enterostomy is used. Temporary enterostomies that use purse-string sutures to hold an indwelling tube or create a short seromuscular tunnel (e.g., Stamm or Witzel enterostomies) are typically created when the tube feeding is expected to last 2–6 months. These enterostomies close "on their own" when the feeding tube is pulled and seldom require further surgery for ostomy closure.[113]

Percutaneous endoscopic gastrostomy (PEG) placement is used in most patients requiring a gastrostomy. Surgical gastrostomy is typically reserved for patients in whom the endoscope cannot be passed, such as those with severe esophageal stricture or obstruction; when the gastrostomy is done as part of a laparotomy for another purpose; or when the PEG procedure is contraindicated for such reasons as [116]:

- Massive ascites.
- Peritoneal dialysis.
- Coagulopathy.
- Hepatomegaly.
- Portal hypertension.
- Gastric varices.
- Morbid obesity.
- A large hiatal hernia.

- Previous subtotal gastrectomy or gastric pull-up.
- Neoplastic or infiltrative disease of the gastric wall.

Massive ascites and coagulopathy may also preclude surgical enterostomy, as may risk of enterocutaneous fistula formation (e.g., Crohn's disease or radiation enteritis). Multiple open surgery methods and laparoscopic surgery are available for gastrostomy formation.[117]

Percutaneous endoscopic jejunostomy (PEJ) placement is more difficult than PEG placement, but its rate of success for feeding patients properly is about 85%.[118] A jejunal tube can be placed through a PEG (JET-PEG) when patients require gastric drainage as well as jejunal feedings. Overall results with JET-PEGs have been disappointing, however, due to relatively high failure rates—especially with respect to preventing aspiration.[118] A gastrostomy for drainage and a separate jejunostomy for feeding may be preferable in many cases. Open and laparoscopic methods are available for placing a jejunostomy surgically.[117]

Percutaneous enterostomies are usually placed under local anesthesia, whereas general anesthesia is used for many surgical enterostomies. Percutaneous placement costs less than surgical placement, but complication rates appear to be similar. Reported morbidity and mortality vary widely for gastrostomy tube placement and it can be difficult to separate the effects of gastrostomy on morbidity and mortality from the effects of malnutrition and the underlying condition leading to gastrostomy. Rates of minor complications appear to average about 5% to 7% for both open surgical gastrostomies and for PEG placement.[116] Complications classified as "minor" include peristomal wound infection, inflammation, leakage around the tube, formation of granulation tissue, tube obstruction, tube breakage, and tube migration into the small bowel. Major complications appear to occur in about 1% to 4% of patients, although procedure-related mortality is under 1% in most studies.[116] Several large studies of PEG placement showed that in patients who developed major complications, however, mortality was 25%.[119] Aspiration, peritonitis, tube migration through the gastric wall, perforation, hemorrhage, necrotizing fasciitis, and gastrocolocutaneous fistula development are considered major complications.

Formula Types and Components

Although many enteral formulas are commercially available, the types are limited. Most facilities include only one or two formulas of a given type on their formulary. Enteral formulas can be classified several ways based on their characteristics and the intended population, but the two major types are polymeric and oligomeric. Their main difference is the degree of digestive function required for absorption.

Formulas can also be classified as general or disease-specific. General formulas can be subdivided by protein content, caloric density, and fiber content. Disease-specific formulas are designed according to patients' alterations in nutrient tolerance or metabolism during specific disease states.

Categories of Medicare Home Enteral Formulas

❑ **Category I:** semisynthetic intact protein or protein isolate.
   Examples (adult): Ensure, Ensure HN, FiberSource HN, Isocal, Isocal HN,
      Jevity, Osmolite, Osmolite HN, ReSource Diabetic, Ultracal
   Examples (pediatric): Pediasure
❑ **Category IB:** natural intact protein or protein isolate.
   Examples (adult): Compleat
   Examples (pediatric): Compleat Pediatric
❑ **Category II:** intact protein or protein isolate, calorically dense.
   Examples (adult): Deliver 2.0, Ensure Plus, Glutasorb, IsoSource 1.5 Cal,
      NovaSource 2.0, TwoCal HN, Respalor
❑ **Category III:** hydrolyzed protein or amino acids.
   Examples (adults): Criticare HN, Isotein HN, Peptamen 1.5, Reabilan, Vital
      HN
   Examples (pediatric): Vivonex Pediatric
❑ **Category IV:** defined formula for special metabolic needs.
   Examples (adult): Advera, AminAid, Choice dm, Crucial, DiabetiSource,
      Glucerna, HepaticAid, Impact, ImmunAid, Nepro, NutriHep, NutriVent,
      Perative, Peptamen, Pulmocare, Replete, Suplena
   Examples (pediatric): Pregestimil
❑ **Category V:** modular components for protein, carbohydrate, fats.
   Examples (protein): Casec, Promix, Propac
   Examples (carbohydrate): Moducal, Polycose liquid or powder
   Examples (fats): Microlipid, MCT oil
❑ **Category VI:** standardized nutrients.
   Examples: Tolerex

Another way to classify enteral formulas is complete versus incomplete. Most are complete sources of nutrition, providing a balance of macronutrients (e.g., protein, carbohydrate, and fat), as well as micronutrients (e.g., vitamins, minerals, and trace elements) required by the human body. Modular components are incomplete formulas that provide a single nutrient and no micronutrients so they can be mixed with other formulas to meet specific needs.

The categories into which Medicare divides enteral formulas (for documentation and reimbursement purposes), along with some formulas in each category, are listed in the sidebar above.[73]

Polymeric Formulas

Most commercially available enteral formulas are polymeric, requiring full digestive function for absorption. They contain intact protein components and relatively complex carbohydrates, and are categorized based on nutrient sources, protein content, caloric density, and fiber content.

Nutrient Sources

In this group there are three categories: blenderized, milk-based, and lactose-free.

Blenderized Products. Blenderized products contain meat, vegetables, and fruit that have been pureed and processed to maintain commercial sterility. Compared to blenderized diets prepared in the home, the commercial products offer more consistent nutrient intake with a lower risk of bacterial contamination, but at a higher price. Blenderized formulas cost about three to four times as much as a standard semi-synthetic formula.[120] Few third-party payers will cover blenderized formulas without clear documentation of medical necessity. Compleat, Compleat Pediatric, and DiabetiSource are among the few commercially available blenderized formulas.

Milk-Based Products. Milk-based formulas (which contain milk and, thus, lactose) tend to be more palatable when taken by mouth than most other formulas. They are often a good option for oral supplementation if the patient does not have lactose intolerance, which causes bloating, abdominal cramps, flatulence and watery diarrhea. Few ethnic groups other than those of northern European descent maintain lactase production through adulthood; thus lactose intolerance is a common condition. Malnutrition and GI tract disease may contribute to lactose intolerance. Most hospitals, therefore, include only lactose-free products on the enteral formulary.

Powdered products designed to mix with milk, such as Meritene or Carnation Instant Breakfast, are typical of the milk-based formulas. Cost tends to be similar to that for standard semisynthetic enteral formulas, but availability may be better because these powdered products are often available at supermarkets.

Lactose-Free Products. Standard enteral formulas—the vast majority of those commercially available—are lactose-free. Casein, caseinates (e.g., sodium, potassium, calcium, or magnesium salts of casein), soy protein isolate, or a combination of these protein sources are used in most lactose-free polymeric formulas. Isolated milk protein, which improves palatability, is also used in several products. Despite the presence of milk proteins (casein, lactalbumin, and whey), these products are lactose-free because they do not contain carbohydrate from milk (i.e., lactose). Patients with a true milk allergy, as opposed to lactose intolerance, should not receive products containing isolated milk protein. If patients express concern about lactose intolerance, you should explain the difference between milk or nonfat dried milk as an ingredient and isolated milk protein.

Protein Content

Polymeric formulas may be categorized by protein content as low, standard, or high nitrogen.

Low Nitrogen. Formulas are considered low nitrogen if they contain less than 11% of calories from protein or if their nonprotein calorie to nitrogen ratio

(NPC:N) is 200:1 or higher. These formulas typically contain other modifications that place them into the category of disease-specific formulas for renal failure.

Standard Nitrogen. Standard nitrogen content corresponds to about 11% to 15% of calories from protein, or a NPC:N of approximately 140:1 to 200:1. Among the many standard nitrogen formulas available are Isocal, IsoSource Standard, Osmolite, Ensure, Ensure Plus, ReSource Standard, and ReSource Plus.

High Nitrogen. High protein formulas contain 16% to 25% of calories from protein, or a NPC:N of 75:1 to 130:1. These formulas are designed for patients with relatively high protein requirements compared to caloric needs. Formulas with 16% to 17% of calories from protein (NPC:N of about 120:1 to 130:1) are often appropriate for elderly patients with good renal function. The higher protein products (20% to 25% of calories from protein) tend to be more appropriate for highly catabolic patients or those with high protein losses, such as patients with closed head injury, long bone fractures, pelvic fractures, large open wounds with drainage, or protein-losing enteropathy.

Many high nitrogen formulas are available, often with names the same as the standard nitrogen product but with "HN" added after the name, such as Isocal HN, IsoSource HN, Osmolite HN, and FiberSource HN. When the initials "VHN" or "VHP" are added they denote very high nitrogen or protein, which correlates with 25% of calories from protein (e.g., IsoSource VHN). Not all high protein products, however, include "HN," "VHN," or "VHP" in the name, despite their high protein content. High nitrogen products may be slightly more expensive than standard nitrogen products, falling into a relative cost of 1.3 when compared to a semisynthetic, standard caloric density (1 kcal/mL), fiber-free formula.[120] Very high nitrogen products may be slightly more expensive than high nitrogen formulas.

Caloric Density

Caloric densities for adult formulas appear in the sidebar on page 256. The more calorically dense the formula, the less free water it provides and the greater the risk of dehydration. Standard calorie polymeric formulas are 80% to 85% free water, meaning that for every liter of formula, 800 mL to 850 mL of water is provided. Formulas with moderate caloric density provide 75% to 79% free water, and calorically dense formulas provide about 70% to 72% free water.

Calorically dense formulas are generally reserved for patients with poor fluid tolerance, such as those with congestive heart failure or renal failure, or patients unable to tolerate the volume of formula necessary to meet nutrient goals. As increased density is fed into the stomach, gastric emptying may be delayed. Also, when it is rapidly infused into the small bowel, the capacity of intestinal enzymes can be overwhelmed.[121]

The names of several moderate calorie products are the same as those for standard calorie products except "plus" is added after the name (e.g., Boost

Caloric Density of Adult Enteral Formulas

Standard: 1 to 1.2 kcal/mL.
Moderate: approximately 1.5 kcal/mL.
Dense: 2 kcal/mL.

Calories are total kilocalories with protein and carbohydrates each providing 4 kcal/g, medium-chain triglycerides providing 8.3 kcal/g, and long-chain fatty acids providing 9 kcal/g.

Plus, ReSource Plus, and Ensure Plus). A few formula names containing "Plus" are only 1.2 kcal/mL; thus "Plus" should not be assumed to mean 1.5 kcal/mL. Calorically dense formulas often contain "two" or "2.0" in the name (e.g., TwoCal HN, NovaSource 2.0, and Deliver 2.0). Nonspecialized moderate caloric density and calorically dense products often cost about the same per 1000 calories as standard caloric density products.[120]

Fiber Content

Polymeric formulas, with the exception of blenderized formulas, are low residue unless fiber is added. Few patients actually require a low residue diet, but in most patients requiring short-term EN therapy it is not clear whether fiber provides physiologic benefits. Dietary fiber is composed of polysaccharides and lignin not digested by the endogenous secretions of the human GI tract.[122] The recommended fiber intake for healthy adults is 20–35 g/day, although few people meet this goal.[123] Total dietary fiber content of enteral formulas ranges from about 4 to 15 g/L, as listed in Table 7-6.

Total dietary fiber is divided into two components: insoluble and soluble. Cellulose and soy polysaccharide or soy fiber are examples of primarily insoluble fibers used in enteral formulas. Insoluble fibers absorb water, thereby increasing fecal bulk and improving stool consistency in healthy subjects. Clinical studies are inconclusive, however, about their effect, when added to enteral products, on bowel function in critically ill patients and those with GI disease.[123]

Soluble fibers are associated with improved glycemic control, lowered serum cholesterol in hyperlipidemic patients, and enhanced fluid and electrolyte absorption. In the colon they are fermented to short chain fatty acids (SCFAs), which in turn appear to be a preferred fuel for colon cells and may provide a trophic effect on healthy colonocytes while inhibiting hyperproliferation of preneoplastic cells in the bowel.[124]

Acacia, partially hydrolyzed guar gum, pectin, and oat fiber are used as sources of soluble fiber in enteral products. In addition, soy polysaccharide has demonstrated clinical effects associated with soluble fiber despite being about 94% insoluble fiber.[125] Fructooligosaccharides (FOS) also have clinical effects similar to those of soluble fiber. These short chain oligosaccharides resist digestion in the upper GI tract but are fermented to SCFAs by bifidobacteria in the colon.[126]

TABLE 7-6 Fiber Sources for Selected Enteral Formulas

| Formula Name | Total Dietary Fiber(g/L) | Primarily Insoluble Fiber | | Primarily Soluble Fiber |
		Soy[a]	Cellulose[b]	
Advera	8.9	x		None
Boost with fiber	10	x	x	Acacia
Choice dm	14.4	x	x	Acacia
Complete Modified	4.2			All fiber from fruits and vegetables
DiabetiSource	4.4			All fiber from fruits and vegetables
Ensure with fiber	14.4	x		None
FiberSource	10		x	Partially Hydrolyzed Guar Gum
Glucerna	14.1	x		None
Glucerna OS	8.5	x	x	Gum Arabic
Glytrol	15	x		Gum Arabic, Pectin
Impact with fiber	10	x		Partially Hydrolyzed Guar Gum
IsoSource VHN	10	x		Partially Hydrolyzed Guar Gum
Jevity Plus	12	x	x	Oat Fiber, Gum Arabic, FOS[c]
NuBasics with fiber	14	x		None
Nutren 1.0 with fiber	14	x		None
Nutriflavor	14.2			Gum Arabic, Pectin
ProBalance	10	x		Gum Arabic
Promote with fiber	14.4	x		Oat Fiber
Protain XL	8	x		None
Replete with fiber	14	x		None
ReSource Diabetic	12.7		x	Partially Hydrolyzed Guar Gum
Ultracal	14.4	x		Oat Fiber

a. Soy fiber or soy polysaccharide.
b. Cellulose gum or gel, or microcrystalline cellulose.
c. Fructooligosaccharides.

Although adequate fiber intake is promoted for healthy adults, the requirements and balance between potential benefits and risks in patients with ongoing disease processes are less clear. Potential adverse effects include diarrhea with excess fiber intake and increased flatulence and abdominal discomfort with rapid advancement of fiber intake.[127,128] Likewise, diarrhea has been reported with excessive intake (> 45 g/day) of FOS.[129] Such symptoms could be mistaken as tube feeding intolerance.

Bezoars formed from fiber have been reported when fluid provision is inadequate and GI motility is poor.[128,130] Decreased absorption of some minerals has been reported in healthy subjects receiving fiber-augmented liquid diets, although the minerals affected were not consistent between studies.[123] Little work has been done in actual patients, and the clinical significance is unclear when a patient is receiving at least the RDA or RDI for a mineral.[43,79]

Fiber-containing formulas may be difficult to administer through small feeding tubes (< 8 French) or by gravity methods because they have higher viscosity than similar formulas without fiber. Soluble fibers' tendency to gel makes them difficult to incorporate into liquid formulas in large quantities.

FOS have physiochemical characteristics that are more favorable for incorporation into liquid formulas than those of most soluble fibers.

Patients most likely to benefit from fiber-containing formulas and least likely to experience adverse effects appear to be those requiring long-term tube feeding who are relatively stable and without significant ongoing GI pathology. You should carefully consider risks versus benefits when selecting a fiber-containing enteral formula for patients who are critically ill or who have significant GI pathology, especially motility problems. Fiber-containing formulas are slightly more expensive than fiber-free formulas (the relative cost compared to a standard caloric density, semisynthetic, fiber-free formula is 1.2 to 1.3), but cost should not be a determining factor in selection.[120]

Oligomeric Formulas

Oligomeric formulas are designed for patients with reduced pancreatic function, impaired small bowel mucosal function, or malabsorption. Their protein component requires minimal digestive action prior to absorption, and the content of long chain fatty acids tends to be low compared to polymeric formulas. Other terms used for oligomeric formulas include chemically defined, monomeric, elemental, or peptide formulas. True "elemental" formulas contain free amino acids as the protein source. Formulas that are "peptide-based" contain a mixture of free amino acids, di- and tri-peptides, and oligopeptides from a hydrolyzed protein source. The percent of peptides more complex than tripeptides determines the extent to which hydrolytic function is required prior to absorption. Di- and tri-peptides are absorbed by specific sodium-independent, noncompetitive carriers located in the small bowel mucosa and do not require further hydrolysis prior to absorption.[131] Free amino acids are absorbed by a separate sodium-dependent active transport mechanism. Most peptide formulas contain a significant proportion of oligopeptides that require hydrolysis before they can be absorbed. The longer peptide units, however, tend to reduce the osmolality of peptide formulas as compared to the osmolality of true elemental formulas. The longer peptides may also improve taste somewhat. Despite attempts to improve palatability of oligomeric formulas by adding flavorings and reformulating, as a whole these products remain quite unpalatable. An aftertaste described as "chemical" and bitter is typically described by people taking oligomeric formulas by mouth.

For most patients, there is no benefit of oligomeric over polymeric formulas, although they may be better for patients with severe pancreatic insufficiency or short bowel syndrome.[132] Even in such conditions, however, the superiority of oligomeric formulas has not been conclusively demonstrated in well-designed studies. Patients with pancreatic insufficiency who would normally use an oligomeric formula may be able to use a polymeric formula if they receive pancreatic enzyme supplementation. In general, oligomeric formulas should be reserved for patients with significant digestive or absorptive impairment for whom an appropriate polymeric formula failed to work.

There are limited data on clinical differences between elemental and peptide-based formulas for patients in whom an oligomeric formula is appropriate. Fat content of elemental formulas tends to be lower than that of peptide-based formulas, which may be a consideration in patients with severe fat malabsorption. Osmolality of elemental formulas is in the mid 600s, somewhat higher than the 300 to 500 mOsm/kg of peptide-based formulas. Currently available elemental formulas, including Tolerex and Vivonex Plus, are powders that must be mixed before use, raising concerns about bacterial contamination and inappropriate preparation. Some peptide-based formulas, such as Vital HN and AlitraQ, also require reconstitution before use, but most are ready to use, including Crucial, Peptamen products, Reabilan, Subdue, and SandoSource Peptide. This may be a significant consideration in some settings, such as the home. Most health care facilities place only one oligomeric product on the enteral formulary for adult patients because the indications for their use are limited and most cost 12 to 15 times more than polymeric formulas.[120] You typically must document the medical necessity for using an oligomeric rather than polymeric formula to obtain third-party reimbursement. Oligomeric formulas are found under three different Medicare categories for home enteral formulas—Categories III, IV, and VI[73]—each of which has a set reimbursement rate per 100 kcal provided.

Specialized Formulas

Formulas designed for patients with specific disease states or conditions are classified as specialized—a grouping that includes both polymeric and oligomeric formulas. For Medicare purposes, specialized formulas fall into Categories I, II, III, and IV for home enteral nutrition.[73] Protein is the most common formula component to be altered, although the carbohydrate-to-fat ratio and the fat sources may also be altered to achieve specific effects. Specialized formulas are often based on a biochemical premise with good theoretical rationale but lacking conclusive evidence of clinical relevance. Well designed, controlled studies of adequate size that support the superiority of specialized formulas over more standard polymeric formulas are rare.

Depending on the components altered, the cost of specialized formulas ranges from slightly more expensive to more than 25 times that of standard formulas.[120] Subcategories of specialized formulas are based on the target disease or condition, including glycemic control, pulmonary disease, renal dysfunction, hepatic disease, stress or critical care, and immune-modulation. Each subcategory of specialized formula is discussed here briefly.

Glycemic Control

Formulas designed for patients with hyperglycemia have relatively minor alterations compared to standard enteral formulas. The percent of calories from carbohydrates tends to be somewhat less than standard formulas, at 35% to 40%, and calories from fat are higher, at 40% to 50% (also higher than the 30% of calories from fat recommended by the American Diabetes Association).[133]

Canola oil and/or high oleic oils provide a reasonable balance of polyunsaturated and monounsaturated fatty acids. Fiber sources associated with positive effects on glycemic control, including various soluble fibers and/or soy polysaccharide, are components of all the formulas designed for glycemic control (see Table 7-6). The amount of fiber in the volume of formula needed to meet 100% of most RDIs ranges widely. DiabetiSource provides only 6.5 g and Choice dm about 15 g, while Glucerna, Glytrol, and ReSource Diabetic provide 20 to 23 g of fiber.[78-81]

A low-carbohydrate, fiber-containing formula showed a blunted glycemic response in initial studies of simulated tube feeding.[134] Follow-up studies noted that the glycemic response varied in each patient.[135] Only small amounts of formula were ingested over several hours in these studies, making it difficult to extrapolate findings to tube-fed patients. No studies have demonstrated a difference in outcome with formulas designed for improved glycemic control, but well-designed clinical trials are scarce.[136] Given the lack of efficacy data, these formulas should be used only after carefully evaluating potential benefits versus the known effect of slowed gastric emptying from a high-fat diet. These formulas cost roughly two to three times more than standard enteral formulas and, for reimbursement purposes, fall into Medicare categories I, II, and IV for home enteral formulas.[73]

Pulmonary Disease

Most formulas for patients with pulmonary disease differ from standard formulas mainly in the carbohydrate-to-fat ratio, containing from 40% to 55% of calories as fat. Theoretically, the high fat content reduces the lungs' work to eliminate carbon dioxide (CO_2), because fat oxidation is associated with a lower respiratory quotient (RQ) than carbohydrate oxidation. The RQ is a measure of CO_2 produced per volume of oxygen consumed; thus fat's lower RQ means less CO_2 is produced that must subsequently be eliminated. High carbohydrate feedings have been reported to precipitate respiratory failure and to prolong or prevent weaning from mechanical ventilation.[136,137]

In addition, ambulatory patients with chronic obstructive pulmonary disease (COPD) and hypercapnia receiving higher carbohydrate, lower fat enteral formulas have demonstrated higher RQs and higher CO_2 production than those receiving a low carbohydrate, high fat formula.[138] Many patients requiring mechanical ventilation, however, do not retain CO_2 and are not hypercapnic, and are unlikely to have the same response to altering the calorie source as COPD patients. For mechanically ventilated patients, in fact, overfeeding is more likely to be detrimental to respiratory status than is the percent of calories from carbohydrate.[139] When total caloric intake approximates caloric requirements, the clinical benefit of manipulating the calorie source is unclear.[93] Patients without CO_2 retention and hypercapnia appear less likely to benefit from a high fat formula. In all cases, you must balance potential risks from the delayed gastric emptying associated with high fat feedings against effects of the caloric source on respiratory status. Adverse effects on diaphragmatic distention and thoracic expansion have been reported in patients who have abdominal distention from delayed gastric emptying.[140]

A relatively new development in pulmonary formulas is inclusion of high omega-3 fatty acid (n-3 FA) content. Oxepa contains deionized sardine oil and borage oil in addition to the canola oil and medium chain triglyceride (MCT) oil found in NutriVent, NovaSource Pulmonary, Respalor, and Pulmocare. As a class, the n-3 FA are precursors to less inflammatory and less thrombotic products than the omega-6 fatty acids (n-6 FA) found in such oils as corn and soybean. Oxepa, therefore, is marketed for patients with an inflammatory response, such as acute respiratory distress syndrome, rather than hypercapnia alone. The use of n-3 FA is discussed further under immune-modulating formulas. The relative cost of products such as Oxepa is several times higher than that of typical pulmonary formulas, where relative cost is about 2.5 times that of a standard semisynthetic, polymeric formula.[120]

Renal Dysfunction

Specialized formulas for renal dysfunction fit into two categories based on protein composition: enriched with essential amino acids (EAAs) and standard amino acid formulas with minerals and electrolytes adjusted for renal dysfunction. All formulas for renal dysfunction are calorically dense (2 kcal/mL) and contain only 70% to 74% free water to minimize fluid administration.

Formulas enriched with EAAs, such as Amin-Aid and Renalcal, are based on the concept that urea nitrogen can be recycled for nonessential amino acid synthesis.[120,136] Theoretically, this would reduce accumulation of urea nitrogen in the blood and avoid azotemia. Recycling of nitrogen and incorporation into amino acids, however, does not appear to occur in clinically significant amounts. Another problem with formulas high in EAAs, when used for more than a couple of weeks, is ammonia accumulation in the bloodstream. Amin-Aid provides only EAAs plus histidine as the protein source, and contains only sodium as a micronutrient, so vitamin and mineral supplementation is necessary. Renalcal contains selected non-EAAs and whey protein concentrate in addition to EAAs, and provides some water-soluble vitamins. Formulas high in EAAs are not appropriate for most patients with renal dysfunction, including those with acute renal failure or receiving renal replacement therapy (i.e., dialysis) of any type. Only patients with chronic renal failure who are receiving a very low protein diet and are not candidates for dialysis should be considered for an EAA formula, and supporting data even for these patients are poor. Palatability of EAA formulas is very poor due to the free amino acid content and associated aftertaste, so they generally must be supplied via tube feeding. Formulas enriched with EAAs tend to be quite expensive, their cost on a par with that of oligomeric formulas.

Standard amino acid formulas with minerals and electrolytes adjusted for renal dysfunction, including Nepro and Suplena, provide a balance of EAAs and non-EAAs from common protein sources. The potassium, phosphorus, and magnesium content of these formulas per 1000 kcal is typically less than half that of standard formulas. In addition, the content of fat-soluble vitamins, especially vitamin A, is reduced compared to standard formulas. Nepro is designed for patients with protein losses or catabolism, supplying 14% of calories as protein. Most hospitalized patients receiving frequent dialysis require 1.2 to 1.8 g protein/kg/day to replace protein losses and heal wounds.[49] Suplena, for patients requiring protein restriction, supplies only 6% of calories from protein. These products are more expensive than standard formulas, with a relative cost of 3 to 3.9, but are much less expensive than formulas enriched with EAAs. All formulas for renal dysfunction are in Category IV for Medicare reimbursement of qualified home care patients. Thus, the Medicare reimbursement per 100 kcal is the same for all the formulas in this category, regardless of their cost.[73]

Hepatic Disease

The hallmark of specialized formulas designed for patients with hepatic disease is enrichment to between 45% and 50% of protein from the branched-chain amino acids (BCAAs), leucine, isoleucine, and valine. Standard formulas contain about 15% to 20% BCAAs. In addition, methionine and the aromatic amino acids (AAAs) phenylalinine, tryrosine, and tryptophan are reduced in the hepatic formulas. These specialized formulas were developed to balance the abnormal plasma amino acid pattern associated with hepatic encephalopathy, in which the normal molar ratio between BCAAs and AAAs drops more than three-fold.[141] The theory on which they were developed is that the common transport mechanism allowing BCAAs and AAAs to cross the blood-brain barrier favors AAAs in patients with hepatic dysfunction, and excess AAAs in the brain contribute to an imbalance of neurotransmitters, such as serotonin, for which the AAAs serve as precursors. The theory of amino acid imbalances causing hepatic encephalopathy has never been proven.

Use of hepatic formulas remains controversial. Few well designed studies exist, and most using control diets were conducted before it was recognized that cirrhotic patients tolerate vegetable better than animal proteins, and that severe protein restriction may be detrimental. Most studies show no advantage of hepatic formulas,[72,120] which are better than giving no protein but generally are not better than conventional therapy with lactulose or neomycin. Specialized hepatic formulas do not appear to improve survival and most patients with hepatic disease can use formulas composed of the standard protein sources.[93] Specialized formulas should be reserved for the select few patients who are compliant with conventional therapies and diets but cannot take adequate protein without precipitating hepatic encephalopathy. Given the high cost of these specialized formulas, the benefit to the patient should be clearly documented if the formula is to continue beyond a trial period. Medicare coverage of home enteral nutrition with a specialized hepatic formula can be problematic, so medical necessity and costs should be carefully evaluated. Because the free amino acid content makes palatability poor, oral supplementation is rarely appropriate—especially considering that patients are typically anorexic, as well. Hepatic-Aid II, a nutritionally incomplete powder formula, requires reconstitution and supplementation with appropriate vitamins and minerals. NutriHep is a liquid formula that includes vitamins and minerals.

Stress or Critical Care Formulas

Formulas designed for metabolic stress (also referred to as critical care formulas) may be enriched with BCAAs but are not the therapeutic equivalent of specialized hepatic formulas. The two types of formulas should not be interchanged in clinical practice. Formulas designed for stressed patients are high in nitrogen (NPC:N typically 100:1 or less) and contain standard amounts of AAAs. They are based on the theory that providing exogenous BCAAs will reduce breakdown of skeletal muscle and improve protein synthesis, since BCAAs appear to be a preferred energy source for skeletal muscle in critically ill patients.[120,136] In a few studies, various nutritional markers improved when enteral or parenteral BCAAs were used in the critically ill, but no difference was seen in morbidity or mortality. Other investigators have failed to find a difference in parameters when comparing formulas enriched with BCAAs to isonitrogenous provision of standard proteins. Studies are generally small and difficult to compare because the amounts of BCAAs and other nutrients provided are not consistent. In addition, patients included in the studies are often not well defined in terms of critical illness.

Formulas enriched with BCAAs are not the current standard of practice in critical care.[4,93] In fact, few formulas marketed for critical care are truly enriched with BCAAs; most contain only a slightly higher percentage of BCAAs than regular high nitrogen products do (see Table 7-7).

Immune-Modulating Formulas

Several formulas marketed for critical care contain components to enhance wound healing and immune function or to reduce the inflammatory response. Such formulas are generally classified as immune-modulating formulas. Some are altered by enriching them with specific amino acids, including glutamine or arginine, adding nucleotides, or manipulating the n-6 FA and n-3 FA ratios. Formulas differ in the number of components altered and the extent of alteration, as shown in Table 7-7. Although immune-modulating components offer promise for improved response to specialized nutrition support in certain situations, none can be considered standard of practice at this time. The rationale for components used in immune-modulating formulas is discussed below.

Glutamine.   Glutamine is a non-EAA that was reclassified in recent years as "conditionally" essential. Decreased skeletal muscle and blood glutamine concentrations are associated with catabolic states. Under such conditions, including metabolic stress and injury, the amount of glutamine released from skeletal muscle may be inadequate to meet demands and an exogenous source may be necessary.[142] Due to stability problems in solution, free glutamine is found only in powdered enteral formulas. For the same reason,

TABLE 7-7 Selected Critical Care and Immune-Modulating Enteral Formulas

Formula	kcal per mL	% kcal as Protein	% Protein as BCAA	ARG g/L[a]	GLU g/L[b]	Dietary Nucleotide g/L	% kcal as Fat	MCT:LCT Ratio	% kcal as LCT	n-6:n-3 Ratio	n-6 FA g/L	n-3 FA g/L
AlitraQ	1	21	18.5	4.5	15.5	none	13	53:47	6.1	>10:1	6.6	0.02
Crucial	1.5	25	17.6	15	7.2	none	39	50:50	19.5	2:1	7.7	3.6
Immun-Aid	1	32	36	14	9	1	20	50:50	10	2.1:1	2.4	1.1
Impact	1	22	17.1	12.5	5.9	1.2	25	27:63	15.7	1.4:1	2.5	1.7
Impact 1.5	1.5	22	17.1	18.7	8.8	1.8	40	55:45	22	1.4:1	3.6	2.6
Impact Oral	1	22	NA[c]	14	NA[c]	1.3	25	25:75	18.7	0.9:1	2.9	3.2
Optimental	1	20.5	NA[c]	5.5	NA[c]	none	25	28:62	15.5	0.86:1	4.2	4.8
Oxepa	1.5	16.7	NA[c]	NA[c]	NA[c]	none	55	25:75	41.2	2:1	18.8	9.4
Peptamen 1.5	1.5	16	NA[c]	NA[c]	NA[c]	none	33	70:30	77	7:1	NA[c]	NA[c]
Peptamen VHP	1	25	21	1.9	4.6	none	33	70:30	77	8:1	NA[c]	NA[c]
Perative	1.3	20.5	18.2	6.5	5.4	none	25	40:60	15	4.8:1	7.5	1.6
Reabilan HN	1.33	17	21	1.9	9.3	none	35	50:50	17.5	5:1	NA[c]	NA[c]
SandoSource Peptide	1	20	30	5	4.7	none	15	54:46	6.3	7:1	NA[c]	NA[c]
Vivonex Plus	1	18	30	5	10	none	6	No MCT	6	7:1	NA[c]	NA[c]

a. ARG = Arginine.

b. GLU = Glutamine.

c. NA = Not Available.

Source: Data compiled from manufacturer's information.

parenteral amino acid solutions do not contain glutamine. Liquid enteral formulas with an intact protein component contain protein-bound glutamine, generally at less than 14% of the total protein.[143] Protein in the normal diet contains about 10% glutamine.[144]

Glutamine functions in multiple metabolic pathways, having a role in synthesis of nucleic acid, nucleotides, glycogen and urea, as well as in gluconeogenesis, ammoniagenesis, and ammonia reduction.[144,145] In specialized nutrition support, interest has focused on the role of glutamine in the small bowel. Glutamine serves as a preferred oxidative fuel for several groups of rapidly dividing cells, including the intestinal mucosa. Animal studies with glutamine supplementation have shown increased nutrient absorption, improved mucosal integrity, and reduced translocation of bacteria from the GI tract.[136] Administering glutamine orally in humans has decreased methotrexate-induced enterocolitis and improved the rate of GI tract recovery following whole abdominal radiation.[144] In one study of critically ill patients, improvement in indicators of protein catabolic rate and immune function were attributed to administration of glutamine-enhanced enteral formula, but no improvement was noted in nitrogen balance, visceral protein status, or outcome.[146] Reduction in hospital costs due to prevention of secondary infections for patients in intensive care has also been attributed to glutamine supplementation.[147] In another study, there were fewer cases of pneumonia and bacteremia and fewer septic events when patients received an enteral formula supplemented with glutamine at about 16 g/L, as compared with the standard formula, which contained glutamine at about 2 g/L.[148]

In bone marrow transplant (BMT) patients, oral glutamine supplementation showed no benefit compared to placebo, but the dose actually consumed may have been inadequate.[149] Several other studies have failed to show a difference in length of stay, oral mucositis, or dependence on parenteral nutrition in BMT patients receiving glutamine supplementation,[149-151] despite earlier reports of shorter hospital stays and decreased infections (but no decrease in antibiotic use) for BMT patients receiving IV glutamine supplementation, as compared with nonsupplemented patients.[152,153] Because these earlier studies lacked objective criteria for hospital discharge and failed to analyze on an "intent to treat" basis, their clinical applicability is questionable. In addition, both studies were small and showed no difference in total antibiotic use, oral mucositis, dependence on parenteral nutrition, or survival. Today many BMT patients not receiving glutamine supplementation have shorter hospital stays than those reported in these studies.

Although glutamine appears promising as an adjuvant to nutrition therapy in critically ill patients, its role has not been clearly defined. Glutamine supplementation, either oral or intravenous, cannot be considered the standard of care for any patient population at this time. Supplementation with up to 40 g per day (0.57 g/kg/day)—at least four times the usual dietary intake—does appear to be well tolerated and safe,[144,154] but the potential effect of large glutamine doses on other amino acids that share transport mechanisms and metabolic pathways is unclear, and whether the impact of intravenous glutamine differs from that of oral supplementation is unknown. It's important to be cautious with critically ill patients because ammonia is produced during intestinal glutamine metabolism. Release of the excess ammonia into the portal vein has been demonstrated in dogs, and is expected to occur in humans.[155] Until carefully monitored clinical trials show that glutamine supplementation is safe in patients with renal or hepatic dysfunction or with abnormalities in ammonia homeostatis, these conditions should be considered at least a relative contraindication to both oral and intravenous glutamine supplementation.

Even when the clinical role of glutamine supplementation has been defined, pharmaceutical issues related to glutamine stability are likely to remain barriers to its routine use. From the enteral standpoint, the role of protein-bound glutamine versus free glutamine must be answered, and the role of glutamine-containing compounds that are more stable should be investigated for both enteral and parenteral application. A few studies suggest that dipeptides containing glutamine may offer alternatives for parenteral administration. Enhanced absorption of oral D-xylose has been demonstrated in critically ill patients receiving alanine-glutamine dipeptides compared with standard parenteral amino acids.[156] In addition, increased villus height and decreased intestinal permeability in patients with stable intestinal disease has been noted with glycl-L-glutamine dipeptides compared with controls receiving standard parenteral amino acids.[157] Glutamate may be another option for providing a source of glutamine, but further study is needed.

Arginine.   Typically, about 5.4% of protein intake is arginine.[144] Under normal conditions, the remainder of arginine the body needs is synthesized via the urea cycle, where it is involved in ammonia detoxification. Endogenous synthesis of arginine may be inadequate during periods of metabolic stress; thus it is considered a "conditionally" essential amino acid. Arginine is important in the production of nitric oxide and polyamines involved in cell growth and differentiation. Many animal studies have demonstrated favorable effects of arginine administration on nitrogen balance, immune function, and wound healing.[136] Human studies have also shown improvement in wound healing and in vitro markers of immune function. In both healthy subjects and the elderly, arginine supplementation improved wound healing.[158] The elderly subjects also showed improvement in markers of immune function, which has been reported following arginine administration after surgery in cancer patients.[158,159] In addition, burn patients randomized to receive an enteral formula supplemented with 2% arginine had fewer wound infections, decreased mortality, and reduced hospital stays based on burn size compared to patients receiving a standard enteral formula.[160]

As with glutamine, the potential for improved outcomes with arginine supplementation is exciting. Routine supplementation with either enteral or parenteral arginine cannot, however, be considered the standard of practice at this time. Individual amino acids often compete with several others for shared mechanisms for absorption, transport, and renal tubular reabsorption. Providing unbalanced amounts of an individual amino acid can result in metabolic abnormalities. Arginine competes with lysine for tubular reabsorption; therefore, excess arginine administration may result in inadequate lysine retention.[161] An EEA required for protein synthesis, lysine can limit the use of other amino acids when intake is inadequate. When and how much arginine should be administered for optimal immune modulation and minimal adverse consequences must still be determined for given conditions, and patients likely to benefit versus those likely to suffer undesirable effects must be identified.

Because arginine enhances immune response, its administration could be a problem—for example, in patients receiving immunosuppressive therapy for autoimmune conditions or following organ transplant. In addition, arginine's role in enhancing replication of cancer cells and promoting septic shock is of concern.[144] Further research is needed to determine the role of arginine alone compared to combinations of immune-modulating components. Many combinations of immune-modulating components are currently available in enteral formulas supplemented with arginine, but most have not been thoroughly studied (see Table 7-7).

Nucleotides. Animal research has stimulated interest in the role of dietary nucleotides in immune response and infection, particularly in relation to neonatal/infant nutrition and supplementation of pediatric formulas with RNA and DNA. Evidence primarily from mouse studies suggests that lack of dietary nucleotides may be detrimental at any age. When challenged with either *Candida* or *Staphylococcus aureus*, animals fed a nucleotide-restricted diet showed decreased phagocytosis and reduced survival when compared with those fed a nucleotide-supplemented diet.[162,163]

Fat Components. Fat, an important dietary component, is an energy substrate and it supplies precursors to metabolically active compounds. Triglycerides, organic esters consisting of three fatty acids (FAs) attached to a glycerol backbone, are the primary form of fat.[17] The source of fat determines the specific content of FAs. Fats can even be designed in the laboratory to carry a specific FA at each of the three ester linkages to glycerol. These fats, known as structured lipids, generally contain a combination of FA molecules that are not found in nature. Different types of FAs exhibit different physiologic effects and absorption characteristics. There are several methods of classifying FAs, including the carbon chain length, the number of double bonds (i.e., degree of saturation), and the location of double bonds. When the location of the first double bond is counted from the methyl end, it is described by an omega (n) number. The numeric identification of FAs includes information for all three classification methods. Linoleic acid, for example, is identified as 18:2n-6. This indicates an 18-carbon (C18) FA containing 2 double bonds with the first being at the 6th carbon from the methyl end, or an omega-6 (n-6) FA.

Based on carbon chain length, FAs are considered short chain (SCFAs), medium chain (MCFAs), or long chain (LCFAs). The possible role of SCFAs, such as butyrate, in maintaining colonic cells was previously mentioned on page 256, under fiber. The MCFAs, a component in many enteral formulas, are most often present as medium chain triglycerides (MCTs); they may also constitute part of the FAs in structured lipids. Coconut oil is the major commercial source of MCTs; palm kernel oil also provides MCFAs. The shorter the carbon chain, the more water-miscible the FA; thus, MCFAs are less hydrophobic than LCFAs.

Absorption of MCTs is less dependent on pancreatic enzymes and bile salts than is absorption of LCFAs; thus, MCTs are used in enteral formulas to improve fat absorption. In addition, MCTs provide a readily available energy source that is an alternative to glucose in patients at risk of glucose intolerance, such as the critically ill. MCTs are generally transported via the portal system to the liver, where they undergo rapid, carnitine-independent metabolism that provides an immediate energy source. Smaller amounts of MCTs may be converted to ketones that the muscles can use for energy. In contrast, LCFAs are reesterified after absorption and are transported as chylomicrons via the lymphatic system to the thoracic duct. Thus, LCFAs are delivered to the peripheral circulation, rather than the liver, and most are stored in adipose tissue for later use. Because MCFAs are C6 to C12 FAs, they only provide about 8.3 kcal/g versus the 9 kcal/g from C14 to C22 LCFAs. Some intact protein formulas contain MCTs, most often at less than 10% of total calories, or 20% to 30% of fat calories. Many oligomeric formulas, including critical care and immune-modulating formulas, and a few polymeric formulas contain 50% or more of their fat calories as MCTs. The percent of total calories as MCTs in these formulas ranges from 7% to 23%. Formulas with 50% or more of fat calories as MCTs include: Lipisorb Liquid, NuBasic 2.0, Nutren 2.0, Nutren 1.5, IsoSource VHN, Crucial, Peptamen products, Reabilan products, Subdue, SandoSource Peptide, Impact 1.5, and Immun-Aid. Of these, NuBasics 2.0, Nutren 2.0, the Peptamen products and Impact 1.5 contain 20% to 25% of total calories as MCTs.

All nutritionally complete enteral formulas contain LCFAs, ranging from 3% to 49% of total calories. Minimum intake of LCFAs to prevent essential FA deficiency is 2% to 4% of total caloric requirements as linoleic acid (18:2n-6) and alpha-linolenic acid (18:3n-3).[17,57] The fat source influences the amount of essential FAs provided. Safflower oil contains approximately 75% of FAs as linoleic acid, while corn oil and soybean oil contain 55% and 51%, respectively.[164]

With safflower oil as the fat source, Vivonex TEN—at 3% of total calories from fat—actually provides about 2% of total calories as linoleic acid. Safflower oil and corn oil only contain trace amounts of linolenic acid and thus are often used in combination with soybean oil, in which 7% of FAs are linolenic acid.[164] Canola oil also provides reasonable amounts of linolenic acid.

Critical care and immune-modulating formulas typically contain less than 20% of total calories from LCFAs. Studies have suggested that substrate utilization in critically ill patients is 20% fat, 60% carbohydrate, and 20% protein.[165] When burn patients receive 15% of calories from fat, through either enteral or parenteral nutrition, they appear to develop pneumonia less often, heal more rapidly, and have better indices of respiratory and nutrition status than when they receive 35% of calories as fat.[166] Lower fat provision may be beneficial due to possible immunosuppressive, inflammatory, and throm-botic effects of certain ecosanoids derived from polyunsaturated FAs (PUFAs).[167,168]

The number of double bonds in LCFAs defines the degree of saturation, with polyunsaturated denoting two or more double bonds, monounsaturated indicating one double bond, and saturated denoting none. The more double bonds present, the more pliable or fluid the FA when incorporated into cell membranes, and the greater the risk of oxidation, or rancidity. A balance between intake of PUFAs and monounsaturated FAs (MUFAs) appears war-ranted for minimizing cardiovascular disease, and potentially for limiting inflammatory responses. About a third of fat intake, or 10% of total calories, from each source is recommended for healthy people.[17] The correct amount of PUFAs and MUFAs for various disease states and injuries, however, must still be determined. Common PUFA sources used in enteral formulas include plant oils that provide linoleic acid (18:2n-6), including oils from corn, soy-beans, and safflower and sunflower seeds. MUFA sources used in enteral formulas are typically high-oleic safflower oil, high-oleic sunflower oil, or canola oil. Oleic acid (18:1n-9) is abundant in nature, occurring in many fats and oils, but the high-oleic oils are selectively developed for the higher content of oleic acid, and are distinct from the "regular" version of the oil.[17,164] Canola oil contains about two-thirds MUFAs, compared to less than one-fourth in the typical plant oils from corn, soybeans, and safflower and sunflower seeds.

There are three groups of LCFAs based on the omega number: omega-9 (n-9 FA), omega-6 (n-6 FA), and omega-3 (n-3 FA). The ecosanoids produced differ among the categories of LCFAs, with n-6 FA and n-3 FA being of most interest. Common plant oils included in enteral formulas as a source of essential FAs, including those from corn, soybean, safflower, and sunflower seed, contain predominantly n-6 PUFAs. Linoleic acid (18:2n-6) is a precursor to arachidonic acid (20:4n-6), which is incorporated into tissue lipids, includ-ing those of the heart and brain, and into phospholipids of cell membranes. From the cell membranes, arachidonic acid becomes a substrate for cyclooxygenase and lipoxygenase, resulting in production of two-series prostaglan-dins and thromboxanes, and four-series leukotrienes. Many of these com-pounds have potent physiologic effects, including mediation of inflammatory responses by prostaglandin E_2 (PGE$_2$) and leukotriene B_4 (LTB$_4$), platelet aggregation by thromboxane A_2 (TXA$_2$), and vasoconstriction.[167-170] Numer-ous immunosuppressive effects of PGE$_2$ have been demonstrated in vitro.[171]

Fish oils, such as sardine and menhaden oil used in immune-modulating enteral formulas, contain eicosapentaenoic acid, or EPA (20:5n-3), and docosahexaenoic acid, or DHA (22:6n-3). Linolenic acid (18:2n-3) is a precur-sor to EPA and DHA. These n-3 FAs are incorporated into tissue lipids and cell membranes in competition with the n-6 FAs. In addition, they are com-petitive substrates with n-6 FAs for elongation enzymes, as well as cyclooxygenase and lipoxygenase, but produce three-series prostaglandins and thromboxanes, plus five-series leukotrienes. As a group, the three- and five-series compounds from n-3 FAs are less inflammatory and less thrombotic than the two- and four-series products from n-6 FAs.[144,168]

Decreased PGE_2 secretion by Kupffer cells and improved survival have been noted in animals when fish oil was incorporated into the diet before a septic challenge.[172,173] In guinea pigs fed a diet containing 100% of fat as fish oil following endotoxin challenge, however, survival was only 9% compared to 21% in animals fed a diet rich in linoleic acid (n-6 FA) and 39% in those fed a 50:50 mixture of the fats.[174] The difference in outcome between these studies suggests that responses may differ when n-3 FAs have been in the diet long enough to be incorporated into cell membranes. All commercially available enteral formulas intended as complete nutritional products provide some n-6 FAs, since these are required to prevent essential fatty acid deficiency. The optimum ratio of n-3 FAs and other FAs, including n-6 PUFAs and MUFAs, has not been determined for any disease state. Formulas containing fish oil typically exhibit an n-6 to n-3 ratio of 2:1 or less; ratios over 10:1 and as low as 2.1:1 can be found in critical care formulas without fish oil. All available immune-modulating formulas, however, contain alterations in other components as well as changes in FA ratios. The role of antioxidants in preventing oxidation of the highly unsaturated n-3 FAs, the necessary antioxidant components, the optimal supplementation schedule, and potential risks of cellular damage from oxidized FAs are unclear.

Immune-Modulating Components in Combination.   Commercially available enteral formulas classified as immune modulating typically contain alterations in multiple components, as shown in Table 7-7. The components altered and the degree of alteration, however, are not consistent from formula to formula. Arginine content of immune-modulating formulas is typically between 12.5 and 19 g/L, or about 10 to 15 g/1000 kcal, compared to under 8 g/L in most other oligomeric and polymeric formulas. As a rule, the n-6 to n-3 ratio is under 2.5:1, compared with 4:1 or higher in most other formulas.[175] Immun-Aid is a BCAA-enriched product with 36% of protein as BCAAs; Vivonex Plus and SandoSource Peptide each contain 30% of protein as BCAAs. This compares with 17% to 18% BCAAs in other arginine-supplemented formulas and under 25% for most others, including critical care formulas. The low n-6 to n-3 ratio in Immun-Aid is accomplished using canola oil in a 50:50 ratio with MCT; no fish oils are included. The combination of arginine, glutamine, and BCAA-enrichment with a low n-6 to n-3 ratio has not been adequately studied for effects on immune modulation.

Oxepa is marketed as a pulmonary formula, but is intended for immune-modulation in pulmonary disease. The fat content is much higher than is typically found in immune-modulating formulas, although the n-6 to n-3 ratio is low. Crucial and Optimental are high protein products with arginine as the only specific amino acid supplemented. Fish oil is used to achieve a low n-6 to n-3 ratio in Crucial; canola oil and structured lipids from sardine oil and MCT are used in Optimental. Fructooligosaccharides are also included in Optimental. Structured lipids from palm kernel oil (MCFAs) and sunflower oil are included in all Impact products, as are menhaden oil, dietary nucleotides, and a high protein content.

Many studies using immune-modulating enteral formulas of various composition have been published. The immune-modulating components in Impact probably represent the best-studied combination available commercially. The influence of fiber, MCT oil, and glutamine on the immune-modulating effects of the Impact formula, however, have not been well studied. Variance in the composition of immune-modulating and control formulas, differences in study design, heterogeneity in study populations, and inconsistencies in data make comparisons between studies difficult. Many studies are small, although a few have been larger. In a study of 326 intensive care patients, reductions in infections and length of stay were reported with the immune-modulating formula.[176] The differences were not significant, however, until the randomization code was broken and extensive subgroup analysis was completed.

The effect of immune-modulating formulas on multiple organ failure shows promise, but studies have been conflicting.[177] Some subgroups of patients may actually suffer more harm than good with immune-modulating formulas.[178] Because decreased mortality has not been demonstrated in any study, the efficacy of immune-modulating components remains in doubt, and their potential benefit, if any, appears to be a reduction in infections that occur several days after injury or surgery. At this time, immune-modulating formulas cannot be considered standard of care in any population and should probably be reserved for patients entering clinical trials. Nonetheless, close attention should be paid to the data accumulating on these formulas.

Modular Components

Although listed as a category of enteral formulas, modular components are not true formulas but instead are single nutrients that supplement the content of foods or enteral formulas. Modular components do not contain the appropriate micronutrients to maintain health and should never be used as the sole source of nutrition. Adding large quantities of modular components may alter the texture and viscosity of enteral formulas. It is best to select a formula that provides most of a patient's calorie and protein requirements and make small increases in a particular nutrient by adding a modular component.

Protein modulars contain 3 to 4 g of protein per tablespoon of powder. Casec, Promod, Procel, and ReSource Instant Protein Powder are intact protein powders. Elementra is a powdered peptide-based protein. Glutamine is available as an individual additive from various companies. Arginine is available as ReSource Arginaid from Novartis.

Carbohydrate modular components contain glucose polymers, as found in Polycose, or maltodextrin, as found in Moducal. These are relatively complex carbohydrate sources that mix well with formulas or food to provide calories without significantly increasing osmolality or sweetness. Additional calories can also be provided by MCT oil. Microlipid provides a source of calories from LCFAs, along with essential FAs, in an emulsified form that mixes with enteral formulas or food. Regular vegetable oils that are not emulsified mix poorly and tend to separate from the formula or food in an oily layer.

Tube Feeding Regimens

The four basic regimens for tube feeding are continuous infusion, cyclic infusion, intermittent administration, and bolus administration. The most appropriate regimen depends on such factors as site of delivery (i.e., gastric versus small bowel), anticipated duration of tube feeding, the patient's location (i.e., home, hospital, nursing home, etc.), formula characteristics, and patient tolerance. Because of limited research, prevailing practices are often minimally "evidence-based," but a few basic concepts are important to consider when selecting a feeding regimen.

Although the stomach provides a reservoir to hold large amounts of food given over a short time, the small bowel has no reservoir. The general rule, therefore, is to use continuous infusion via an enteral pump for administration into the small bowel. Over time, the small bowel may adapt to larger volumes administered over a shorter period, allowing a cyclic schedule. A pump is used so that formula is administered at a consistent rate without the fluctuations that can occur with rate controllers or gravity drip. Unless a jejunal "reservoir" has been created during placement of a surgical jejunostomy, intermittent or bolus feeding into the small bowel is not appropriate. Signs of intolerance include abdominal pain, cramping, and diarrhea. Intermittent and bolus feedings into the stomach are acceptable if the patient tolerates the schedule without nausea, vomiting, significant gastric distention, or reflux of stomach contents into the esophagus.

Patients are typically started on a continuous infusion regimen in the hospital and transitioned to another regimen if the tube feeding is to continue after hospital discharge. Small bowel feedings may be changed to a cyclic schedule for home, especially when tube feeding is supplementing inadequate oral intake or when the patient is ambulatory and will require feedings for more than a few weeks. With cyclic schedules, the prescribed volume of formula is infused by enteral pump at a set rate for a specified period under 24 hours; for example, 1440 mL/day infused at 90 mL/hour for 16 hours/day.

Gastric feedings are commonly converted from continuous infusion to intermittent or bolus feedings–usually several per day of a specified volume. For instance, 1440 mL/day can be provided as six feedings of 240 mL each. Intermittent feedings of 200 to 300 mL are typically provided over 30 to 60 minutes, while bolus feedings are administered more rapidly. The bolus rate should not exceed 60 mL/minute, but administration at 20 to 30 mL/minute is more common.[179] Signs of intolerance to the administration rate may include nausea, vomiting, gastric distention, cramping, and diarrhea. Intermittent and bolus schedules are more physiologic than continuous infusion, and are often easier to manage for patients in a nursing home or at home.

Formula characteristics may influence the feeding regimen. Osmolality, fiber content, and fat content are most likely to affect tolerance. High osmolality formulas may result in nausea, cramping, and diarrhea when fed into the distal duodenum or jejunum, since normal mechanisms of osmoregulation have been bypassed at these sites. Diluting the formula to an osmolality of approximately 300 mOsm/kg may improve tolerance in such cases, but routinely diluting hyperosmolar formulas is not recommended; nor is dilution of isotonic formulas. Initiating tube feeding with a diluted formula tends to limit the nutrition provided without significantly affecting tolerance in most patients.

Rapid administration of high osmolality formulas can result in nausea, cramping, and diarrhea, which can be addressed by increasing the administration time, improving rate control via a pump, or changing to continuous infusion. When a continuous infusion regimen is already in use, tolerance may improve by temporarily decreasing the infusion rate and then gradually increasing over a few days, changing to a calorically dense formula, or selecting a formula with different substrates, such as less fat or altered fiber content. Formulas containing fiber may be thicker than fiber-free formulas and so may need to be administered over a longer period with the aid of an enteral pump when using a small-bore feeding tube.

High fat content in enteral formulas can result in nausea, vomiting, gastric distention, abdominal pain, bloating, and diarrhea due to delayed gastric emptying and/or fat malabsorption. Formulas with a high content of LCFAs, such as the specialized pulmonary formulas, tend to delay gastric emptying. When given in large quantities, either LCFAs or MCTs can overwhelm the small bowel's hydrolytic and absorptive capacity, resulting in fat malabsorption. In such cases you can try formulas with a lower fat content or administer pancreatic enzymes, especially in patients with known pancreatic insufficiency.

Monitoring and Complications

Patients receiving EN therapy should be monitored to detect gastrointestinal, metabolic, and mechanical complications. The frequency of monitoring depends on the patient's condition and risk factors for complications, as well as how long the patient has been receiving tube feedings. Monitoring tends to be more intense initially, then decrease as tolerance to the feedings is established. Protocols and clinical pathways that help determine monitoring frequency and complexity have been published elsewhere, as have tables of complications along with probable causes and prevention or treatment strategies.[2,73,120,180-182]

Gastrointestinal Complications

The most common type of complications noted with tube feeding are gastrointestinal, which can be minimized by selecting patients carefully before starting EN therapy and placing the tube appropriately. Nausea and vomiting occur in about 20% of patients receiving tube feeding,[180] usually due to delayed gastric emptying.[181,183] The risk of these problems can be reduced by identifying patients in advance who have poor gastric emptying and subsequently placing the feeding tube into the small bowel. Medications that can contribute to slowed gastric emptying include opiates and anticholinergic medications, which slow motility throughout the GI tract.[184-186] To improve GI motility and tolerance to EN therapy you can minimize doses or change to therapeutic equivalents in another drug class. Abdominal distention, bloating, and cramping occur when formula is administered too fast, as previously discussed. Ileus and obstruction, however, can also cause these symptoms, and are a contraindication to tube feeding. Patients should be assessed for distention and bloating every few hours with continuous infusion EN therapy or before each feeding with bolus or intermittent schedules, especially those patients unable to tell you about their abdominal discomfort. GI complications involving bowel transit time, including both diarrhea and constipation, are common in patients receiving EN therapy.

Diarrhea

Causes of diarrhea in patients receiving EN therapy are often multifactorial.[180,181,187] Disease processes such as diabetes, malabsorption, pancreatic insufficiency, and GI tract inflammation, as well as enteric pathogens, formula characteristics, and patient characteristics can all be issues. In addition, medications frequently contribute to diarrhea, and should be evaluated. GI motility may be affected by direct pharmacologic actions, as occurs with metoclopramide or erythromycin,[184] or medications may cause diarrhea through indirect effects on GI flora, as occurs with broad spectrum antibiotics. The high osmolality associated with many medications, especially liquid dosage forms, contributes to diarrhea, and the sweeteners and solubilizing agents used in liquid medications tend to increase osmolality. Multiple doses of several liquid medications are often administered through a feeding tube daily, with osmolality frequently above 2000 mOsm/kg for each medication and electrolyte dose.[188,189] In addition, the cumulative daily sorbitol dose administered with medications in liquid dosage forms often exceeds cathartic doses.[184,190]

Constipation

Constipation is less common than diarrhea in patients receiving EN therapy, but can be a significant problem for some patients and is associated with two enteral formula components, fluid and fiber. Adequate fluid is important to avoid dehydration, but also to allow fiber to soften stool properly, which it does by binding water. Otherwise, constipation or fecal impaction may result. In other words, if fiber intake is excessive the usual fluids will not be able to hydrate it, but if fiber intake is too low, constipation may result from inadequate stool hydration and bulk. The minimum fluid intake generally recommended with fiber-containing formulas is 1 mL/kcal.[180] Daily weights and intake/ouput records provide an indicator of fluid status in hospitalized patients, but are less likely to be available in nonhospitalized patients—thus other methods should be used such as skin turgor or moistness of mucous membranes, especially if thirst is not a reliable indicator. Medications that decrease GI motility can contribute to constipation as well.[184] A routine bowel regimen that includes a stool softener, stimulant laxative, or cleansing enema may be appropriate if therapies contributing to constipation are required and alternatives with less effect on GI motility are not an option.

Metabolic Complications

Complications related to fluid and electrolyte imbalances, acid-base disturbances, and nutrient deficiencies or excesses are classified as metabolic. The patient's risk for these is largely determined by underlying disease state and degree of metabolic instability. To minimize complications related to fluids, electrolytes, and acid-base status, laboratory tests must be monitored frequently in unstable patients (e.g., those in intensive care or just starting EN) and fluid status must be monitored.

Selecting an enteral formula with the appropriate balance of macronutrients can reduce metabolic complications. A calorically dense formula is usually appropriate for fluid restricted patients, and one with lower-than-standard potassium, phosphorus, magnesium, and vitamin A is generally desirable for patients with renal failure. Anabolic patients, on the other hand, frequently require a high nitrogen formula with higher amounts of potassium, phosphorus, and magnesium. Patients with high sodium losses may need salt added to the enteral formula, since most formulas are designed for moderate sodium restriction. The RDIs for essential micronutrients are provided in a specified volume of enteral formula.[78-81] Because patients receiving less than the specified volume may not get adequate micronutrients to prevent vitamin and mineral deficiencies during long-term tube feeding, a vitamin-mineral supplement may be necessary. They may require additional supplementation when micronutrient losses are excessive and to correct documented micronutrient deficiencies.

Mechanical Complications

Complications associated with feeding tube placement, feeding site, and tube patency are classified as mechanical. Examples include nasal or pharyngeal irritation or necrosis, skin breakdown around feeding ostomies, pneumothorax, pneumonitis, aspiration, tube displacement, and feeding tube occlusion. Good nursing technique, such as caring for the insertion site properly, frequently assessing tube position, raising the head of the bed during gastric feedings, and adhering to flushing protocols, are critical to minimize mechanical complications.

Avoiding Occlusion

Feeding tube occlusion is a particular concern from the pharmacy standpoint, since medication administration is often via the tube. Feeding tube occlusion is associated with such factors as pump malfunction, inadequate tube flushing, high formula viscosity (as occurs with high fiber formulas), small-bore tubes, intact protein formulas, and medication administration through the tube.[191] Flushing the feeding tube every 4 to 6 hours with 20 to 30 mL of warm water during continuous infusion or before and after intermittent or bolus feedings is important to maintain tube patency.[184,192] Water, the preferred flush solution, is as effective as carbonated beverages or other fluids and is less likely to interact adversely with formula components.[192]

Declogging Tubes

Occluded feeding tubes can be difficult to salvage, but chances of restoring patency are better when the occlusion is fresh. Warm water is the first choice of fluids to use when attempting to declog a feeding tube, but if it fails, pancreatic enzymes plus sodium bicarbonate appear to be most effective in disrupting the clot.[193] Carbonated beverages are minimally effective, as are meat tenderizer and unbuffered pancreatic enzymes. Cranberry juice should not be used to irrigate or flush the tube because it may cause enteral formulas to coagulate.[192] If patency cannot be restored the feeding tube must be replaced, which, depending on the type of tube, can be difficult and expensive.

Medication Issues

Administering medication via the feeding tube can result in clogged tubes, inappropriate doses, and alteration in pharmacokinetic parameters. In addition, the enteral formula may alter bioavailability or activity of medications. Whenever possible, an administration route other than the feeding tube should be used to reduce the risk of tube occlusion. Patients may be able to take medications by mouth even when EN therapy is required to meet nutritional requirements, and sometimes rectal, sublingual, dermal (i.e., creams and ointments), and transdermal routes may be available.

If medications must be administered via the feeding tube, the enteral formula should be stopped and the feeding tube flushed with 10 to 30 mL of warm water before and after administering medication via the tube.[184] Each medication should be administered individually with at least 5 mL of water between medications. Solid dosage forms must be pulverized to a fine powder and mixed with a few mL of water, and soft gelatin capsules must be dissolved completely, before being administered through the feeding tube.

Immediate-release dosage forms must generally be used for administration via the feeding tube. Most prolonged-acting dosage forms should not be administered through a feeding tube because crushing them destroys the prolonged-action mechanism and a large dose is released immediately rather than over several hours.[194] Likewise, crushing of enteric-coated tablets is not advised when the tube tip is in the stomach because acid-labile medications may be destroyed.

Few studies have examined the effect of delivery site on pharmacokinetic parameters, including bioavailability, of medications administered through a feeding tube. Absorption may be delayed or reduced due to poor dissolution when the stomach is bypassed, and metabolism may be altered when medications are delivered to the small bowel, bypassing salivary enzymes and gastric acidity. Bypassing the stomach may result in less hydrolysis of the medication and a concomitant increase in bioavailability.

When medications' availability is affected by the presence of food, tube feedings are likely to have a similar effect, but continuous feedings may affect medications differently than intermittent feedings.[184] Some medications minimally affected by food appear to have reduced bioavailability when administered to patients receiving EN therapy. Of particular concern are phenytoin and carbamazipine, which require that the tube-fed patient's serum concentrations be monitored closely to avoid subtherapeutic levels.[184] To reduce this risk you can avoid administering enteral formula for 1–2 hours on either side of medication administration, but this is frequently ineffective.

Reversal of warfarin anticoagulation by enteral formula is a serious pharmacologic interaction that may involve two separate mechanisms. The first mechanism involves interference of vitamin K in the formula with the action of warfarin. It cannot be prevented by separating administration of warfarin and formula, but careful selection of enteral formulas and awareness of vitamin K content can reduce the risk of the interaction. Some enteral formulas contain higher amounts of vitamin K than others (see Table 7-8). Tube fed patients receiving antibiotic therapy may obtain little vitamin K from GI flora, which under normal circumstances produce a significant proportion of daily vitamin K intake. The second mechanism by which enteral formula may interfere with warfarin anticoagulation is binding of warfarin to a component of the formula, most likely to protein. To reduce this interaction, you can avoid administering enteral formula for 1–2 hours on either side of warfarin administration. Patients receiving warfarin should be monitored for adequate response to therapy, and should receive additional monitoring when an enteral formula is started or stopped.

You should assess patients' tolerance to EN therapy frequently, especially when therapy is initiated and when the patient's overall status changes. Recognizing a problem early can often avoid or minimize complications. At times, however, adequate enteral feeding may not be possible because of intolerance or a change in the functional status of the GI tract. If specialized nutrition support is appropriate but EN therapy is contraindicated or cannot supply the patient with adequate nutrition, PN is indicated. Because the GI tract should be used to the extent possible, a patient may receive both EN and PN therapy.

PARENTERAL NUTRITION

Intravenous Access

Access is essential for PN therapy and can be provided through two possible routes: peripheral and central (see Figure 7-3). Peripheral parenteral nutrition (PPN) is generally reserved for short-term therapy in patients with good fluid tolerance and low to moderate metabolic stress. Patients with poor peripheral venous access (which often includes those who are elderly, chronically ill, or receiving long-term corticosteroid therapy) are not good candidates for PPN. Vein status must be assessed by a person knowledgeable in venous access.

Compared to PN therapy delivered to the central venous system, PPN requires more volume and a higher percentage of calories as fat. Although the osmolarity of PPN is limited to minimize peripheral vein damage, administration is often hindered by vein irritation, phlebitis, and thrombophlebitis. Most patients receive PN therapy through a central venous access device (CVAD). According to infusion nursing standards, the distal tip of the catheter must be advanced to the superior vena cava to be considered central

TABLE 7-8 Vitamin K Content of Selected
Enteral Formulas

Formula (Manufacturer)	Vitamin K (mcg/1000 kcal)[a]
Pediatric Formulas	
Nutren Junior (Nestle)	30
Peptamen Junior (Nestle)	30
Compleat Pediatric (Novartis)	38
Pediasure [with or without fiber] (Ross)	38
Vivonex Pediatric (Novartis)	50
Polymeric Formulas	
NuBasics (Nestle)	37.6
NuBasics Plus (Nestle)	37.6
NuBasics VHP (Nestle)	37.6
Ensure Plus (Ross)	38
Osmolite (Ross)	41
NovaSource 2.0 (Novartis)	42
TwoCal HN (Ross)	43
Boost Plus (Mead Johnson)	45
NuBasics 2.0 (Nestle)	50
Nutren Products: 1.0, 1.5, 2.0 (Nestle)	50
Nutren 1.0 with fiber (Nestle)	50
Replete [with or without fiber] (Nestle)	50
Perative (Ross)	54
Ensure Plus HN (Ross)	57
IsoSource 1.5 (Novartis)	57
Jevity (Ross)	58
Osmolite HN (Ross)	58
Compleat (Novartis)	62.7
FiberSource HN (Novartis)	66.7
IsoSource HN (Novartis)	66.7
IsoSource Standard (Novartis)	66.7
ProBalance (Nestle)	66.7
Jevity Plus (Ross)	67
Osmolite HN Plus (Ross)	67
Ensure (Ross)	80
Carnation Instant Breakfast (Nestle) with 2% Milk	80
Ensure High Protein (Ross)	89
Carnation Instant Breakfast (Nestle) Ready to Drink	100
Carnation Instant Breakfast (Nestle) No Sugar Added Sugar with 2% Milk	105
Isocal HN (Mead Johnson)	100
Deliver 2.0 (Ross)	125
Isocal (Mead Johnson)	125
Boost (Mead Johnson)	127
Boost High Protein (Mead Johnson)	238

TABLE 7-8   Vitamin K Content of Selected
Enteral Formulas (continued)

Formula (Manufacturer)	Vitamin K (mcg/1000 kcal)[a]
Specialized Formulas	
Critical Care/Immune Modulation	
Crucial (Nestle)	50
Impact 1.5 (Novartis)	53
Impact (Novartis)	67
Impact with fiber (Novartis)	67
TraumaCal (Mead Johnson)	85
Protain XL (Mead Johnson)	120
Glucose Control	
Glytrol (Nestle)	50
Glucerna (Ross)	57
DiabetiSource (Novartis)	67
Choice dm (Mead Johnson)	120
Pulmonary Function	
Respalor (Mead Johnson)	37
NutriVent (Nestle)	50
NovaSource Pulmonary (Novartis)	57
Pulmocare (Ross)	57
Oxepa (Ross)	68
Renal Dysfunction	
Nepro (Ross)	43
Oligomeric Formulas	
Vivonex T.E.N. (Novartis)	40
Tolerex (Novartis)	44
Vivonex Plus (Novartis)	44
Peptamen VHP (Nestle)	50
Reabilan (Nestle)	50
Optimental (Ross)	85
Subdue (Mead Johnson)	85

[a] Vitamin K content of enteral formulas can change. Always confirm current vitamin K content with the product label and current manufacturer's data.

Compiled from manufacturers' information.

access; catheters with the tip short of this point are peripheral, and should be treated as such for PN therapy.[73,195] Among the types of CVADs available are peripherally inserted central catheters (PICCs), temporary internal jugular (IJ) or subclavian catheters, long-term tunneled catheters, and implanted ports.[73,196] Specific protocols for care and maintenance of the various types of CVADs are generally included in nursing policies and procedures.[196]

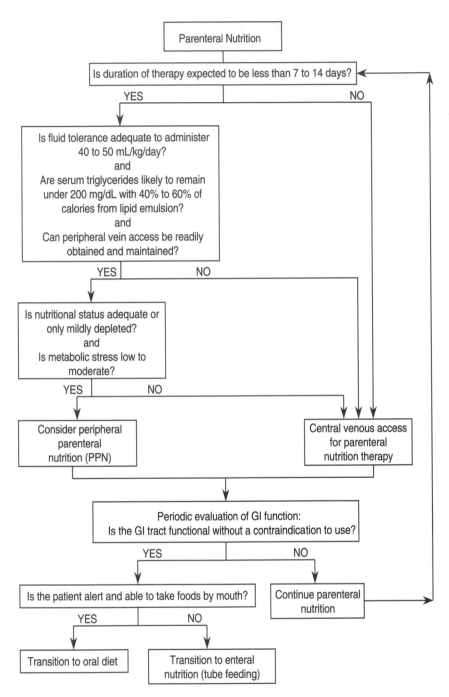

FIGURE 7-3 Parenteral Nutrition Algorithm

Components and Substrates

Because PN therapy is delivered directly into the bloodstream, aqueous or water-compatible components are required. PN formulations must be in an "elemental" form because all digestive mechanisms are bypassed. Complex carbohydrates, fiber, intact proteins, and dietary fats cannot be used.

Protein

Crystalline amino acids provide the protein, or nitrogen, source in PN formulations. As with enteral products, the protein contribution to total calories is 4 kcal/g. Standard amino acid solutions contain an amino acid profile patterned after Food and Agriculture Organization (FAO)/World Health Organization (WHO) protein standards for an optimal EEA pattern, plus additional amounts of arginine and histidine, which are conditionally essential, along with non-EAAs.[197] A listing of commercially available amino acid solutions can be found elsewhere.[198,199]

Standard amino acid solutions of the same concentration are therapeutic equivalents rather than generic equivalents. Specific amino acid content varies somewhat between products, resulting in differences in the percent of AAAs and BCAAs. In addition, chloride and acetate content differs between brands, as does the pH of products.

Specialized amino acid solutions designed for renal failure, hepatic failure, and stress or critical care are available. The rationale for each category of specialized amino acid is the same as that discussed for the enteral counterpart (see page 261).[120,136,200] Solutions for renal failure, including Aminess and NephrAmine, contain only EAAs plus histidine. Aminosyn-RF includes EAAs, histidine, and arginine. RenAmin is an EAA-enriched solution composed of 60% EAAs and 40% non-EAAs. HepatAmine is a high BCAA, low AAA solution for hepatic failure. BranchAmin, which provides only leucine, isoleucine, and valine, is designed to supplement BCAA content of standard amino acid solutions for patients with high metabolic stress. Other amino acid solutions for stress, including FreAmine-HBC and Aminosyn-HBC, are intended as the sole source of amino acids. Well designed clinical studies have failed to support a superiority of specialty amino acid solutions over standard products, so their use is usually difficult to justify given the significantly higher cost.[120,136,200] Specialized amino acid solutions available for neonates and infants, including TrophAmine and Aminosyn-PF, are patterned after amino acid blood concentrations during breastfeeding. Studies do support the use of these solutions in neonates and infants, especially when PN is expected to be more than a few days.[200,201]

Carbohydrates

Dextrose monohydrate is the major caloric source in PN formulations. In the monohydrate form, dextrose supplies only 3.4 kcal/g, as opposed to 4 kcal/g for dietary carbohydrates. Commercially available concentrations of dextrose in water range from 2.5% to 70%. Because dextrose is generally derived from hydrolysis of corn starch, patients allergic to corn may experience an allergic reaction to dextrose solutions. Other carbohydrate sources, including fructose, xylitol, sorbitol, and glycerol, have been investigated as caloric sources, but only glycerol, which provides 4.3 kcal/g, is commercially available in the United States. Glycerine, or glycerol, is used as a 3% final concentration in a premixed solution (ProcalAmine) with 3% amino acids that is intended for PPN, but it is not available commercially for compounding PN formulations. The alcohol structure of glycerine permits the premixed product to be sterilized without the browning reaction that occurs with dextrose in the presence of amino acids.

Lipid (Fat) Emulsion

The only fat sources for intravenous administration commercially available in the United States are oil-in-water emulsions of LCFAs. They can be purchased in 10%, 20%, and 30% concentrations. Fat emulsions contain egg phosphatides as the emulsifier for soybean oil (Intralipid and Lyposyn III) or soybean oil plus safflower oil (Liposyn II). Therefore, patients with a severe allergy to egg, or to soybeans or other legumes, may experience an allergic reaction to lipid emulsion.

Glycerol is added to all lipid emulsions to adjust osmolarity and to provide adequate tonicity to 10% and 20% emulsion for infusion into peripheral veins. The size of fat particles is 0.4 to 0.5 microns, or about the size of chylomicrons formed from absorbed dietary fats.[200] Lipid emulsions provide a source of essential fatty acids and calories. As with dietary fats, each gram of LCFAs provides 9 kcal; however, calories are also contributed by the glycerol. The result is that total calories in lipid emulsions, quoted on the basis of grams of fat, are 11 kcal/g for 10% emulsions and 10 kcal/g for both 20% and 30% emulsions. On a volume basis, 10% lipid emulsion provides 1.1 kcal/mL, 20% provides 2 kcal/mL, and 30% emulsion is 3 kcal/mL. Both the 10% and 20% emulsion can be administered by peripheral vein, co-infusion with the PN formulation, or admixture in the PN formulation. The 30% emulsion is only for admixture.

Micronutrients

Electrolytes, vitamins, minerals, and trace elements are included in PN formulations to provide a complete source of nutrition and to avoid potentially life-threatening imbalances or deficiencies. As a general rule, PN formulations should not be made without appropriate micronutrients. Table 7-5 includes guidelines for parenteral micronutrient requirements. The electrolyte guidelines listed are typical requirements for adults with normal organ function and no excessive losses. Acid-base status, organ function, GI losses (e.g., vomiting, nasogastric suction, diarrhea, fistulas, and ileostomy output), medications, and the patient's underlying condition influence individual requirements and may fluctuate from day to day. Managing PN therapy on a daily basis is, therefore, largely fluid and electrolyte management, rather than nutrition per se.

A thorough understanding of fluids and electrolytes is important to the clinician managing PN therapy. Discussion of such a broad topic is, however, beyond the scope of this chapter. Electrolytes for PN admixture are available as concentrated solutions containing sodium, potassium, calcium, magnesium, chloride, and acetate in varying concentrations, and as single electrolyte salts. All amino acid solutions contain chloride and acetate, some contain phosphate, and there are also solutions containing multiple electrolytes. The amount of each electrolyte added to the PN formulation should be individualized based on patient-specific requirements. Multiple electrolyte products are best suited to patients with normal organ function and serum electrolytes that are within normal limits.

Because vitamins are involved in the metabolism of all substrates and in many enzyme systems of the body, they are indispensable to multiple metabolic functions. For safe and efficacious PN therapy, a multivitamin preparation that follows AMA-NAG guidelines and FDA conditions for marketing an effective parenteral multivitamin must be provided daily. [38,82,86] Several of the vitamins in injectable multivitamin products are not available as single-entity preparations for IV administration, so appropriate supplementation cannot be achieved with single-entity vitamins, but the vitamins most likely to cause significant harm or death when omitted short-term are available as single entities. Both thiamin and folic acid deficiency have been reported during injectable multivitamin shortages, as occurred in 1988 and 1997. If supplies of injectable multivitamin are not adequate to provide a full daily dose, it is imperative that adequate thiamin and folic acid be provided to all patients to avoid serious complications and, potentially, death.[87-89,200,202-204] Ascorbic acid, vitamin B_6, niacin, riboflavin, and vitamin B_{12} are other water-soluble vitamins available as single-entity parenteral products.[200] Fat-soluble vitamins in parenteral form, although not necessarily formulated for addition to intravenous fluids or PN, include vitamins A, D, E, and K. It is not acceptable to substitute oral multivitamin products for parenteral multivitamins in patients requiring PN therapy except during parenteral vitamin shortages, and even then oral supplements should be reserved only for patients capable of adequate vitamin absorption.

Due to stability issues, vitamins should be added to the PN formulation shortly before use. Therefore, when PN therapy is administered at home, the vitamins must be added there rather than at the pharmacy when the PN admixture is compounded.[205] Both deficiency and solubility problems have been reported when multivitamins were added during batch compounding that included addition of vitamins.[91,205,206]

Trace elements, which function as cofactors in numerous enzyme systems, are required dietary components. Table 7-5 lists recommendations for parenteral trace elements, assuming normal organ function and no excessive losses. Zinc requirements increase with stress and GI losses, including diarrhea and fistula output.[207] Copper and manganese are eliminated via the biliary route and may accumulate in cholestasis.[200] Manganese may also accumulate in the brain of patients receiving long-term PN therapy, causing neurologic symptoms.[208-210] In patients with Wilson's disease, copper should, of course, be avoided. To allow the dose of each trace element to be adjusted, some patients may need to receive single-entity trace element products, especially those receiving long-term PN therapy. Multiple trace element products can be safely used in most patients receiving short-term PN therapy, with the exceptions noted above.

Administration Regimens

For adults, PN is generally initiated with partial support and increased to meet goal calories and protein within 24 hours. One of the two common methods of initiating PN therapy is to provide half the goal volume and nutrients the first day, then increase to meet goals the next day. For a goal of 100 g protein, 350 g dextrose, and 50 g fat in 2000 mL/day, the PN order the first day would be for 50 g protein, 175 g dextrose, and 25 g fat in 1000 mL to infuse over 24 hours at 42 ml/hr. This is equivalent to final concentrations of 5% amino acids, 17.5% dextrose, and 2.5% fat if mixed as a total nutrient admixture (TNA). The order for the next day would be for goal nutrients and goal volume, although the plan might be modified if the patient is hyperglycemic. Using this method, the final concentrations of macronutrients do not change day to day. The full volume and goal nutrients could also be compounded on the first day, allowing the PN rate to increase to goal more quickly. Many facilities start PN at approximately half the goal rate and increase to goal rate after 6 to 8 hours if glucose tolerance, assessed by fingerstick, is acceptable.

The second common method of initiating PN is to provide the goal volume of PN with nutrients at approximately 50% of goal for the first day. With the same goals as above, the initial order would be for 50 g protein, 175 g dextrose, and 25 g fat in 2000 mL to infuse over 24 hours at 84 mL/hr. This is equivalent to final concentrations of 2.5% amino acids, 8.75% dextrose, and 1.25% fat if mixed as a TNA, which would be outside the limits of stability. The lipid emulsion must be omitted or given as a separate infusion, at least for the first day. The order the next day would be for goal amounts of nutrients (100 g protein, 350 g dextrose, and 50 g fat) in the 2000 mL volume. You must use caution with this method because stability and compatibility of certain PN components depend on macronutrient final concentrations. As a safety measure, clinicians writing PN orders and pharmacists compounding PN should be able to calculate final concentrations of substrates. Electrolytes are generally adjusted in proportion to the macronutrients and fluid.

The PN formulation can be administered as a continuous infusion or on a cyclic schedule, but either method should use a pump to control the infusion rate. Patients are generally started on a continuous infusion and changed to a cyclic schedule if PN therapy is to continue after discharge from an acute care facility. Cyclic administration is discontinuous: infusion is on for part of a 24-hour period and off for the other part. Time on PN depends on the patient's need for time off and tolerance for higher dextrose loads and volume during the PN infusion. The main advantage of cyclic schedules is convenience for patients who are ambulatory. There may also be some benefit in terms of PN-related liver dysfunction for patients requiring long-term therapy.[201]

Complications

Metabolic Complications

Parenteral nutrition is a complex therapy that can be life-sustaining for patients with gut failure, yet can cause life-threatening complications during both short-term and long-term therapy. The major complications short-term are metabolic, including hyperglycemia, hypertriglyceridemia, and electrolyte imbalances. Daily monitoring of serum glucose, triglycerides, and electrolytes after initiating PN therapy can minimize serious metabolic complications. Fingerstick glucose tests every 6 hours may be necessary for patients with glucose abnormalities. Once patients have been stabilized, less frequent monitoring is appropriate. Glucose control may involve modifying the dextrose infusion rate, using sliding scale insulin coverage, adding insulin to the PN admixture, or administering insulin as a drip. Hypertriglyceridemia is generally managed by reducing the lipid emulsion dose and/or increasing infusion time when PN is administered over less than 24 hours. Electrolyte imbalances are managed by adjusting the electrolyte content of the PN formulation or administering separate electrolyte doses. A thorough understanding of disease states' and medications' effects and of patient-specific responses to electrolyte replacement help you determine the appropriate management method and monitoring frequency.

Venous Access-Related Complications

Intravenous access device complications are a concern during both short-term and long-term PN therapy. As previously noted, vein irritation, phlebitis, and thrombophlebitis often impede PPN administration. Infection, thrombosis, and occlusion are risks with CVADs. Infections are most often associated with the lumen of the CVAD, but may occur at the exit site, in the tunnel of long-term tunneled catheters, or in the pocket of implantable ports. The latter two sites are particularly difficult to treat, and about three-fourths of catheters must be removed.[73]

Intralumenal colonization is denoted by positive blood cultures drawn through the CVAD, but an asymptomatic patient. Catheter-related bloodstream infections, on the other hand, are indicated by signs and symptoms of infection with no other apparent cause. In addition, blood cultures drawn through the CVAD and a peripheral vein must be positive for the same organism, but with at least a five times higher count in the sample from the CVAD.[73] Positive cultures from the tip of the removed CVAD also indicate a catheter-related bloodstream infection. The patient should be treated aggressively with antibiotics or the catheter should be removed because catheter-related bloodstream infections can be life threatening. Temporary CVADs are typically removed, but catheter salvage is likely to be attempted with tunneled CVADs or implanted ports.

Factors influencing the risk of catheter-related infection include contamination during insertion, catheter materials and design, poor compliance or inappropriate techniques with catheter care protocols, and hematogenous spread from other sites of infection. For home PN patients, Staphylococcus species account for about 80% of catheter-related bloodstream infections, with an equal split between *S. epidermidis* and *S. aureus*.[73] The Centers for Disease Control and Prevention reports *S. epidermidis*, *S. aureus*, enterococci, and *Candida albicans* as the most common pathogens.[211] Maintaining aseptic technique and adhering to catheter care protocols are critical to minimize catheter-related infections.

Endothelial damage during CVAD placement initiates thrombosis at the vessel wall (mural thrombosis), while presence of the CVAD in the vessel promotes thrombosis. Fibrin deposits on the outer surface of the CVAD begin almost immediately after insertion. The fibrin forms a sheath around the CVAD that can extend beyond the tip to form a fibrin tail, which can occlude the CVAD if the fibrin tail is pulled into or over the end of the CVAD. In addition, the fibrin sheath can serve as an origination point for thrombus formation around the CVAD. This thrombus can grow and, potentially, extend to the mural thrombus, totally occluding the vessel in which the CVAD is located.

Superior vena cava syndrome refers to the signs and symptoms associated with occlusion of a major vessel emptying into the superior vena cava, such as a subclavian vein. Symptoms include swelling in the face, neck, and arm on the side of the body where the vessel occludes; pain, numbness or tingling in that arm; and chest, shoulder, and neck pain on that side of the body.[73] Tachycardia and shortness of breath may develop. Superficial collateral veins generally develop on the chest to allow limited blood flow around the occlusion. Thrombolytic therapy may be used as treatment, and anticoagulation is generally initiated to prevent extension of the thrombus.

Occlusion of the CVAD may result in loss of venous access if not recognized and treated promptly. Impending occlusion may be signaled by sluggish flow through the CVAD and pressure/occlusion alarms sounding on the pump used to administer the PN formulation.[73] No flow will occur through the CVAD if complete occlusion occurs. Most occlusions are thrombotic, with less than 10% caused by mechanical obstruction, precipitate within the CVAD, or lipid residue.[73,212,213]

The first choice of treatment for an occlusion of uncertain etiology is a thrombolytic agent, such as alteplase. Bleeding is a minimal risk with the small doses needed for CVAD clearance. Proper technique involves instilling into the CVAD a volume of thrombolytic that fills the lumen; the thrombolytic should not be infused through the CVAD into the patient. The thrombolytic instillation may be repeated once or twice if the first attempt does not clear the occlusion. If repeated thrombolytic instillation does not clear the occlusion, the thrombus is probably old or the occlusion is nonthrombotic. Temporary CVADs are often replaced if the occlusion does not clear with a thrombolytic, but for long-term CVADs, further attempts at salvage are likely.

Obvious mechanical obstructions, such as clamped or kinked administration set tubing and clogged filters, should be evaluated before ordering a thrombotic agent. Less obvious mechanical occlusions, including CVAD malposition or migration, require radiographic confirmation of CVAD position. Before further clearance attempts, the position of the CVAD should be confirmed.

Calcium phosphate precipitation can cause nonthrombotic occlusion in a CVAD used for PN infusion, especially when calcium and phosphate are maximized in the PN formulation, as is typical in PN for neonates. Instillation of 0.1 N hydrochloride acid or cysteine hydrochloride into the occluded CVAD lumen may dissolve the calcium phosphate precipitate, thereby clearing the occlusion.[73,212,213] Medications can also cause nonthrombotic CVAD occlusion. For example, 100 unit/mL heparin, which is used to maintain patency in many CVADs, is incompatible with numerous medications and can form precipitates if the CVAD is not flushed with saline or dextrose in water before medication is administered.[73,214] Reducing the pH in the CVAD lumen with 0.1 N hydrochloric acid or cysteine hydrochloride may dissolve precipitates of acidic medications, while increasing the pH with sodium bicarbonate may dissolve precipitates of basic (alkaline) medications. Occlusion secondary to lipid residue may be removed from the CVAD with 70% to 100% ethanol.[73,212,213]

Hepatic Complications

Hepatic dysfunction associated with PN therapy ranges from a mild increase in liver function tests to life-threatening hepatic failure. Hepatic steatosis is generally the first step in PN-associated hepatic dysfunction in adults; cholestasis commonly occurs in neonates and infants.[201,215] At this stage, hepatic dysfunction is generally reversible if PN therapy can be discontinued soon. When PN therapy cannot be discontinued, the dysfunction progresses to necrosis and cirrhosis in a small percentage of patients. Adults receiving short-term PN therapy are unlikely to experience anything more than minor elevations in liver function tests. Increased aminotransferases are associated with steatosis, while increased alkaline phosphatase, followed later by increased bilirubin, is associated with cholestasis.[201] Risk of hepatic dysfunction is increased in adults requiring PN therapy for months to years. Other risk factors for progression of hepatic dysfunction include infection, especially sepsis, and absence of enteral stimulation. Absence of food in the GI tract can affect GI tract motility, secretion of cholecystokinin and secretin, and integrity of intestinal mucosa, precipitating events leading to hepatic dysfunction.[201,215] Cytokines released during severe infection may contribute to hepatic dysfunction through effects on inflammation and amino acid metabolism. Duration of PN, lack of enteral stimulation, and infection are also associated with biliary sludge and gallstones in patients receiving PN therapy.

Infections, medications, the underlying disease process, the extent of malnutrition, lack of enteral stimulation, and PN therapy may all contribute to hepatic dysfunction, but because it is difficult to separate the effect of PN therapy from the other factors, the etiology of PN-associated hepatic dysfunction remains uncertain. It is likely that PN-associated hepatic dysfunction results from more than a single factor and that different factors may be involved in different patients or populations.

Amino acid composition may play a role in PN-associated hepatic dysfunction, at least in some patient populations. Because metabolic pathways involving trans-sulfuration are immature in neonates, taurine and cysteine production may be impaired.[201] This in turn, may influence the risk of cholestasis through alterations in bile acids, since taurine is required for bile acid metabolism in the neonate.[216,217] Cysteine may also be important.[218] Specialized amino acid solutions for pediatrics contain taurine, as well as other amino acid alterations, and cysteine may be added during PN compounding. Using specialized pediatric amino acid solutions appears to reduce the risk of PN-associated hepatic dysfunction in neonates and infants receiving PN therapy.[201]

Amino acids are not currently implicated in adult PN-associated hepatic dysfunction.[201] Lack of glutamine has, however, been suggested as a possible contributing factor based on rat studies.[219]

Dextrose and lipid emulsion have been suggested as factors contributing to hepatic dysfunction, as have compounds involved in lipid clearance, such as choline and L-carnitine. The diet and most enteral formulas contain choline and L-carnitine, which are not typically present in PN formulations. Thus, with long-term dependence on PN therapy, serum choline and L-carnitine concentrations decrease. Supplementation with intravenous L-carnitine was shown to improve low serum carnitine concentrations but leave steatosis unaffected in home PN patients.[220] Choline supplementation in the form of lecithin, on the other hand, was reported to decrease fatty infiltration of the liver and improve serum choline concentrations in patients with low levels receiving long-term PN therapy.[221] Studies are needed in a much larger population to confirm these results before lecithin (choline) supplementation can be routinely recommended.

Lipid emulsion itself does not appear to be responsible for fatty infiltration and hepatic dysfunction; nor does the caloric source per se, but the balance between caloric sources and administration regimen may be important.[222,223] Liver function tests were reported to be higher when patients received minimal lipid emulsion on a twice weekly schedule versus 40% of nonprotein calories as lipid daily.[224] The investigators suggested that overfeeding may contribute to increased liver function tests in patients receiving PN therapy. Others studies have reported a significant correlation between liver abnormalities and high caloric provision.[225]

Bacterial overgrowth in the GI tract has been implicated in hepatic dysfunction. Endotoxin and lithocholic acid produced by the bacteria may be transported across the GI mucosa and induce hepatic dysfunction.[226,227] Although bacterial translocation and endotoxin transport have never been proven in humans, decontaminating the GI tract does appear to be beneficial in PN-associated cholestasis.[228] Metronidazole has had some success in preventing or mitigating cholestasis in patients with bacterial overgrowth, suggesting that anaerobic bacteria may be involved.[227,229]

Other potential etiologies of PN-associated hepatic dysfunction include oxidation-induced damage and contaminants. Photo-oxidation of certain amino acids by riboflavin in the injectable multivitamin preparation may result in products that are hepatotoxic, as strongly suggested by animal studies.[201] Although clinical data are lacking, this may be a mechanism contributing to PN-associated hepatic dysfunction. The PUFAs of lipid emulsion are prone to autoxidation that results in a free-radical chain reaction and hydroperoxide formation. High concentrations of hydroperoxides in lipid emulsions are evidence of oxidation.[230] Cell membrane lipids may also be damaged by the oxidative reaction, which may contribute to cholestasis.[230,231]

Lipid emulsion contamination by plant sterols may also contribute to hepatic dysfunction. These compounds may accumulate in hepatocytes, and elevated concentrations have been reported in children with cholestasis.[232]

Aluminum is yet another contaminant in PN formulations that may result in liver damage. Although calcium and phosphate salts are significant contributors to the overall aluminum load, many products used to compound PN are contaminated with aluminum.[233-235] The greatest risk of aluminum accumulation is in neonates and patients with renal failure due to reduced elimination by the kidneys.

Patients receiving long-term PN therapy may be at risk of aluminum toxicity due to cumulative effects from continual exposure. Over time, aluminum can accumulate in the brain, bones, and liver. Neurotoxicity, encephalopathy, anemia, bone disease, and hepatic abnormalities have been reported.[236-239] Thus, aluminum may be a factor in both PN-associated metabolic bone disease and hepatic dysfunction. To limit aluminum exposure, the FDA has issued labeling requirements for aluminum content of products used in compounding PN formulations that take effect on January 26, 2003.[240,241] All large volume parenterals, such as crystalline amino acid solutions and dextrose solutions, must contain no more than 25 mcg of aluminum per liter. Small volume parenterals, such as calcium and phosphate salts, must list their aluminum content on the label. The rule states that no one should receive more than 5 mcg/kg/day of aluminum, which is considered a safe amount.[237,240]

Treatment of PN-associated hepatic dysfunction depends on the extent of damage. The best treatment—and possibly a preventive measure—is to use the GI tract to the extent possible and limit administration of PN to the lowest duration necessary. For those who must receive PN therapy for months to years, avoid overfeeding and provide a balance between dextrose and lipids. Cyclic administration of the PN formulation may also be helpful. Oral antibiotics to prevent bacterial overgrowth, phenobarbital, ursodeoxycholic acid, and cholecystokinin are other potential options in treating PN-associated hepatic dysfunction.[201] Preventing CVAD infection and treating sepsis aggressively may also be useful strategies to minimize the risk of PN-associated hepatic dysfunction.

Metabolic Bone Disease

Metabolic bone disease is a serious complication of PN therapy that can occur within a few months of initiating PN therapy. Those with malabsorption syndromes, intestinal disease, or corticosteroid therapy are at greatest risk, perhaps reflecting a pre-existing bone disease when PN therapy is initiated. Patients with PN-associated metabolic bone disease develop patchy osteomalacia and an insidious onset of pain in the long bones and weight-bearing joints.

Defective bone mineralization has been reported with PN therapy,[242] although other studies have reported decreased bone matrix formation, not a mineralization defect.[243] Excess urinary calcium loss is noted in patients with PN-associated bone disease but the etiology is uncertain,[242,243] perhaps involving a negative calcium balance or altered parathyroid hormone function. Calcium excretion may be increased by a number of factors, including excess protein intake, high sodium loads, excess fluid administration, and hyperglycemia.[244] Aluminum contamination may also increase calcium losses and play a role in bone disease. After the heavily contaminated protein hydrolysates were changed to crystalline amino acids in 1981, urinary calcium losses in patients receiving PN decreased.[245] An inverse relationship was noted between bone formation and aluminum in both plasma and bone. Excess vitamin D may alter parathyroid hormone activity, thereby altering bone formation and bone resorption.[73] Because vitamin D is required for bone formation and remodeling, the 5 mcg/day provided as a component of the daily injectable multivitamin product should be administered (see Table 7-5). To help minimize the risk of metabolic bone disease, additional vitamin D supplementation should be avoided and adequate calcium supplementation should be provided to prevent a negative calcium balance. Also, aluminum administration should be minimized.

The PN Formulation

The PN formulation, whether a traditional 2+1 formulation or TNA, is a complex admixture of components in a single container. Traditional formulations consist of dextrose, amino acids, and micronutrients in one container and lipid emulsion administered from a separate container. This dextrose-based, or 2+1, formulation is easier to prepare without automated compounding equipment and has greater stability than TNAs. The TNAs, also known as 3-in-1 or fat-based formulations, contain all components of the PN formulation, including lipid emulsion, in a single container that generally holds the volume needed for 24 hours at the prescribed infusion rate. Automated compounding equipment is most often used to prepare TNAs, as manual preparation can be tedious and inflexible. At least a moderate number of PN formulations must be prepared daily for automated compounding equipment to be economical; many health care facilities rely on the 2+1 system. An extra pump and administration set for lipid administration in the 2+1 system adds to the cost.[246] Most suppliers of home care products prepare TNAs because administration costs are lower and they are more convenient in the home setting. In addition, microbial growth occurs less readily in TNAs than in lipid emulsion alone.[247] The TNA, however, is extremely complex and requires attention to multiple pharmaceutical issues to be stable and safe.

Total Nutrient Admixtures

Lipid emulsions are inherently unstable systems in which lipid particles are dispersed in an aqueous phase. The egg yolk phospholipid emulsifier maintains particle dispersion by forming an interfacial film around each lipid particle.[184,248,249] The film serves as a mechanical barrier to particle coalescence and imparts a negative surface charge, or zeta potential, to the lipid particle. Electrostatic repulsion between the negative charges further impedes particle coalescence. Anything that disturbs the negative charge or disrupts the mechanical barrier can destabilize the lipid emulsion.

Stability of a TNA parallels that of the lipid emulsion, except the TNA destabilizes more rapidly due to the complex environment in which the admixed lipid emulsion is placed. Unstable lipid emulsions or TNAs are unsafe and may cause significant harm if administered to a patient. Enlarged lipid particles or oil droplets that form as destabilization proceeds can clog small blood vessels and pulmonary arterioles, resulting in fat emboli.[250]

Stable lipid emulsions and TNAs have a uniform white to off-white appearance throughout. Creaming is the term applied when a thin, slightly whiter, layer forms at the top of the lipid emulsion or TNA. The cream layer consists of electronically destabilized particles that maintain their individual identity and small particle size. Gentle agitation readily disperses the cream layer, which stays dispersed for at least several hours. Although creaming is the first step in destabilization, products can be safely used if the cream layer is redispersed by gentle agitation.[249]

The next step in destabilization, aggregation, is clumping of individual lipid particles. Although aggregation is not readily visible, the cream layer may be larger and may reappear more quickly than usual after gentle agitation. If the lipid particles are close together during aggregation they may coalesce, causing the number of lipid particles to decrease while their size increases. The merging of individual particles during coalescence is an irreversible process that represents the beginning of terminal destabilization. The enlarged lipid particles may float on top of the remaining TNA components, causing an opaque white upper layer with a semitransparent yellowish to gray lower layer, or a large cream layer may reappear within seconds after dispersing the cream layer by gentle agitation. At other times, coalescence is not evident until the mechanical barrier totally fails and oil droplets appear on the surface of the TNA, or as streaks through the TNA, a process known as cracking or oiling-out of the emulsion. Oil droplets do not generally appear until several hours after the TNA is compounded.

Limits of stability for TNAs may differ somewhat between brands of lipid emulsion, but a few general guidelines apply to all products. The amino acid solution used for PN compounding influences TNA stability significantly because amino acids are a major stabilizing force in TNAs. Lipid emulsions are pH sensitive, and the final pH of TNAs is very near that of the amino acid solution used for admixture.[184,248,249] Freshly manufactured lipid emulsion has a pH between 8 and 8.3, although this decreases with time.[200] At a pH of around 5 to 5.3, the egg phospholipid emulsifier begins to degrade, thereby destabilizing the emulsion or TNA.[73] Amino acids must be present in adequate quantity to provide an effective buffer. Low final amino acid concentrations in TNAs are associated with more rapid destabilization.[73,184,248,249]

Low final concentrations of dextrose and lipid emulsion in TNAs are less stable than higher concentrations. The concentration of divalent cations influences stability to a greater extent than the concentration of monovalent cations. Order of mixing, time since admixture, additive pH and electrical charge, and storage conditions are other factors influencing TNA stability. To assure stability and safety, the pharmacist responsible for PN formulations must establish limits of stability for TNA compounding based on specific manufacturer data and available published literature. Much of the data available has been generated by manufacturers using their own brand of amino acids and lipid emulsion, so amino acids and lipid emulsion from different manufacturers should not be mixed in a TNA without further study of compatibility. The same concentrations of amino acid solutions and lipid emulsions from different manufacturers are therapeutic equivalents, yet they are not generic equivalents.

Degradation of PN Components

Although TNAs have unique pharmaceutical issues related to the lipid component, they also have multiple issues in common with 2+1 formulations. For safe and effective products, both the clinician writing PN orders and the compounding pharmacist must be familiar with the pharmaceutical issues related to PN components and admixtures. Improperly prepared PN formulations have resulted in fatalities.[38] Both traditional 2+1 formulations and TNAs are subject to degradation, which may be related to physiochemical interactions among components, heat, or light.

Certain amino acids and vitamins are most susceptible to degradation. Arginine, methionine, and tryptophan are relatively unstable at room temperature after mixing with dextrose, yet they may be stable for weeks when the admixture is kept cold (4°C) and in the dark.[251] Although cold slows the reaction, some loss of tryptophan may occur in the dark through enzymatic oxidation.[201] Prolonged exposure of tryptophan to light results in photo-oxidation and development of an indigo blue coloration when riboflavin is present in the admixture.[251,252] In addition, photo-oxidation occurs with cysteine, methionine, histidine, and tyrosine.[201] Tryptophan and tyrosine form potentially toxic degradation products when irradiated with riboflavin present.[201]

Vitamin losses occur in all PN formulations from physiochemical interactions. Pyridoxine (vitamin B_6), nicotinamide, pantothenic acid, and folic acid are reported to be relatively stable in PN formulations during storage.[253,254] Cyanocobalamin (vitamin B_{12}) is essentially stable, except in strong light.[253] Riboflavin is stable when protected from light.[254] Photodegradation occurs with riboflavin, as well as vitamins A, E, and C.[205,254-256] Ultraviolet light and sunlight are primarily responsible for photodegradation, and fluorescent lighting generally has minimal effect. Eight hours of exposure to direct sunlight has resulted in complete loss of riboflavin from PN formulations, while indirect daylight resulted in 47% loss.[254,256] Vitamin A loss due primarily to photodegradation has resulted in vitamin A deficiency.[91] In this case, multivitamin for injection was added to the PN formulation when the formulation was compounded for a home PN patient, a practice now known to be inappropriate. Up to 90% of the vitamin A content can be lost within 4 hours of initiating a PN infusion exposed to daylight.[90,254] Losses of 30% to 50% for vitamin E have been reported with exposure of PN to sunlight during administration.[257] The opaque nature of TNAs provides significant protection from photodegradation for vitamins A, E, and riboflavin, but not vitamin C.[255,258] Riboflavin loss is reduced to between 10% and 20% during indirect exposure of a TNA to daylight versus 47% loss without lipid emulsion present.[254,256] Vitamin D is also protected from losses by the presence of lipid emulsion.[92,253] Thiamin is relatively stable to light; minor loss may occur to sunlight, but not to fluorescent light.[256,259]

Loss of thiamin can be substantial due to hydrolytic degradation,[255,256,259] which is most pronounced at low pH and in the presence of strong reducing substances, such as the bisulfites found in some amino acid solutions. Presence of bisulfites also increases ascorbic acid loss, but a low pH is favorable to ascorbic acid stability, as is the presence of cysteine.[256] Ascorbic acid, the least stable vitamin in solution,[254] is progressively lost over time at room temperature, with 50% loss reported within four hours, and 80% by 24 hours.[254] Loss is reduced when the PN formulation is stored in the refrigerator.[254,256] Copper accelerates loss of ascorbic acid, with up to 60% of vitamin C being lost during infusion of PN when copper is present.[84,254] Oxygen dissolved in the PN formulation during compounding and via permeation through the container appears to be responsible for vitamin C loss, making losses highly variable.[260] Oxalate is a product of vitamin C degradation, and formation of insoluble calcium oxalate has been reported in PN formulations.[206]

Fat soluble vitamins, as well as lipid emulsion, may interact with plastics (such as polyvinyl chloride [PVC] and ethylene vinyl acetate [EVA]) used in bags serving as delivery containers for PN formulations and IV administration sets. Diethylhexylphthalate (DEHP), a plasticizer and potential carcinogen used in some PVC plastics, can be extracted into the PN formulation by lipid emulsion and may adsorb fat soluble vitamins, at least vitamin A, into the plastic matrix. Therefore, non-DEHP plastics should be used with lipid emulsion and TNAs. Adsorption or sorption of vitamin A into the plastic matrix of the PN container has contributed to vitamin A deficiency when the multivitamin was added well in advance of PN infusion.[91] Up to 30% loss of retinol acetate can occur during storage in PVC containers, although loss of retinol palmitate to plastics appears to be minimal.[90,92]

To limit vitamin loss to plastics, the multivitamin should be added shortly before infusing PN formulations. Even so, vitamin A loss can be substantial during a 24-hour infusion period. In one study only 31% of the initial vitamin A concentration was present in the effluent from administration tubing when a 24-hour infusion was simulated.[92] Vitamins D and E fared somewhat better, with effluent concentrations at 68% and 64% of the initial concentrations, respectively. Based on the pattern of vitamin concentrations in the effluent over time, adsorptive loss was apparent. Vitamin K has been reported to be stable when EVA containers are used for PN.[261]

Calcium Phosphate Solubility

Calcium phosphate solubility is a major pharmaceutical issue for PN formulations. Both calcium and phosphate are necessary nutrients, but calcium readily forms insoluble salts with phosphate, oxylate, and bicarbonate. High calcium and phosphate requirements in the face of fluid restriction, common in the neonatal population, poses the greatest risk of calcium-phosphate precipitation. To avoid serious adverse effects or death, the clinician writing PN orders and the compounding pharmacist must be familiar with the factors influencing calcium-phosphate solubility.[38] Calcium phosphate is most soluble in an acidic environment where the relatively soluble (1800 mg/dL) monobasic calcium-phosphate predominates.[184] Dibasic phosphate becomes more predominate as pH increases, causing formation of insoluble (30 mg/dL) dibasic calcium phosphate. Factors associated with a favorable pH for calcium phosphate solubility include compounding PN formulations with a more acidic amino acid solution; a final amino acid concentration of at least 2%; adding cysteine to the PN formulation, using the 2+1 system rather than TNAs, and a high final concentration of dextrose.[73,184,200,254]

The concentrations of calcium and phosphate and the amount of each that has dissociated from its salt form also influence the risk of calcium phosphate precipitation. Solubility graphs showing calcium versus phosphate concentrations in relation to precipitation are available as a guide to solubility limits under various conditions.[262] The calcium phosphate product can be used as an alternative to the solubility graphs.

Because many equations can be used to calculate a calcium phosphate product, multiple products (i.e., critical values) represent the upper limit of safety for calcium and phosphate concentrations.[184] Multiple products arise because calcium and phosphate concentrations can be expressed by several different units, including mg, mEq, or millimoles (mM) of the elemental electrolyte, mg of the salt form, or mEq of the cation associated with phosphate.[184] The units used for calculating the calcium phosphate product must be properly matched with the "safe" product.

When using mM calcium/L times mM phosphate/L to calculate the solubility product, a "safe" product is considered to be 75 mM^2/L^2 or less.[263] If mEq calcium/L is used rather than mM calcium/L, 150 or less would be an equivalent "safe" product or critical value. The calcium phosphate product considered safe is also influenced by the calcium salt selected for PN compounding. Easily dissociated calcium salts have a lower "safe" calcium phosphate product than the more tightly bound calcium gluconate. Calcium chloride and calcium acetate dissociate readily, so the risk of calcium binding to phosphate and forming a precipitate is higher than for calcium gluconate.[184,254] These salts may be selected as the calcium source in PN for patients at risk of aluminum toxicity, since calcium gluconate tends to have greater aluminum contamination.[233,234] When these salts are used, you must be extremely cautious because infusing a calcium phosphate precipitate into a patient can be fatal.[38] An appropriate solubility product or graph for the more dissociated calcium salt must be used to determine the "safe" upper limit for calcium and phosphate concentrations.[184,214]

Magnesium concentration, temperature, time since admixture, rate of administration, and order of mixing also influence calcium phosphate solubility and risk of precipitation. Magnesium may reduce the risk of calcium phosphate precipitation by forming more soluble salts with phosphate, especially with increased pH.[254] Cooler temperatures lessen the risk of calcium phosphate precipitation.[184] As temperature increases, calcium dissociates from its salt, as does phosphate, resulting in more opportunities for the two to bind. Furthermore, dissociation of salts increases with time, which means that the more time elapsed since admixture, the greater the risk of calcium phosphate precipitation.[184,254]

Administering the PN formulation very slowly, as sometimes occurs with neonatal and pediatric patients, increases fluid loss through the administration tubing, which can increase calcium and phosphate concentrations to the point of precipitation. Order of mixing probably influences precipitation due to the concentration of commercial calcium salts versus the concentration of commercial phosphate salts used for PN admixture.[184] Phosphate salts are more concentrated than calcium salts and may be present in commercial amino acid solutions. Adding phosphate salts to the PN formulation first allows the concentrated phosphate to be diluted before calcium is added. If calcium is added first, precipitation may occur as the concentrated phosphate salt contacts the calcium in the PN formulation.

Admixture and Co-Infusion of Medications

Admixture with either 2+1 formulations or TNAs is generally limited to a few medications, including insulin and H^2 antagonists. Low concentration heparin (1–3 units/mL) is a routine PN additive in some health care facilities, but an interaction with calcium may occur in TNAs and with co-infused lipid emulsion.[261] Before admixing any medication with a PN formulation, you must document compatibility and stability of both the medication and PN components over the 24-hour infusion period. In addition, be sure the medication is safe and effective when administered by continuous infusion.

An alternative to admixture of medication with PN formulations is to co-infuse the medication via the same administration tubing and CVAD lumen. This is often referred to as Y-site administration when the side port of the administration tubing is used to administer the medication. Standard of practice is to dedicate the CVAD or one lumen of a multiple lumen device solely to PN. Co-infusing medications with the PN formulation should be reserved for patients in whom adequate venous access cannot be obtained and when the risks associated with co-infusion are justified.[184] Risks include infection, increased CVAD occlusion, and potential loss or altered activity of the medication or a PN component. Consult specialized references on medication compatibility before co-infusing medications with PN formulations.[214] Pay attention to the concentration of medication, PN components in the test

Overview of Key Points

❑ Nutrition assessment is used to determine nutritional status, risk of malnutrition, appropriate options for nutrition intervention, and estimated nutrient requirements.

❑ When specialized nutrition support is indicated, EN therapy is the route of choice if there are no contraindications to using the GI tract. In general, tube feeding is considered safer, more physiologic, and more cost-effective than PN therapy.

❑ The GI tract should be used to whatever extent it can be used.

❑ When EN alone cannot meet the patient's nutrient requirements, both EN and PN should be administered.

❑ Using PN as the sole source of nutrition should be reserved for patients in whom use of the GI tract is contraindicated or appropriate GI access cannot be achieved.

❑ Comprehensive literature are published periodically that summarize supporting data for when to feed, what to feed, and the most appropriate route for feeding.[4,93,106]

❑ Because patients requiring specialized nutrition support tend to be complex, it can be difficult to isolate nutrition support effects from those of the primary disease process and its therapies.

❑ Although much has been learned about specific nutrients and feeding routes, much is still unknown.

❑ Because specialized nutrition support can be both life-sustaining and life-threatening, potential benefits must always be carefully evaluated against potential harm. A team approach is encouraged to make the most of the expertise of pharmacists, nurses, dietitians, and physicians and to minimize the risk of complications.

formulation, whether data is for y-site or admixture, whether chemical stability was evaluated, and physical compatibility.

Two relatively large compatibility studies with medications and PN formulations have been reported in the past few years; one with traditional 2+1 formulations and one with TNAs.[265,266] Both focused on physical compatibility and only a few selected PN formulations were tested. You must be prepared to use professional judgment about the acceptability of co-infusing a particular medication with a particular PN formulation based on clinical and scientific data, not on convenience.

Safety Issues

Parenteral nutrition formulations are high-risk products when it comes to preparation, so a proper environment is essential to limit the risk of contamination. A class 100 environment, which limits particles of 0.5 micron or larger to less than 100 per cubic foot of air volume, is appropriate for PN compounding.[73] Quality assurance should include environmental monitoring, quality checks of automated compounding equipment, and assessment of personnel's competence in using the equipment and adhering to aseptic technique. Labels should be clear and readable because patient deaths have occurred when PN labels were misinterpreted.[38]

The ASPEN National Advisory Group on Standards and Practice Guidelines for Parenteral Nutrition published recommendations on "Safe Practices for Parenteral Nutrition Formulations" in 1998 that included labeling recommendations.[38] Because these guidelines have not been universally adopted, be cautious when interpreting PN orders from labels and evaluate the appropriateness of nutrients ordered outside of typical requirements before you start compounding. For a patient receiving 2000 mL of PN daily with 420 g dextrose, the label may be in a final concentration (21%), mL of stock solution per liter (300 mL of 70% dextrose/L or 420 mL of 50% dextrose/L), mL of stock solution per day (600 mL of 70% dextrose/day or 840 mL of 50% dextrose/day), grams dextrose per liter (210 g dextrose/L), or grams dextrose per day (420 g dextrose/day). Electrolytes may be labeled as individual electrolytes (Na^+, K^+, Cl^-, etc.) or as the salt form ($NaCl$, KCl, etc.). The units may be mEq/L, mM/L, mEq/day, or mM/day. Phosphate may be listed as mEq of the cation, either per liter or per day, or as mM phosphate per liter or per day. Occasionally components are ordered in mL/L or mL/day, a practice that is especially prone to misinterpretation.

The "Safe Practices" document recommends that labels include the amount of each component per day, or amount/kg/day for pediatric patients.[38] Brand name should also be included on the label for the amino acid solution and the lipid emulsion, since different brands are not generic equivalents and may have different solubility or compatibility profiles.

In-line filtration reduces the risk of infusing particulate matter or precipitate—a potentially life-threatening event—into patients. The "Safe Practices" document recommends use of an in-line filter during administration of all PN formulations.[38] Standard antimicrobial filters (0.2 micron) can be used for dextrose-based PN but 1.2 or 5 micron filters must be used with TNAs.

REFERENCES

1. Sanderson I, Basi SS, Deitel M. History of nutrition in surgery. In: Deitel M, ed. *Nutrition in Clinical Surgery*. 2nd ed. Baltimore: Williams & Wilkins; 1985:3-13.
2. A.S.P.E.N. Board of Directors. *Clinical Pathways and Algorithms for Delivery of Parenteral and Enteral Nutrition Support in Adults*. Silver Spring, MD: American Society for Parenteral and Enteral Nutrition; 1998.
3. American Academy of Family Physicians, the American Dietetic Association and the National Council on the Aging, Inc. *Nutrition Interventions Manual for Professionals Caring for Older Americans*. Washington, DC: The Nutrition Screening Initiative; 1992.
4. Klein S, Kinney J, Jeejeebhoy K, et al. Nutrition support in clinical practice: review of published data and recommendations for future research directions. *J Parenter Enteral Nutr.* 1997;21:133-56.
5. Institute of Medicine, Food and Nutrition Board, Standing Committee on the Scientific Evaluation of Dietary Reference Intakes. *Dietary Reference Intakes: Applications in Dietary Assessment*. Washington, DC: National Academy Press; 2001.
6. Shronts EP, Fish JA, Hammond KP. Nutrition assessment. In: Merritt RJ, ed. *The A.S.P.E.N. Nutrition Support Practice Manual*. Silver Spring, MD: American Society for Parenteral and Enteral Nutrition; 1998:1.1-1.17.

7. Charney P. Nutrition assessment in the 1990's: where are we now? *Nutr Clin Pract.* 1995;10:131-9.

8. James WPT, Ferro-Luzzi A, Waterlow JC. Definition of chronic energy deficiency in adults: report of a working party of the International Dietary Energy Consultative Group. *Eur J Clin Nutr.* 1988;42:969-81.

9. Howell WH. Anthropometry and body composition. In: Matarese LE, Gottschlich MM, eds. *Contemporary Nutrition Support Practice: A Clinical Guide.* Philadelphia: WB Saunders Company; 1998:33-46.

10. Kushner RF. Bioelectrical impedance analysis: a review of principles and applications. *J Am Coll Nutr.* 1992;11:199-209.

11. National Institutes of Health. *Bioelectrical Impedance Analysis in Body Composition Measurement.* NIH Technol Assess Statement. NIH Office of Medical Applications of Research; December 14, 1994:3-28.

12. Hammond K. The nutritional dimension of physical assessment. *Nutrition.* 1999;15:411-9.

13. Shopbell JM, Hopkins B, Shronts EP. Nutrition screening and assessment. In: Gottschlich MM, ed. *The Science and Practice of Nutrition Support: A Case-Based Core Curriculum.* Dubuque, IA: Kendall/Hunt Publishing Company; 2001:107-40.

14. Konstantinides FN. Nitrogen balance studies in clinical nutrition. *Nutr Clin Pract.* 1992;7:231-8.

15. Burge JC, Choban P, McKnight T, et al. Urinary ammonia plus urinary urea nitrogen as an estimate of total urinary nitrogen in patients receiving parenteral nutrition support. *J Parenter Enteral Nutr.* 1993;17:529-31.

16. Sargent J, Gotch F, Borah M, et al. Urea kinetics: a guide to nutritional management of renal failure. *Am J Clin Nutr.* 1978;31:1696-702.

17. Claudio VS, Lagua RT. *Nutrition and Diet Therapy Dictionary.* 3rd ed. New York: Van Norstrand Reinhold; 1991.

18. Rothschild MA, Oratz M, Schreiber SS. Albumin synthesis. *N Engl J Med.* 1972;286:748-57.

19. Igenbleek Y, Van Den Schrieck HG, De Nayer P, et al. Albumin, transferrin and the thyroxine-binding prealbumin/retinol-binding protein (TBPA-RBP) complex in assessment of malnutrition. *Clin Chim Acta.* 1975;63(1):61-7.

20. Spiekerman AM. Proteins used in nutritional assessment. *Clin Lab Med.* 1993;13:353-69.

21. Fletcher JP, Little JM, Gust PK. A comparison of serum transferrin and serum prealbumin as nutritional parameters. *J Parenter Enteral Nutr.* 1987;11:144-7.

22. Doweiko JP, Nompleggi DJ. The role of albumin in human physiology and pathophysiology. Part III: albumin and disease states. *J Parenter Enteral Nutr.* 1991;15:476-83.

23. Fleck A, Raines G, Hawker F, et al. Increased vascular permeability: a major cause of hypoalbuminemia in disease and injury. *Lancet.* 1985;325(1):781-4.

24. Reilly JJ, Hull SF, Albert N, et al. Economic impact of malnutrition: a model system for hospitalized patients. *J Parenter Enteral Nutr.* 1988;12:371-6.

25. Anderson CF, Wochos DN. The utility of serum albumin values in the nutritional assessment of hospitalized patients. *Mayo Clin Proc.* 1982;57:181-4.

26. Randle NW, Hubert-Hartmann K, Mulheran LC. Serum albumin levels: relationship to length of hospital stay. *Hosp Pharm.*1984;19:802-5.

27. Swails WS, Samour PQ, Babineau TJ, et al. A proposed revision of current ICD-9-CM malnutrition code definitions. *J Am Diet Assoc.* 1996;96:370-3.

28. Cano N, DiCostanzo-Dufebel J, Calaf R, et al. Prealbumin-retinol-binding-protein-retinol complex in hemodialysis patients. *Am J Clin Nutr.* 1988;47:664-7.

29. Hunt DR, Rowlands BJ, Johnson D. Hand grip strength: a simple prognostic indicator in surgical patients. *J Parenter Enteral Nutr.* 1985;9:701-4.

30. Kalfarentzos F, Spiliotis J, Velimezis G, et al. Comparison of forearm muscle dynamometry with nutritional prognostic index as a preoperative indicator in cancer patients. *J Parenter Enteral Nutr.* 1989;13:34-6.

31. Detsky AS, McLaughlin JR, Baker JP, et al. What is subjective global assessment of nutritional status? *J Parenter Enteral Nutr.* 1987;11:9-13.

32. Detsky AS, Baker JP, O'Rourke K, et al. Predicting nutrition-associated complications for patients undergoing gastrointestinal surgery. *J Parenter Enteral Nutr.* 1987;11:440-6.

33. Detsky AS, Mendelson RA, Baker JP, et al. The choice to treat all, some, or no patients undergoing gastrointestinal surgery with nutritional support: a decision analysis approach. *J Parenter Enteral Nutr.* 1984;8:245-53.

34. Ottery FD. Definition of standardized nutritional assessment and interventional pathways in oncology. *Nutrition.* 1996;12:S15-9.

35. Hasse J, Strong S, Gorman MA, et al. Subjective global assessment: alternative nutrition assessment technique for liver-transplant candidates. *Nutrition.* 1993;9:339-43.

36. Guigoz Y, Vellas B, Garry PJ. Assessing the nutritional status of the elderly: The Mini Nutritional Assessment as part of the geriatric evaluation. *Nutr Rev.* 1996;54:S59-65.
37. The Veteran's Affairs Total Parenteral Nutrition Cooperative Study Group. Perioperative total parenteral nutrition in surgical patients. *N Engl J Med.* 1991;325:525-32.
38. National Advisory Group on Standards and Practice Guidelines for Parenteral Nutrition, A.S.P.E.N. Board of Directors. Safe practices for parenteral nutrition formulations. *J Parenter Enteral Nutr.* 1998;22:49-66.
39. Ireton-Jones CS. Evaluation of energy expenditures in obese patients. *Nutr Clin Pract.* 1989;4:127-9.
40. Ireton-Jones CS, Francis C. Obesity: nutrition support practice and application to critical care. *Nutr Clin Pract.* 1995;10:144-9.
41. Saltzman E, Robert SB. The role of energy expenditure in energy regulation: findings from a decade of research. *Nutr Rev.* 1995;53:209-20.
42. Forbes GB, Brown MR, Welle SL, et al. Deliberate overfeeding in women and men: energy cost and composition of weight gain. *Br J Nutr.* 1986;56:1-9.
43. National Research Council. *Recommended Dietary Allowances.* 10th ed. Washington, DC: National Academy Press; 1989.
44. Young VR, Borgonha S. Adult human amino acid requirements. *Curr Opin Clin Nutr Metab Care.* 1999;2:39-45.
45. Campbell WW, Crim MC, Dallal GE, et al. Increased protein requirement in elderly people: new data and retrospective reassessments. *Am J Clin Nutr.* 1994;60:501-9.
46. Millward DJ, Fereday A, Gibson N, et al. Aging, protein requirements, and protein turnover. *Am J Clin Nutr.* 1997;66:774-86.
47. McMahon M, Miles JM. Common errors in parenteral and enteral nutrition. *Semin Gastrointest Dis.* 1993;4:127-36.
48. Shaw JHF, Wildbore M, Wolfe RR. Whole body protein kinetics in severely septic patients: the response to glucose infusion and total parenteral nutrition. *Ann Surg.* 1987;205:288-94.
49. Macias WL, Alaka KJ, Murphy MH, et al. Impact of the nutritional regimen on protein catabolism and nitrogen balance in patients with acute renal failure. *J Parenter Enteral Nutr.* 1996;20:56-62.
50. Levey AS, Adler S, Caggiula AW, et al. Effects of dietary protein restriction on the progression of advanced renal disease in the Modification of Diet in Renal Disease Study. *Am J Kidney Dis.* 1996;27:652-63.
51. McCullough AJ, Mullen KD, Tavill AS, et al. In vivo differences between the turnover rates of leucine and leucine's ketoacid in stable cirrhosis. *Gastroenterology.* 1992;103:571-8.
52. Butterworth RF. Complications of cirrhosis Part III. Hepatic encephalopathy. *J Hepatol.* 2000;32(Suppl 1):171-80.
53. Gabuzda GJ, Shear L. Metabolism of dietary protein in hepatic cirrhosis: nutritional and clinical considerations. *Am J Clin Nutr.* 1970;23:479-87.
54. Fulton S, McCullough AJ. Treatment of alcoholic hepatitis. *Clin Liver Dis.* 1998;2:799-820.
55. Garrel DR, Jobin N, De Jonge L. Should we still use the Harris and Benedict equations? *Nutr Clin Pract.* 1996;11:99-103.
56. Spady DW, Payne PR, Picou D, et al. Energy balance during recovery from malnutrition. *Am J Clin Nutr.* 1976;29:1073-88.
57. Frakenfield D. Energy and macrosubstrate requirements. In: Gottschlich MM, ed. *The Science and Practice of Nutrition Support: A Case-Based Core Curriculum.* Dubuque, IA: Kendall/Hunt Publishing Company; 2001:31-52.
58. Heshka S, Feld K, Yang MU, et al. Resting energy expenditure in the obese: a cross-validation and comparison of prediction equations. *J Am Diet Assoc.* 1993;93:1031-6.
59. Swinamer DL, Grace MG, Hamilton SM, et al. Predictive equation for assessing energy expenditure in mechanically ventilated critically ill patients. *Crit Care Med.* 1990:657-61.
60. Daly JM, Heymsfield SB, Head CA, et al. Human energy requirements: overestimation by widely used prediction equation. *Am J Clin Nutr.* 1985;42:1170-4.
61. Harris JA, Benedict FG. *Biometric Studies of Basal Metabolism in Man.* Washington, DC: Carnegie Institute of Washington; 1919. Pub No. 297.
62. Mifflin MD, St. Jeor ST, Hill LA, et al. A new predictive equation for resting energy expenditure in healthy individuals. *Am J Clin Nutr.* 1990;51:241-7.
63. Owen OE, Holup JL, D'Allessio DA, et al. A reappraisal of the caloric requirements of healthy men. *Am J Clin Nutr.* 1987;46:875-85.
64. Owen OE, Kavle E, Owen RS, et al. A reappraisal of the caloric requirements of healthy women. *Am J Clin Nutr.* 1986;44:1-19.

65. Long CL, Schaffer N, Geiger JW, et al. Metabolic response to injury and illness: estimation of energy and protein needs from indirect calorimetry and nitrogen balance. *J Parenter Enteral Nutr.* 1979;3:452-6.

66. Baker JP, Detsky AS, Stewart S, et al. Randomized trial of total parenteral nutrition in critically ill patients: metabolic effects of varying glucose lipid ratios as the energy source. *Gastroenterology.* 1984;87:53-9.

67. Hunter DC, Jaksic T, Lewis D, et al. Resting energy expenditure in the critically ill: estimations versus measurement. *Br J Surg.* 1988;75:875-8

68. Quebbeman EJ, Ausman RK, Schneider TC. A re-evaluation of energy expenditure during parenteral nutrition. *Ann Surg.* 1982;195:282-6.

69. Caldwell FT, Wallace BH, Cone JB, et al. Control of the hypermetabolic response to burn injury using environmental factors. *Ann Surg.* 1992;215:485-90.

70. Rutan TC, Herndon DN, VanOsten T, et al. Metabolic rate alterations in early excision and grafting versus conservative treatment. *J Trauma.* 1986;26:140-2.

71. Kopple J. Dietary protein and energy requirements in ESRD patients. *Am J Kidney Dis.* 1998;32:975-1045.

72. Teran JC, McCullough AJ. Nutrition in liver disease. In: Gottschlich MM, ed. *The Science and Practice of Nutrition Support: A Case-Based Core Curriculum.* Dubuque, IA: Kendall/Hunt Publishing Company; 2001:537-52.

73. Rollins CJ. Home care issues in nutrition support. In: *Pharmacotherapy Self-Assessment Program, Module 8: Gastroenterology/Nutrition.* 3rd ed. Kansas City: American College of Clinical Pharmacy; 1999:185-226.

74. Cahill GF. Starvation in man. *N Engl J Med.* 1970;282:668-75.

75. Skipper A, Millikan KW. Parenteral nutrition implementation and management. In: Merritt RJ, ed. *The A.S.P.E.N. Nutrition Support Practice Manual.* Silver Spring, MD: American Society for Parenteral and Enteral Nutrition; 1998:9.1-9.9.

76. Baumgartner TG. Parenteral macronutrition. In: Baumgartner TG, ed. *Clinical Guide to Parenteral Micronutrition.* 3rd ed. Gainesville, FL: Fujisawa USA, Inc; 1997:27-51.

77. Randall HT. Water, electrolytes and acid-base balance. In: Shils ME, Young VR, eds. *Modern Nutrition in Health and Disease.* 7th ed. Philadelphia: Lea and Febiger; 1988:108-41.

78. Institute of Medicine, Food and Nutrition Board, Standing Committee on the Scientific Evaluation of Dietary Reference Intakes. *Dietary Reference Intakes for Vitamin A, Vitamin K, Arsenic, Boron, Chromium, Copper, Iodine, Iron, Manganese, Molybdenum, Nickel, Silicon, Vanadium, and Zinc.* Washington, DC: National Academy Press; 2001.

79. Institute of Medicine, Food and Nutrition Board, Standing Committee on the Scientific Evaluation of Dietary Reference Intakes. *Dietary Reference Intakes for Calcium, Phosphorus, Magnesium, Vitamin D, and Fluoride.* Washington, DC: National Academy Press; 1999.

80. Institute of Medicine, Food and Nutrition Board, Standing Committee on the Scientific Evaluation of Dietary Reference Intakes. *Dietary Reference Intakes for Thiamin, Riboflavin, Niacin, Vitamin B_6, Folate, Vitamin B_{12}, Pantothenic acid, Biotin, and Choline.* Washington, DC: National Academy Press; 2000.

81. Institute of Medicine, Food and Nutrition Board, Standing Committee on the Scientific Evaluation of Dietary Reference Intakes. *Dietary Reference Intakes for Vitamin C, Vitamin E, Selenium, and Carotenoids.* Washington, DC: National Academy Press; 2000.

82. American Medical Association, Department of Foods and Nutrition, 1975. Multivitamin preparations for parenteral use: a statement by the nutrition advisory group. *J Parenter Enteral Nutr.* 1979;3:258-62.

83. Schiano TD, Klang MG, Quesada E, et al. Thiamin status in patients receiving long-term home parenteral nutrition. *Am J Gastroenterol.* 1996;91:2555-9.

84. Shils ME, Baker H, Frank O. Blood vitamin levels of long-term adult total parenteral nutrition patients: the efficacy of the AMA-FDA parenteral multivitamin formulation. *J Parenter Enteral Nutr.* 1985;9:179-88.

85. Greene HL, Moore MEC, Phillips B, et al. Evaluation of a pediatric multiple-vitamin preparation for total parenteral nutrition. Part II. Blood levels of vitamins A, D, and E. No 297. *Pediatrics.* 1986;77:539-47.

86. Food and Drug Administration. Parenteral multivitamin products; drugs for human use; drug efficacy study implementation; amendment, *Federal Register* 21200-1 (2000) (codified at 21 CFR § 5.7) 65(77).

87. Romanski SA, McMahon MM. Metabolic acidosis and thiamin deficiency. *Mayo Clin Proc.* 1999;74:259-63.

88. Centers for Disease Control and Prevention. Lactic acidosis traced to thiamin deficiency related to nationwide shortage of multivitamins for total parenteral nutrition: United States, 1997. *MMWR Morb Mortal Wkly Rep.* 1997;46:522-8.

89. Zak J III, Burns D, Lingenfelser T, et al. Dry beriberi: unusual complication of prolonged parenteral nutrition. *J Parenter Enteral Nutr.* 1991;15:200-1.

90. Billion-Rey F, Guillaumont M, Frederich A, et al. Stability of fat-soluble vitamin A (retinol palmitate), E (tocopherol acetate), and K_1 (phylloquinone) in total parenteral nutrition at home. *J Parenter Enteral Nutr.* 1993;17:56-60.

91. Howard L, Chu R, Feman S, et al. Vitamin A deficiency from long-term parenteral nutrition. *Ann Intern Med.* 1980;93:576-7.

92. Gillis J, Jones G, Penchary P. Delivery of vitamins A, D, and E in total parenteral nutrition solutions. *J Parenter Enteral Nutr.* 1983;7:11-4.

93. A.S.P.E.N. Board of Directors. Guidelines for the use of parenteral and enteral nutrition in adult and pediatric patients. *J Parenter Enteral Nutr.* 1993;17:SA1-52.

94. Archer SB, Burnett RJ, Fischer JE. Current uses and abuses of total parenteral nutrition. *Adv Surg.* 1996;29:165-89.

95. Buchman AL, Moukarzel AA, Bhuta S, et al. Parenteral nutrition is associated with intestinal morphologic and functional changes in humans. *J Parenter Enteral Nutr.* 1995;19:453-6.

96. Kudsk DA, Croce MA, Fabian TC, et al. Enteral versus parenteral feeding: effect on septic morbidity after blunt and penetrating abdominal trauma. *Ann Surg.* 1992;215:503-13.

97. Moore FA, Moore EE, Jones TN, et al. TEN versus TPN following major abdominal trauma: reduced septic morbidity. *J Trauma.* 1989;29:916-23.

98. Suchner U, Senftleben U, Eckart T, et al. Enteral versus parenteral nutrition: effects on gastrointestinal function and metabolism. *Nutrition.* 1996;12:13-22.

99. McClave SA, Greene LM, Snider HL, et al. Comparison of the safety of early enteral vs parenteral nutrition in mild acute pancreatitis. *J Parenter Enteral Nutr.* 1997;21:14-20.

100. Cerra FB, Benitez MR, Blackburn GL, et al. Applied nutrition in ICU patients: a consensus statement of the American College of Chest Physicians. *Chest.* 1997;111:769-78.

101. Gottschlich MM. Early and perioperative nutrition support. In: Matarese L, Gottschlich MM, eds. *Contemporary Nutrition Support Practice: A Clinicians Guide.* Philadelphia: WB Saunders Company; 1998:265-78.

102. Carr CS. Randomized trial of safety and efficacy of immediate postoperative enteral feeding in patients undergoing gastrointestinal resection. *Br Med J.* 1996;312:869-71.

103. Heyland DK. Do critically ill patients tolerate early intragastric enteral nutrition. *Clinical Intensive Care.* 1996;7:68-73.

104. Heyland DK, Konopad E, Alberda C, et al. How well do critically ill patients tolerate early, intragastric enteral feeding: results of a prospective, multicenter trial. *Nutr Clin Pract.* 1999;14:23-8.

105. McDonald WS, Sharp CW, Deitch EA. Immediate enteral feeding in burn patients is safe and effective. *Ann Surg.* 1991;213:177-83.

106. A.S.P.E.N. Board of Directors. Guidelines for the use of parenteral and enteral nutrition in adult and pediatric patients. *J Parenter Enteral Nutr.* 2002;26(Suppl):1-138.

107. Dive A, Moulan M, Jonard P, et al. Gastroduodenal motility in mechanically ventilated critically ill patients: a manometric study. *Crit Care Med.* 1994;22:441-7.

108. Lazarus BA, Murphy JB, Culpepper L. Aspiration associated with long-term gastric versus jejunal feeding: a critical analysis of the literature. *Arch Phys Med Rehabil.* 1990;71:46-53.

109. Spain DA, DeWeese C, Reynolds MA, et al. Transpyloric passage of feeding tubes in patients with head injuries does not decrease complications. *J Trauma.* 1995;39:1100-2.

110. Levy H, Esparza JE, Hartshorne M. Aspiration pneumonia rates in gastric vs jejunal feeding [abstract from Society of Critical Care Medicine 21st Educational and Scientific Symposium, San Antonio, TX; May 25-29, 1992].

111. Kirby DF, DeLegge MH, Fleming CR. American Gastroenterological Association technical review on tube feeding for enteral nutrition. *Gastroenterol.* 1995;108:1282-301.

112. American Gastroenterological Association. American Gastroenterological Association Medical Position Statement: guidelines for the use of enteral nutrition. *Gastroenterol.* 1995;108:1280-1.

113. Levy H. Nasogastric and nasoenteric feeding tubes. *Gastrointest Endosc Clin N Am.* 1998;8:529-49.

114. Methany N, Dettenmeier P, Hampton K, et al. Detection of inadvertent respiratory placement of small-bore feeding tubes: a report of 10 cases. *Heart Lung.* 1990;19:631-8.

115. DeLegge MH. Enteral access: the foundation of feeding. *J Parenter Enteral Nutr.* 2001;25:S8-13.

116. Safadi BY, Marks JM, Ponsky JL. Percutaneous endoscopic gastrostomy. *Gastrointest Endosc Clin N Am.* 1998;8:551-68.

117. Georgeson K, Owings E. Surgical and laparoscopic techniques for feeding tube placement. *Gastrointest Endosc Clin N Am.* 1998;8:581-92.

118. Shike M, Latkany L. Direct percutaneous endoscopic jejunostomy. *Gastrointest Endosc Clin N Am.* 1998;8:569-80.

119. Foutch PG. Complications of percutaneous endoscopic gastrostomy and jejunostomy: recognition, prevention, and treatment. *Gastrointest Endosc Clin N Am.* 1992; 2:231-4.

120. Rollins CJ. Adult enteral nutrition. In: Koda-Kimble MA, Young LY, eds. *Applied Therapeutics: The Clinical Use of Drugs.* 7th ed. Philadelphia: Lippincott, Williams & Wilkins; 2001:34.1-34.34.

121. Kelly DG, Fleming CR. Physiology of the gastrointestinal tract as applied to patients receiving tube enteral nutrition. In: Rombea JL, Rolandelli RH, eds. *Clinical Nutrition: Enteral and Tube Feeding.* 3rd ed. Philadelphia: WB Saunders Company; 1997:12-22.

122. Trowell H. Definitions of fibre [letter]. *Lancet.* 1974;303(1):503.

123. Slavin J. Dietary fiber. In: Matarese LE, Gottschlich MM, eds. *Contemporary Nutrition Support Practice: A Clinical Guide.* Philadelphia: WB Saunders Company; 1998:174-82.

124. Evans MA, Shronts EP. Intestinal fuels: glutamine, short chain fatty acids, and dietary fiber. *J Am Diet Assoc.* 1992;92:1239-46.

125. Slavin J. Commercially available enteral formulas with fiber and bowel function measures. *Nutr Clin Pract.* 1990;5:247-50.

126. Molis C, Fourie B, Ouarne F, et al. Digestion, excretion, and energy value of fructooligosaccharides in healthy humans. *Am J Clin Nutr.* 1996;64:324-8.

127. Saibil F. Diarrhea due to fiber overload [letter]. *N Engl J Med.* 1989;320:599.

128. Cooper SG, Tracey EJ. Small bowel obstruction caused by oat bran bezoar. *N Engl J Med.* 1989;320:1148-9.

129. Speigel JE, Rose R, Karabell P, et al. Safety and benefits of fructooligosaccharides as food ingredients. *Food Technol.* 1994;48:85-9.

130. McIvor AC, Mequid MM, Curtas S, et al. Intestinal obstruction from cecal bezoar: a complication of fiber-containing tube feedings. *Nutrition.* 1990;6:115-7.

131. Zologa GP. Physiologic effects of peptide-based enteral formulas. *Nutr Clin Pract.* 1990;5:231-4.

132. Silk DBA, Grimble GK. Relevance of physiology of nutrient absorption to formulation of enteral diets. *Nutrition.* 1992;8:1-12.

133. American Diabetes Association. Nutrition recommendations and principles for people with diabetes mellitus. *Diabetes Care.* 1995;18:16-9.

134. Peters AL, Davidson MD, Isaac RM. Lack of glucose elevation after simulated tube feeding in patients with type I diabetes. *Am J Med.* 1989;87:178-82.

135. Peters AL, Davidson MD. Effects of various enteral feeding products on postprandial blood glucose response in patients with type I diabetes. *J Parenter Enteral Nutr.* 1992;16:69-74.

136. Matarese LE. Rationale and efficacy of specialized enteral and parenteral formulas. In: Matarese LE, Gottschlich MM, eds. *Contemporary Nutrition Support Practice: A Clinical Guide.* Philadelphia: WB Saunders Company; 1998:265-78.

137. Covelli HD, Black JW, Olsen MS, et al. Respiratory failure precipitated by high carbohydrate loads. *Ann Intern Med.* 1981;95:579-81.

138. Angellillo VA, Bedi S, Durfee D, et al. Effects of low and high carbohydrate feedings in ambulatory patients with chronic obstructive pulmonary disease and chronic hypercapnia. *Ann Intern Med.* 1985;103:883-5.

139. Talpers SS, Romberger DJ, Bunce SB, et al. Nutritionally associated increased carbon dioxide production: excess total calories vs high proportion of carbohydrate calories. *Chest.* 1992;102:551-5.

140. Akrabawi SS, Mobarhan S, Stoltz RR, et al. Gastric emptying, pulmonary function, gas exchange, and respiratory quotient after feeding a moderate versus high fat enteral formula meal in chronic obstructive pulmonary disease patients. *Nutrition.* 1996;12:260-5.

141. Fischer JE, Funovics JM, Aguirre A, et al. The role of plasma amino acids in hepatic encephalopathy. *Surgery.* 1975;78:276-90.

142. Savy GK. Enteral glutamine supplementation: clinical reviews and practical guidelines. *Nutr Clin Pract.* 1997;12:259-62.

143. Swails W, Bell SJ, Borlase BC, et al. Glutamine content of whole proteins: implications for enteral formulas. *Nutr Clin Pract.* 1992;7:77-80.

144. Schloerb PR. Immune-enhancing diets: products, components, and their rationales. *J Parenter Enteral Nutr.* 2001;25:S3-7.

145. Smith RJ. Glutamine metabolism and its physiologic importance. *J Parenter Enteral Nutr.* 1990;14:S40-4.

146. Jensen GL, Miller RH, Talabiska DG, et al. A double-blind, prospective, randomized study of glutamine-enriched compared with standard peptide-based feeding in critically ill patients. *Am J Clin Nutr.* 1996;64:615-21.

147. Jones C, Palmer TE, Griffiths RD. Randomized clinical outcome study of critically ill patients given glutamine-supplemented enteral nutrition. *Nutrition.* 1999;15:108-15.

148. Houdijik AR, Rijnsburger ER, Jansen J, et al. Randomized trial of glutamine-enriched enteral nutrition on infectious morbidity in patients with multiple trauma. *Lancet.* 1998;352(2):772-6.

149. Dickson TMC, Wong RM, Negrin RS, et al. Effect of oral glutamine supplementation during bone marrow transplantation. *J Parenter Enteral Nutr.* 2000;24:61-6.

150. Schloerb PR, Skikne BS. Oral and parenteral glutamine in bone marrow transplantation: a randomized, double-blind study. *J Parenter Enteral Nutr.* 1999;23:117-22.
151. Jebb SA, Marcus R, Elia M. A pilot study of oral glutamine supplementation on patients receiving bone marrow transplantations. *Clin Nutr.* 1995;14:162-5.
152. Ziegler TR, Young LS, Benfell K, et al. Clinical and metabolic efficacy of glutamine-supplemented parenteral nutrition after bone marrow transplantation: a randomized, double-blind, controlled study. *Ann Intern Med.* 1992;116:821-8.
153. Schloerb RR, Amare M. Total parenteral nutrition with glutamine in bone marrow transplantation and other clinical applications: a randomized, double-blind study. *J Parenter Enteral Nutr.* 1993;17:407-13.
154. Ziegler TR, Benfell K, Smith RJ, et al. Safety and metabolic effects of L-glutamine administration in humans. *J Parenter Enteral Nutr.* 1990;14:S137-46.
155. Weber FL, Veach GL. The importance of small intestine in gut ammonia production in the fasting dog. *Gastroenterology.* 1979;77:235-40.
156. Tremel H, Kienle B, Weilemann LS, et al. Glutamine dipeptide supplemented TPN maintains intestinal function in the critically ill. *Gastroenterology.* 1994;107:1595-601.
157. Van der Hulst RRW, Van Kreel BK, Meyenfeldt MF, et al. Glutamine and the preservation of gut integrity. *Lancet.* 1993;341(1):1363-5.
158. Kirk SJ, Hurson M, Regan MC, et al. Arginine stimulates wound healing and immune function in elderly human beings. *Surgery.* 1993;114:155-60.
159. Daly JM, Reynolds JV, Thom A, et al. Immune and metabolic effects of arginine in surgical patient. *Ann Surg.* 1988;208:512-23.
160. Alexander JW, Gottschlich MM. Nutritional immunomodulation in burn patients. *Crit Care Med.* 1990;18:S149-53.
161. Vinnars E, Furst P, Hallgren B, et al. The nutritive value in man of non-essential amino acids infused intravenously: together with the essential ones. Individual non-essential amino acids. *Acta Anaesthesiol Scand.* 1970;14:147-72.
162. Kulkarni AD, Fanslow WC, Rudolph FB, et al. Effects of dietary nucleotides on response to bacterial infections. J *Parenter Enteral Nutr.* 1986;10:169-71.
163. Fanslow WC, Kulkarni AD, VanBuren CT, et al. Effects of nucleotide restriction and supplementation on resistance to experimental murine candidiasis. *J Parenter Enteral Nutr.* 1988;12:49-52.
164. Jones JH, Kubow S. Lipids, sterols, and their metabolites. In: Shil ME, Olson JA, Shike M, et al., eds. *Modern Nutrition in Health and Disease.* 9th ed. Philadelphia: Lea and Febiger; 1999:67-94.
165. Long CL, Nelson KM, Akin JM Jr, et al. A physiologic basis for the provision of fuel mixtures in normal and stressed patients. *J Trauma.* 1990;30:1077-86.
166. Garrel DR, Razi M, Lariviere F, et al. Improved clinical status and length of care with low-fat nutrition support in burn patients. *J Parenter Enteral Nutr.* 1995;19:482-91.
167. Furst P. Old and new substrates in clinical nutrition. *J Nutr.* 1998;128:787-96.
168. Ulrich H, Pastores SM, Katz DP, et al. Parenteral use of medium-chain triglycerides: a reappraisal. *Nutrition.* 1996;12:231-8.
169. Gottschlich MM. Selection of optimal lipid sources in enteral and parenteral nutrition. *Nutr Clin Pract.* 1992;7:152-65.
170. Kinsella JE, Lokesh B. Dietary lipids, eicosanoids, and the immune system. *Crit Care Med.* 1990;18:S94-113.
171. Ayala A, Chaudry IH. Dietary n-3 polyunsaturated fatty acid modulation of immune cell function before and after trauma. *Nutrition.* 1995;11:1-11.
172. Barton RG, Wells CL, Carlson A, et al. Dietary omega-3 fatty acids decrease mortality and Kupffer cell prostaglandin E2 production in a rat model of chronic sepsis. *J Trauma.* 1991;31:768-74.
173. Johnson JA, Griswold JA, Muakkassa FF. Essential fatty acids influence survival in sepsis. *J Trauma.* 1993;35:128-31.
174. Peck MD, Ogle CK, Alexander JW. Composition of fat in enteral diets can influence outcome in experimental peritonitis. *Ann Surg.* 1991;214:74-82.
175. Cresci GA. Special appendix: immune enhancing formula product comparison. *J Parenter Enteral Nutr.* 2001;25:S63.
176. Bower RH, Cerra FB, Bershadky B, et al. Early enteral administration of a formula (Impact) supplemented with arginine, nucleotides, and fish oil in intensive care unit patients: results of a multicenter, prospective, randomized, clinical trial. *Crit Care Med.* 1995;23:436-49.
177. Moore FA. Effects of immune-enhancing diets on infectious morbidity and multiple organ failure. *J Parenter Enteral Nutr.* 2001;25:S36-43.
178. Heyland DK, Novak F. Immunonutrition in the critically ill patient: more harm than good? *J Parenter Enteral Nutr.* 2001;25:S51-6.

179. Lord L, Trumbore L, Zologa G. Enteral nutrition implementation and management. In: Merritt RJ, ed. *The A.S.P.E.N. Nutrition Support Practice Manual.* Silver Spring, MD: American Society for Parenteral and Enteral Nutrition; 1998:5.1-5.16.

180. Russell M, Cromes M, Grant J. Complications of enteral nutrition therapy. In: Gottschlich MM, ed. *The Science and Practice of Nutrition Support: A Case-Based Core Curriculum.* Dubuque, IA: Kendall/Hunt Publishing Company; 2001:189-209.

181. Beyer PL. Complications of enteral nutrition. In: Matarese LE, Gottschlich MM, eds. *Contemporary Nutrition Support Practice: A Clinical Guide.* Philadelphia: WB Saunders Company; 1998:216-26.

182. Main BJ, Morrison DL. Development of a clinical pathway for enteral nutrition. *Nutr Clin Pract.* 1998;13:20-4.

183. Hammaoui E., Kodsi R. Complications of enteral feeding and their prevention. In: Rombeau JL, Rolandelli RH, eds. *Clinical Nutrition: Enteral and Tube Feeding.* 3rd ed. Philadelphia: WB Saunders Company; 1997:554-74.

184. Rollins CJ. General pharmacologic issues. In: Matarese LE, Gottschlich MM, eds. *Contemporary Nutrition Support Practice: A Clinical Guide.* Philadelphia: WB Saunders Company; 1998:303-24.

185. Orlando R. Gastrointestinal motility and tube feeding. *Crit Care Med.* 1998;26:1472.

186. Bosschak K, Nieuwenhuijs VB, Vos A, et al. Gastrointestinal motility and gastric tube feeding in mechanically ventilated patients. *Crit Care Med.* 1998;26:1510-7.

187. Williams MS, Harper R, Magnuson B, et al. Diarrhea management in enterally fed patients. *Nutr Clin Pract.* 1998;13:225-9.

188. Dickerson RN, Melnick G. Osmolality of oral drug solutions and suspensions. *Am J Hosp Pharm.* 1988;45:832-4.

189. Niemec PW, Vanderveen TW, Morrison JL, et al. Gastrointestinal disorders caused by medication and electrolyte solution osmolality during enteral nutrition. *J Parenter Enteral Nutr.* 1983;7:387-9.

190. Johnston KR, Govel LA, Andritz MH. Gastrointestinal effects of sorbitol as an additive in liquid medications. *Am J Med.* 1994;97:185-91.

191. Hofstetter J, Allen L. Causes of nonmedication-induced nasogastric tube occlusion. *Am J Hosp Pharm.* 1992;49:603-7.

192. Metheny N, Eisenberg P, McSweeney M. Effect of feeding tube properties and three irrigants on clogging rates. *Nurs Res.* 1988;37:165-9.

193. Marcuard S, Stegall K, Trogden S. Clearing obstructed feeding tubes. *J Parenter Enteral Nutr.* 1989;13:81-3.

194. Mitchell JF. Oral dosage forms that should not be crushed: 2000 update. *Hosp Pharm.* 2000;35:553-67.

195. Intravenous Nurses Society. Intravenous nursing standards of practice [revised 1998]. *J Intravenous Nurs.* 1998;21:S1-91.

196. Krzywda EA, Edmiston CE Jr. Parenteral access and equipment. In: Merritt RJ, ed. *The A.S.P.E.N. Nutrition Support Practice Manual.* Silver Spring, MD: American Society for Parenteral and Enteral Nutrition; 1998:7.1-7.10.

197. Joint Food and Agriculture Organization (FAO)/World Health Organization (WHO) Expert Group. *Protein requirements: report of a joint FAO/WHO Expert Group.* WHO Tech Report; 1965. Ser No. 301.

198. *American Hospital Formulary Service Drug Information.* Bethesda: American Society of Health-System Pharmacists; 2001.

199. Nutritional Products. In: Short RM, ed. *Drug Facts and Comparisons.* St. Louis: A Wolters Kluwer Company; 2001:1-132.

200. Mirtallo JM. Parenteral formulas. In: Rombeau JL, Rolandelli RH, eds. *Clinical Nutrition: Parenteral Nutrition.* 3rd ed. Philadelphia: WB Saunders Company; 2001:118-39.

201. Shattuck KE, Klein GL. Hepatobiliary complications of parenteral nutrition. In: Rombeau JL, Rolandelli RH, eds. *Clinical Nutrition: Parenteral Nutrition.* 3rd ed. Philadelphia: WB Saunders Company; 2001:140-56.

202. Anonymous. Death associated with thiamine deficient total parenteral nutrition. *MMWR Morb Mortal Wkly Rep.* 1987;38:38-43.

203. Alliou M, Ehrinpreis MN. Shortage of intravenous multivitamin solution in the United States [letter]. *N Engl J Med.* 1997;337:54-5.

204. American Society for Parenteral and Enteral Nutrition. IV multivitamin shortage - update 23, March 20, 1998. Management of chronic shortage of IV multivitamins. Available at: http://www.clinnutr.org/mvi.htm. Accessed January 2001.

205. Rollins CJ. Home care issues with multivitamin therapy. *Nutr Clin Pract.* 2001;16:512-6.

206. Gupta DV. Stability of vitamins in total parenteral nutrient solutions. *Am J Hosp Pharm.* 1986;43:2132.

207. Solomons NW. Zinc. In: Baumgartner TG, ed. *Clinical Guide to Parenteral Micronutrition.* 3rd ed. Gainesville, FL: Fujisawa USA Inc; 1997:293-309.

208. Ono J, Harada K, Kodaka R, et al. Manganese deposition in the brain during long-term total parenteral nutrition. *J Parenter Enteral Nutr.* 1995;19:310-2.

209. Reynolds AP, Kiely E, Meadows N. Manganese in long term paediatric parenteral nutrition. *Arch Dis Child.* 1994;71:527-8.

210. Fredstrom S, Rogosheske J, Gupta P, et al. Extrapyramidal symptoms in a BMT recipient with hyperintense basal ganglia and elevated manganese. *Bone Marrow Transplant.* 1995;15:989-92.

211. Centers for Disease Control, Hospital Infection Control Practice Advisory Committee. Guidelines for the prevention of intravascular device-related infection. *Infect Control Hosp Epidemiol.* 1996;17:438-73.

212. Herbst SL, Kaplan LK, McKinnon BT. Vascular access devices: managing occlusions and related complications in home infusion [monograph]. *Infusion.* 1998; Vol 4.

213. Thompson B, Veal D. Pharmacologic treatment of pediatric catheter occlusions. *Hosp Pharm.* 1992;27:137-41.

214. Trissel LA. *Handbook on Injectable Drugs.* 10th ed. Bethesda: American Society of Health-System Pharmacists Inc; 1999.

215. Quigley EMM, Marsh MN, Shaffer JL, et al. Hepatobiliary complications of total parenteral nutrition. *Gastroenterology.* 1993;104:286-301.

216. Lester R. Bile acid metabolism in the newborn. *J Pediatr Gastroenterol Nutr.* 1983;2:335-6.

217. Drongowski RA, Coran AG. An analysis of factors contributing to the development of total parenteral nutrition-induced cholestasis. *J Parenter Enteral Nutr.* 1989;13:586-9.

218. Sturman JA, Gaull G, Raiha NC. Absence of cystathionase in human fetal liver: is cysteine essential? *Science.* 1970;169:74-6.

219. Li S, Nussbaum MS, McFadden DW, et al. Addition of L-glutamine to total parenteral nutrition and its effects on portal insulin and glucagon and the development of hepatic steatosis in rats. *J Surg Res.* 1990;48:421-6.

220. Bowyer BA, Miles JM, Haymond MW, et al. L-carnitine therapy in home parenteral nutrition patients with abnormal liver tests and low plasma carnitine concentrations. *Gastroenterology.* 1988;94:434-8.

221. Buchman AL, Dubin M, Jenden D, et al. Lecithin increases plasma free choline and decreases hepatic steatosis in long-term total parenteral nutrition patients. *Gastroenterology.* 1992;102:1363-70.

222. Moss RL, Das JB, Raffensperger JG. Total parenteral nutrition associated cholestasis: clinical and histopathologic correlation. *J Pediatr Surg.* 1993;28:1270-5.

223. Wagner WH, Lowry AC, Silberman H. Similar liver function abnormalities occur in patients receiving glucose-based and lipid-based parenteral nutrition. *Am J Gastroenterol.* 1983;78:199-202.

224. Buchmiller CE, Kleiman-Wexler RL, Ephgrave KS, et al. Liver dysfunction and energy source: results of a randomized clinical trial. *J Parenter Enteral Nutr.* 1993;17:301-6.

225. Lowry SF, Brennan MF. Abnormal liver function during parenteral nutrition: relation to infusion excess. *J Surg Res.* 1979;26:300-7.

226. Fouin-Fortunet H, Quernec LL, Erlinger S, et al. Hepatic alterations during parenteral nutrition in patients with inflammatory bowel disease: a possible consequence of lithocholate toxicity. *Gastroenterology.* 1982;82.932-7.

227. Freund HR, Muggia-Sullam M, LaFrance R, et al. A possible beneficial effect of metronidazole in reducing TPN-associated liver function derangements. *J Surg Res.* 1985;38:356-63.

228. Lipman TO. Bacterial translocation and enteral nutrition in humans: an outsider looks in. *J Parenter Enteral Nutr.* 1995;19:156-65.

229. Capron JP, Gineston JL, Herve MA, et al. Metronidazole in prevention of cholestasis associated with total parenteral nutrition. *Lancet.* 1983; 321(1):446-7.

230. Pitkanen O, Hallman M, Andersson S. Generation of free radicals in lipid emulsion used in parenteral nutrition. *Pediatr Res.* 1991;29:56-9.

231. Wispe JR, Bell EF, Roberts RJ. Assessment of lipid peroxidation in newborn infants and rabbits by measurement of expired ethane and pentane: influence of parenteral lipid infusion. *Pediatr Res.* 1985;19:374-9.

232. Clayton PT, Bowron A, Mills KA, et al. Phytoesterolemia in children with parenteral nutrition-associated cholestatic liver disease. *Gastroenterology.* 1993;105:1806-13.

233. Popinskak K, Kierkus J, Lyszkowska M, et al. Aluminum contamination of parenteral nutrition additives, amino acids solutions, and lipid emulsion. *Nutrition.* 1999;15:683-6.

234. Koo WWK, Kaplan LA, Horn J, et al. Aluminum in parenteral nutrition solutions: sources and possible alternatives. *J Parenter Enteral Nutr.* 1986;10:591-5.

235. Klein GL. Aluminum in parenteral solutions revisited: again. *Am J Clin Nutr.* 1995;61:449-56.

236. Committee on Nutrition, American Academy of Pediatrics. Aluminum toxicity in children. *Pediatrics.* 1996;97:413-6.

237. Bishop NJ, Morley R, Chir B, et al. Aluminum neurotoxicity in preterm infants receiving intravenous feeding solutions. *N Engl J Med.* 1997;336:1557-61.

238. Milliner DS, Shinaberger JH, Shuman P, et al. Inadvertent aluminum administration during plasma exchange due to aluminum contamination of albumin-replacement solutions. *N Engl J Med.* 1985;312:165-7.

239. Sedman AB, Klein GL, Merritt RJ, et al. Evidence of aluminum loading in infants receiving intravenous therapy. *N Engl J Med.* 1985;312:1337-43.

240. Department of Health and Human Services, Food and Drug Administration. Aluminum in large and small volume parenterals used in total parenteral nutrition. 65(17) *Federal Register* 4103-11 (2000). 21 CFR 201.323.

241. Department of Health and Human Services, Food and Drug Administration. Aluminum in large and small volume parenterals used in total parenteral nutrition; delay of effective date. 66(18) *Federal Register* 7864-5 (2001). 21 CFR 201 Docket No. 90N-0056, FR DOC 01-2125.

242. Klein GL, Ament ME, Bluestone R, et al. Bone disease associated with total perenteral nutrition. *Lancet.* 1980; 316(2):1041-4.

243. Shike M, Shils ME, Heller A, et al. Bone disease in prolonged parenteral nutrition: osteopenia without mineralization defect. *Am J Clin Nutr.* 1986;44:89-98.

244. Koo WWK. Parenteral nutrition-related bone disease. *J Parenter Enteral Nutr.* 1992;16:386-94.

245. Vargas JH, Klein GL, Ament ME, et al. Metabolic bone disease of total parenteral nutrition: course after changing from casein to amino acids in parenteral solutions with reduced aluminum content. *Am J Clin Nutr.* 1988;48:1070-8.

246. Rollins CJ, Elsberry VA, Pollack KA, et al. Three-in-one parenteral nutrition: a safe and economical method of nutritional support for infants. *J Parenter Enteral Nutr.* 1990;14:290-4.

247. Gilbert M, Gallagher C, Eads M, et al. Microbial growth patterns in a total parenteral nutrition formulation containing lipid emulsion. *J Parenter Enteral Nutr.* 1986;10:494-7.

248. Rollins CJ. Total nutrient admixtures: stability issues and their impact on nursing practice. *J Intravenous Nurs.* 1997;20:297-304.

249. Driscoll DF. Total nutrient admixtures: theory and practice. *Nutr Clin Pract.* 1995;10:114-9.

250. Atik M, Marrero R, Isla F, Manale B. Hemodynamic changes following infusion of intravenous fat emulsions. *Am J Clin Nutr.* 1965;16:68-74.

251. Jurgens RW, Henry RS, Welco A. Amino acid stability in a mixed parenteral nutrition solution. *Am J Hosp Pharm.* 1981;38:1358-9.

252. Kanner JD, Fennema OJ. Photo-oxidation of tryptophan in the presence of riboflavin. *J Agric Food Chem.* 1987;35:71-6.

253. Dahl GB, Jeppson RI, Tengborn HJ. Vitamin stability in a TPN mixture stored in an EVA plastic bag. *J Clin Hosp Pharm.* 1986;11:271-9.

254. Allwood MC, Kearney MCJ. Compatibility and stability of additives in parenteral nutrition admixtures. *Nutrition.* 1998;14:697-706.

255. Smith JH, Canham JE, Wells PA. Effect of phototherapy light, sodium bisulfite, and pH on vitamin stability in total parenteral nutrition admixtures. *J Parenter Enteral Nutr.* 1988;12:394-402.

256. Smith JL, Canham JE, Kirland WD, et al. Effect of Intralipid, amino acids, container, temperature and duration of storage on vitamin stability in total parenteral nutrition admixtures. *J Parenter Enteral Nutr.* 1988; 12:478-83.

257. McGee CD, Mascarwanhas MG, Ostro MJM, et al. Selenium and vitamin E stability in parenteral solutions. *J Parenter Enteral Nutr.* 1985; 5:568-70.

258. Dahl GB, Svensson L, Kennander NJG, et al. Stability of vitamins in soybean oil fat emulsion under conditions simulating intravenous feeding of neonates and children. *J Parenter Enteral Nutr.* 1994;18:234-9.

259. Kearney MCJ, Allwood MC, Hardy G. The stability of thiamine in TPN mixtures stored in EVA and multilayer bags. *Clin Nutr.* 1995;14:295-301.

260. Proot P, DePoureq L, Raymakers AA. Stability of ascorbic acid in a standard total parenteral nutrition mixture. *Clin Nutr.* 1994;13:273-9.

261. Schmutz CW, Martinelli E, Muhlebach S. Stability of vitamin K assessed by HPLC in total parenteral nutrition. *Clin Nutr.* 1992;12:S169.

262. Trissel LA. *Trissel's Calcium and Phosphate Compatibility in Parenteral Nutrition.* Houston, TX: TriPharma; 2001.

263. Baumgartner TG. Calcium. In: Baumgartner TG, ed. *Clinical Guide to Parenteral Micronutrition.* 3rd ed. Gainesville, FL: Fujisawa USA Inc; 1997:109-55.

264. Raupp P, von Kries R, Schmidt E, et al. Incompatibility between fat emulsion and calcium plus heparin in parenteral nutrition of premature babies [letter]. *Lancet.* 1988; 332(2):700.

265. Trissel LA, Gilbert JF, Martinez MB, et al. Compatibility of parenteral nutrient solutions with selected drugs during simulated Y-site administration. *Am J Hosp Pharm.* 1997;54:1295-300.

266. Trissel LA, Gilbert JF, Martinez MB, et al. Compatibility of medications with 3-in-1 parenteral nutrition admixtures. *J Parenter Enteral Nutr.* 1999;23:67-74.

CHAPTER **8**

ENERGY BALANCE AND WEIGHT CONTROL

Sarah J. Miller

More people in the United States are overweight than ever before, and obesity is increasing worldwide. The Behavioral Risk Factor Surveillance System (BRFSS), a telephone survey conducted in 2000 by state health departments, estimated that about 31% of men and 45% of women were attempting to lose weight.[1] People often set unrealistic weight loss goals that result in disappointment and feelings of failure, although even modest weight losses have been shown to benefit health.

Billions of dollars are spent annually in the United States on weight loss products and services, and advertising is often deceptive and misleading. The pharmacist can serve as a knowledgeable and accessible source of information to the patient seeking advice on weight loss.

In 1997, the Federal Trade Commission put together a multidisciplinary panel to formulate voluntary guidelines for providers of weight loss programs. This panel formed the Partnership for Healthy Weight Management (PHWM), which includes representatives from science, health care, government, and the commercial industry. The PHWM lists as its mission "to promote sound guidance on strategies for achieving and maintaining a healthy weight."[2] Guidelines promulgated by this group can be useful to the consumer in choosing a weight management program.

DEFINITIONS OF OVERWEIGHT AND OBESITY

Historically in the United States, weight-for-height tables such as the Metropolitan Life Insurance Company tables have defined normal weight ranges. Tables of this type have limitations such as use of unvalidated estimates of body frame size, lack of ethnic diversity in derivation of the tables, and derivation from mortality data alone.[3]

In 1998, the National Heart, Lung, and Blood Institute (NHLBI) of the National Institutes of Health published clinical guidelines on the identification, evaluation, and treatment of overweight and obesity in adults.[4] These guidelines have become a standard for health care workers dealing with people desiring to lose weight, despite criticisms that they stigmatize too many people as being overweight and ignore the serious health risks associated with low weight.[5]

The guidelines define overweight and obesity in terms of the Quetelet index or body mass index (BMI), which is calculated by taking a person's weight in kilograms and dividing by his or her height in meters squared. Overweight is defined as a BMI between 25.0 and 29.9 kg/m², and obesity is defined as a BMI of 30.0 or more. These cutoffs were chosen based on epidemiological data showing an increase in mortality in patients with a BMI over 25 kg/m², and especially with a BMI above 30 kg/m². The American Heart Association (AHA) and the World Health Organization (WHO) have adopted the same BMI breakpoints for defining overweight and obesity.[6,7]

Another method used to assess overweight and obesity involves waist and hip measurements. People with excess fat stores in the abdomen have a greater risk of chronic diseases, especially cardiovascular disease, compared to those who have excess fat stores in the hips.[8] Those with excess intraabdominal fat are said to have an "apple-shaped" or android body type, while people with excess fat in the hips have a "pear-shaped" or gynecoid body type. Men tend to exhibit the android body type and women tend to exhibit the gynecoid body type.

The *Practical Guide to Identification, Evaluation, and Treatment of Overweight and Obesity in Adults*, a 2000 publication of the NHLBI and the North American Association for the Study of Obesity (NAASO), says men with a waist circumference greater than 40 inches (102 cm) and women whose waist size is greater than 35 inches (89 cm) who also have BMIs of 25 to 34.9 are at risk for type 2 diabetes, dyslipidemia, hypertension, and cardiovascular disease.[8] A limitation of the BMI is that it does not take into account where a person's body fat is primarily distributed.[3]

EPIDEMIOLOGY OF OVERWEIGHT AND OBESITY

Increasing rates of overweight and obesity, with their attendant health risks and costs, are a problem around the world. The WHO estimates that there were about 200 million obese adults worldwide in 1995 and that this number increased to over 300 million by the year 2000.[9]

The problem is not restricted to industrialized nations. In the mid 1990s, the WHO estimated that 10% to 25% of adults in most western European countries and 20% to 25% in some of the American countries are obese.[7] The highest rates of obesity in the world are found in Micronesia, where up to 70% of women and 65% of men are obese. The WHO ascribes this obesity epidemic to sedentary lifestyles and high-fat, energy-dense diets.

In the United States, data on the prevalence of overweight and obesity come from the National Health Examination Survey (NHES - 1960–62), the National Health and Nutrition Examination Surveys (NHANES I, II, and III – 1971–74, 1976–80, and 1988–94) and the BRFSS.[4,10] Whereas incidence of overweight has stayed fairly constant in both men and women in the data (38% to 41% of men and 24% to 25% of women), the prevalence of obesity

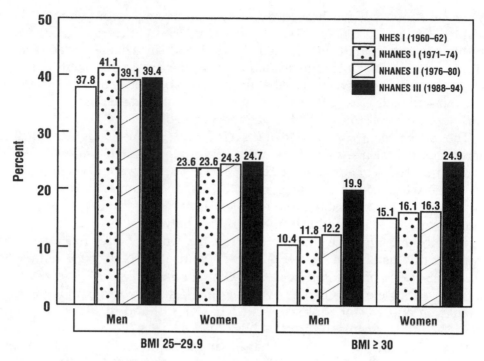

FIGURE 8-1 Age-Adjusted Prevalence of Overweight and Obesity*

* Overweight is a body mass index (BMI) of 25 to 29.9; obesity is BMI ≥ 30.
NHES = National Health Examination Survey.
NHANES = National Health and Nutrition Examination Surveys.
Source: Brown CD, Higgins M, Donato KA, et al. Body mass index and the prevalence of hypertension and dyslipidemia. *Obes Res.* 2000;8:605-19. Reprinted with permission.

increased sharply from NHANES II to NHANES III in both sexes.[4] See Figure 8-1 for a graphic representation of these data from the National Center for Health Statistics, which was included in the NHLBI guidelines.[4] Preliminary data from a 1999 NHANES study show that these trends are continuing, with 26% of Americans being classified as obese as compared to 23% in NHANES III.

The Centers for Disease Control and Prevention has noted that median energy intake (calories consumed) for adults increased from NHANES II to NHANES III, while participation in leisure-time physical activity from the mid-1980s to early 1990s remained fairly stable.[11] Data from the BRFSS showed that leisure-time physical activity also remained relatively unchanged during the period 1990 to 1998. Only about 1/4 of U.S. adults meet the levels of physical activity recommended by the NHLBI guidelines.[12] Decreased energy expenditure in activities such as walking for transportation and less automated household work, as well as increasing time spent watching television and playing computer games, may further explain the prevalence of overweight and obesity.

For several decades, the federal government's Dietary Guidelines for Americans have recommended lower dietary fat intake. Data show that fat intake by Americans has indeed decreased, on average, from about 40% of total calories in the 1960s to 34% in the early 1990s.[6] Since the incidence of obesity has increased during the same period, and since obesity is associated with increasing risk of cardiovascular disease, the AHA points out that lowering fat intake is one way to combat the problem of obesity and help prevent cardiovascular disease. Other recommendations include restricting calories and increasing consumption of fruits and vegetables.[6]

The BRFSS data corroborate the NHES and NHANES data regarding increasing prevalence of obesity in adults in the United States.[10] BRFSS revealed that 12% of adults in 1991 and 17.9% in 1998 were obese. Increases over time were seen in all states; in both men and women; and across age groups, races and educational levels. Data from Great Britain show similar trends, with a rise in obesity from 8% to 15% between 1980 and 1995.[13]

The number of overweight children in the United States has also risen dramatically, as shown by NHANES III and 1999 NHANES data.[14] In NHANES II, 7% of children ages 6 to 11 years and 5% of adolescents ages 12 to 19 years were classified as overweight. These numbers climbed to 11% of children and 11% of adolescents in NHANES III and to 13% of children and 14% of adolescents in the 1999 NHANES.

Recent research data indicate that dieting is common in 9 to 14 year old girls of normal weight, with 27.9% of them reporting that they have dieted to lose weight in the previous year.[15] At least 12.5% reported binge eating monthly. Frequent dieters were significantly more likely to become overweight than those who reported never dieting, even when data were corrected for reported intake of total calories, carbohydrate and fat intake, and physical activity. The authors explain these results by pointing out that it is difficult to adhere to a restrictive diet, and periods of dieting may be interspersed with periods of overeating in these youngsters.

EFFECT OF OVERWEIGHT AND OBESITY ON OVERALL HEALTH

Hippocrates said "sudden death is more common in those who are naturally fat than in the lean."[16] Over 2000 years later, the idea that overweight and obesity increases morbidity and mortality from various diseases continues to interest the medical community. It was recently estimated that approximately 300,000 deaths per year among adults in the United States are attributed to obesity.[17] Relative weight stability since early adulthood has been correlated with lower mortality rates.[18]

The relationship between BMI and prevalence of hypertension as found in NHANES III is shown in Figure 8-2.[19] The International Study of Salt found that a 10 kg higher body weight was associated with a 3.0 mm Hg higher systolic blood pressure and a 2.3 mm Hg higher diastolic blood pressure, values that translate into an estimated 12% increase in risk for coronary heart disease and a 24% increase in risk for stroke.[4] The AHA has added obesity to its list of major modifiable risk factors for coronary heart disease.

Conditions Associated with Higher Morbidity in Overweight or Obese Patients

❑ Coronary Heart Disease.
❑ Endometrial, Breast, and Colon Cancer.
❑ Gallbladder Disease.
❑ Hypertension.
❑ Osteoarthritis.
❑ Sleep Apnea and Respiratory Problems.
❑ Stroke.
❑ Type 2 Diabetes.

Source: National Heart, Lung, and Blood Institute.

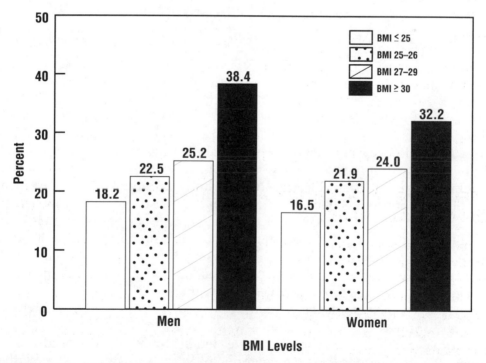

FIGURE 8-2 NHANES III Age-Adjusted Prevalence of Hypertension* According to Body Mass Index (BMI)

*Defined as mean systolic blood pressure ≥ 140 mm Hg, mean diastolic as ≥ 90 mm Hg, or currently taking antihypertensive medication.

Source: Brown CD, Higgins M, Donato KA, et al. Body mass index and the prevalence of hypertension and dyslipidemia. *Obes Res*. 2000;8:605-19. Reprinted with permission.

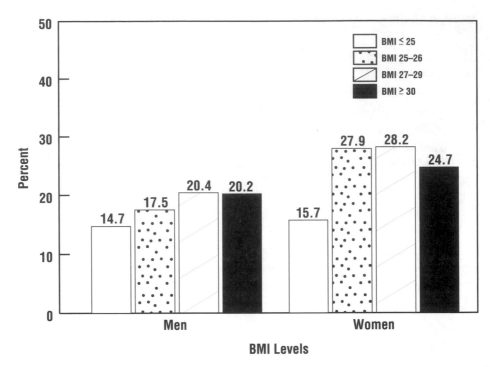

FIGURE 8-3 NHANES III Age-Adjusted Prevalence of High Blood Cholesterol*
According to Body Mass Index (BMI)

*Defined as ≥ 240 mg/dL.
Source: Brown CD, Higgins M, Donato KA, et al. Body mass index and the prevalence of
hypertension and dyslipidemia. *Obes Res.* 2000;8:605-19. Reprinted with permission.

The relationship between BMI and dyslipidemia as found in NHANES
III is illustrated in Figures 8-3 and 8-4.[19] Other studies, including a 20 year
follow-up to the Western Electric Study (a study begun in 1957 which examined the relationship between nutrition and heart disease in about 1800 men)
have shown a clear correlation of overweight and obesity with increasing
total cholesterol levels.[20] People with the abdominal obesity pattern tend to
have higher total cholesterol levels.[21] Increasing BMI has been associated with
increasing triglyceride levels across various age ranges and in both sexes.[4]
The relationship between higher BMI levels and lower high density lipoprotein (HDL) cholesterol levels shown in Figure 8-4 further substantiates the
risk of cardiovascular disease in overweight and obese patients.

Studies from various countries have demonstrated an increased risk of
type 2 diabetes with increasing weight.[4] One study showed that the relative
risk of diabetes in women goes up for each one-unit increase of BMI over 22
kg/m[2]. For example, women with a BMI at age 18 of 29.0 to 30.9 had a 4.5
fold increased risk for diabetes compared to women with a BMI less than
22.0 after a 14-year follow-up.[22] Another study estimated that 27% of new
cases of diabetes were attributable to weight gain of 5 kg or more during
adulthood.[23] Again, the abdominal pattern of obesity is considered a risk

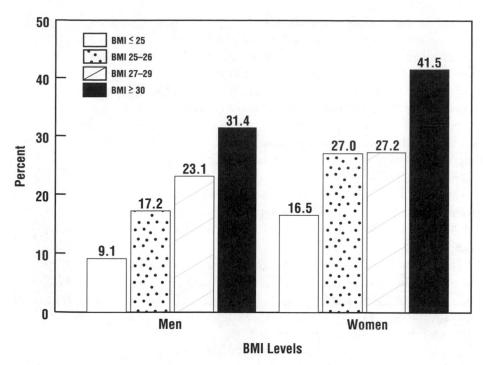

FIGURE 8-4   NHANES III Age-Adjusted Prevalence of Low HDL Cholesterol*
According to Body Mass Index (BMI)

* Defined as < 35 mg/dL in men and < 45 mg/dL in women.
Source: Brown CD, Higgins M, Donato KA, et al. Body mass index and the prevalence of
hypertension and dyslipidemia. *Obes Res.* 2000;8:605-19. Reprinted with permission.

factor for type 2 diabetes. Waist circumference has been positively associated
with risk of diabetes in men.[24]

Higher incidences of hypertension, dyslipidemia, and type 2 diabetes in
overweight people contribute to the increased morbidity and mortality from
coronary heart disease. The risk of nonfatal myocardial infarction and death
from coronary heart disease both go up with increasing BMI.[4] The association
between obesity and coronary heart disease is confounded by cigarette smoking; although smoking is a clear risk factor for coronary heart disease, people
who smoke tend to weigh less.[4] Congestive heart failure has also been associated with obesity; the increased risk of hypertension and type 2 diabetes
in obese patients may facilitate the development of congestive heart failure.[4]
In addition, excess weight appears to increase the risk for ischemic, but not
hemorrhagic, stroke.[3]

A clear relationship between gallstones, cholecystectomy, and excess
weight was demonstrated by NHANES III data for both men and women.[4]
One study showed that there was a substantial risk for cholecystectomy in
middle-aged women with a history of weight gains and losses; risk was
especially high in "severe" cyclers, those who had intentionally lost more
than 20 pounds followed by weight regain.[25]

Overweight and obese individuals are at increased risk of osteoarthritis. Greater weight increases stress on weight-bearing joints such as the knees, although other factors may also be involved.[3] Several studies have demonstrated improvement in osteoarthritis symptoms with weight loss.[4] Increased body weight may also be a risk factor for hyperuricemia and gout.[3]

People with a BMI over 30 are at increased risk of developing sleep apnea; those with large neck girth (circumference of at least 17 inches (43 cm) in men and 16 inches (41 cm) in women) who snore are especially at risk for sleep apnea.[4] This is probably related to anatomic changes in the thorax, such as deposition of fat.[3]

Various cancers have been associated with excess weight, although it is difficult to determine from epidemiologic studies the roles of obesity and high-fat diets. Colon cancer appears to be more common in both obese men and women.[4]

Obesity is a risk factor for postmenopausal breast cancer, although it has actually been inversely related to the incidence of premenopausal breast cancer.[4] Women who gain more than 20 pounds (9 kg) from age 18 to midlife have double the risk of breast cancer compared to women who maintained stable weight during this period of their life.[3] Endometrial cancer is clearly more common in obese women, with adult weight gain again increasing risk.[4]

NHLBI says obesity is associated with increased complications of pregnancy, menstrual irregularities, hirsutism, stress incontinence, and depression.[4] Hypertension is more prevalent in obese women during pregnancy, and incidences of gestational diabetes increase modestly. Obesity is associated with higher rates of induction and primary Cesarean section. The risk of congenital defects, including neural tube defects, increases in offspring of obese women. Abdominal obesity is associated with polycystic ovary syndrome that is manifested by infertility, anovulation and menstrual disturbances, and hirsutism.

Many studies from the 1980s and 1990s have shown that weight reduction can be beneficial to health over the short term.[26] Diabetics have shown improved glycemic control and reduction in hypoglycemic medications with weight reduction and a healthy diet. Losing excess weight reduces blood pressure and antihypertensive drug requirements in hypertensive patients. In several studies, lipid profiles have improved with weight loss in patients with dyslipidemias. Weight loss has been shown to alleviate symptoms of obstructive sleep apnea in some obese subjects. Weight reduction in these studies was often modest (5 to 10 kg).

Even modest weight loss has short-term benefits. An important question is whether weight loss over the longer term is associated with a reduction in major clinical outcomes, such as myocardial infarction, stroke, and cardiovascular death.[26] Cross-sectional and retrospective data suggest that such a reduction may occur, but results of long-term studies have not yet been published.

FACTORS AFFECTING ENERGY EXPENDITURE

In very general terms, increase in weight is related to energy imbalance, where energy intake (food consumption) exceeds energy expenditure. Weight gain following a period of weight maintenance could result from eating more calories, exercising less, or a combination of the two. Since a pound of stored fat represents about 3500 excess kcal, an average excess of only 10 kcal per day in energy intake over energy expenditure can result in approximately a 1-pound (0.45 kg or 3650 kcal) weight gain in a year.

Many factors affect energy expenditure.[27] Typically, the largest proportion of total energy expenditure (TEE) is the resting energy expenditure (REE), which represents the energy expended by someone at rest. The term REE is sometimes used synonymously with basal metabolic rate (BMR), although they are not technically the same. The BMR is the REE measured soon after awakening in the morning and at least 12 hours after a meal.[27]

The second largest proportion of TEE is physical activity. In an era of increasing automation, physical activity would be expected to decrease, making obesity more likely. A third component of TEE is dietary-induced thermogenesis, or the metabolic response to food. This reflects the energy required to utilize consumed food; it reaches a maximum about 1 hour after food is ingested. Another factor influencing the TEE is age; TEE tends to decrease with aging due to loss of lean body mass, the most metabolically active tissue.

Men tend to have higher TEE than women because they have proportionally more muscle mass. Women have proportionally more fat mass. Muscle is more metabolically active than adipose tissue. Energy expenditure is also related to a person's weight, as it takes more energy to move a larger object over a distance than it does to move a smaller object.

Growth and climate are other factors affecting energy expenditure. Growth (in children and during pregnancy) requires energy for synthesis and deposition of body tissue; this is most pronounced during the first year of life. In cold climates, a small increase in energy expenditure accompanies the wearing of extra clothing and footwear; shivering increases energy expenditure as well. People performing heavy work in very hot climates experience increased body temperature and metabolic rate, resulting in slightly higher energy expenditure to maintain optimal thermal balance.

The most common formulas used to estimate BMR are the Harris-Benedict equations. Factors can be applied to the BMR to account for a person's activity level.[27] REE can be measured, most commonly by indirect calorimetry, the measuring of oxygen consumption and carbon dioxide production. From these measurements REE can be calculated.

ETIOLOGY OF OVERWEIGHT AND OBESITY

The etiology of overweight and obesity is complex, involving a combination of physiological, genetic, environmental, and psychological factors. For example, endocrine system pathology is one unusual cause of obesity.[28] An overactive adrenal gland, leading to Cushing's syndrome, is associated with central obesity. Severe hypothyroidism can cause an increase in adipose tissue, but it is an unusual cause of obesity. Hypogonadism may be associated with mild obesity. Hypothalamic lesions caused by tumors, infection, or trauma may affect food intake regulation and lead to obesity.

Harris-Benedict Equations

Basal metabolic rate (BMR) is the resting energy expenditure measured soon after awakening in the morning and at least 12 hours after a meal. BMR is estimated using the Harris-Benedict Equations, the formulas for which are:

Woman (kcal):

Basal metabolic rate = 655 + [4.3 x weight (lb)] + [4.3 x height (in)] − [4.7 x age (yr)]

Man (kcal):

Basal metabolic rate = 65 + [6.2 x weight (lb)] + [12.7 x height (in)] − [6.8 x age (yr)]

Genetics are a major determinant of body weight. The so-called *ob/ob* mouse is an obese rodent with a genetic defect that results in a deficiency of the protein leptin.[28] Study of this and other obesity genes in animals has led to great interest in how genetics affect human obesity. Studies of identical twins raised in separate environments suggest that genetics are an important determinant of human weight; despite environmental differences, the twins often have similar body types.[28]

Ready availability of food, increasing portion sizes, and high fat diets are environmental factors that promote overeating.[29] Psychological factors also affect those with a tendency to obesity. As many as 20% of obese people wanting to lose weight report symptoms of depression.[30] In some cases the patient's obesity may contribute to the depression, whereas in others depression could have contributed to overeating and development of overweight and obesity.

DIETARY THERAPY OF OVERWEIGHT AND OBESITY

A variety of diets are used to treat overweight and obesity. The NHLBI guidelines reviewed three major types of diets: low calorie diets (LCD), very low calorie diets (VLCD), and lower fat diets.[4] These three types of diets will be briefly reviewed here, as will the currently popular low carbohydrate, high fat diet.

Low Calorie Diets (LCD)

LCD typically supply between 1000 and 1500 kcal per day. They are often low in fat to keep calorie counts low. These diets will typically result in a caloric deficit of 500 to 1000 kcal per day in mildly to moderately active people. A 500 kcal per day deficit (3500 kcal per week) will result in about a pound (0.45 kg) of weight lost per week. A 1000 kcal per day deficit (7000 kcal per week) will result in about a 2 pound (0.9 kg) weight loss per week.

The results of studies of LCD reviewed by the NHLBI showed a mean weight loss of about 8% of initial body weight over 3 to 12 months.[4] Studies including long-term weight loss and maintenance phases lasting 3 to 4.5 years reported average weight loss of 4%. From the studies in which waist circumference was reported, weight loss on LCD resulted in decreased waist circumference, or losses of abdominal fat, which should result in decreased risk of coronary heart disease.

Several of the studies included by the NHLBI examined whether weight loss through diet alone (without increased physical activity) improved cardiorespiratory fitness. When compared to control subjects who did not lose weight, people who lost weight but did not increase activity levels did not improve their overall cardiovascular health.

Very Low Calorie Diets (VLCD)

VLCD are generally defined as diets containing no more than 800 kcal per day, but some of these diets may contain as few as 400 to 500 kcal per day. These diets are also known as protein-modified-fasts. Although VLCD produce greater initial weight losses than LCD, weight loss over a year or more tends not to differ, probably due to nonadherence to the VLCD.[4] Regain of lost weight is to be expected unless the subject dramatically alters eating and exercise habits long-term.[31]

People who use these diets should consume adequate amounts of protein, limit fat and carbohydrate, and meet recommended dietary allowances of vitamins, minerals, and electrolytes. It is generally recommended that such diets be used only under the supervision of a physician and dietitian, due to the health risks associated with rapid weight loss.[32]

VLCD were first described in 1929.[33] Experiments over the next decade showed that, even with the limited nutritional knowledge of the day, the approach could be used fairly safely. World War II distracted the public, and fewer tried these diets as weight loss was apparently not a priority during this period. VLCD finally caught on after studies in the late 1950s and early 1960s evaluated complete fasting for weight loss.[32] Because fasting led to large protein and potassium losses and some deaths were reported, people were drawn to safer semi-starvation rather than total starvation diets.

In the mid 1970s, several companies marketed liquid-protein, modified-fast formulas, which contained a protein of poor biologic value (hydrolyzed collagen) and inadequate vitamin, mineral, and electrolyte content. These products led to at least 60 deaths (some of which occurred in otherwise healthy people), probably as a result of arrhythmias. Autopsies of some of these people showed atrophy of cardiac myofibrils.[33]

The more current commercial VLCDs contain proteins of higher biologic value, with recommended protein intake of 50 to 100 gm per day (about 1.5 gm/kg ideal body weight per day).[32] These diets result in rapid initial weight losses, due largely to diuresis and sodium loss. Risks include abnormalities in electrolytes, trace elements, and vitamins; gout; gallstones; cold intolerance; fatigue; light-headedness; euphoria (secondary to ketosis); disturbances in bowel frequency; dry skin; thinning hair; anemia; and menstrual irregularities.[31,32]

The American Dietetic Association states that VLCD may be appropriate for highly motivated people with a BMI over 30 who have failed to lose weight using more conservative methods.[31] Patients with a BMI of 27 to 30 who have comorbid conditions (such as those outlined later as criteria for use of pharmacotherapy for obesity) may also be appropriate for VLCD therapy.

Intermittent VLCD therapy, where the subject uses VLCD for short periods of time and consumes a diet that maintains weight between VLCD periods, may be effective for weight loss. One recent study showed that intermittent VLCD therapy produced weight loss similar to that produced by continuous VLCD over several months.[34]

Low Fat Diets

Does reducing fat in a diet result in weight loss independent of a reduction in total calories?[35-38] Stated another way, are high fat diets more likely to lead to weight gain than low fat diets containing equivalent numbers of calories? High fat diets are usually energy dense and are often associated with high energy intakes; energy intake exceeds energy expenditure, and there is weight gain. Diets high in fat are typically quite palatable, and are associated with lower satiety. People eat more because the food tastes good and they do not feel full. Diets rich in foods containing lower energy densities, like fruits and vegetables, do not have the same appeal.[35]

If high fat content in a diet is independently related to weight gain, should dietary fat be replaced with carbohydrate?[37] This idea could be derived from the widely disseminated Dietary Guidelines for Americans and the Food Guide Pyramid created by the United States Department of Agriculture.[39,40] In a sedentary overweight and obese population there is a high degree of insulin resistance. An increase in the carbohydrate content of the diet could lead to more hyperinsulinemia, hypertriglyceridemia, and lower HDL cholesterol.[37] In the future, recommendations may include more emphasis on the type of fat consumed. For example, diets relatively high in monounsaturated fatty acids may have beneficial effects.

Although artificial fats such as olestra can help lower the fat content of the diet, foods containing these substances may not necessarily have fewer total calories.[41] Many of the foods containing artificial fats contain added sugars, so some low fat foods are high in calories. Foods containing artificial fat could help people lose weight if they choose reduced fat foods that are also low in calories, and do not eat additional food to compensate for the caloric reductions.[41]

The NHLBI guidelines state that there is little evidence that lower fat diets cause weight loss independent of caloric reduction. Lower fat diets coupled with total reduction of calories produce more weight loss than lower fat diets alone.[4] NHLBI recommends low calorie diets for weight loss with the caveat that reducing fat is a practical way to reduce caloric intake.

High Protein Low Carbohydrate Diets

Many so-called "fad" diets become popular at various times. One such diet is the high protein, low carbohydrate diet. In the 1960s, this diet was called the Scarsdale Medical Diet. In the 1970s the name Atkins became associated with this diet, and that name is also associated with some current versions of the diet.[42] Others call this plan the Zone diet.

Different versions of this diet advocate varying degrees of carbohydrate restriction.[42] Some of the diets are very low in carbohydrate, providing 10% to 15% of total calories as carbohydrates, whereas others suggest 40% of calories from carbohydrate. General recommendations advocate about 55% of calories from carbohydrate. Total calorie content for the diets is typically 1200 to 1700 calories per day, depending on the particular diet and the stage of the diet.

Low carbohydrate diets do lead to weight loss in many patients. One factor contributing to weight loss may be the induction of a mild ketosis, enhanced production of ketones, when carbohydrate is ingested at a level less than 40 g per day.[43] This ketosis may lead to a decrease in appetite.

People strictly following these diets do significantly decrease their overall energy intake. This may seem paradoxical, since the diets are relatively high in fat. However, when one considers the practical ramifications of severely restricting carbohydrate intake, it is not so surprising. Patients following these diets may need to consume sandwiches without the bread, a meat entrée without a potato, or tomato sauce without pasta, for example.[42]

Water loss also contributes to early weight loss on low carbohydrate diets.[42] Glycogen is stored in the body with water in a 1 to 3 ratio; as glycogen stores are utilized at the beginning of a low carbohydrate diet, water stores are also used.

A third factor that may explain the weight loss seen with low carbohydrate diets is the decrease in insulin levels.[44] Insulin enhances lipogenesis and inhibits lipolysis, thus the lower insulin levels seen in patients on low carbohydrate diets might be useful in reducing fat stores in the body. This theory requires further study.

The National Weight Control Registry was established by the University of Colorado Health Sciences Center and Brown University to gather information on people who have successfully maintained weight losses long-term.[45] To be eligible for the registry, a person must have lost at least 30 pounds and kept it off for at least a year. The average registrant to date has lost about 60 pounds (27 kg) and maintained the loss for 5 years.

Of 2681 subjects in the registry, 204 (8%) reported eating less than 90 g of carbohydrates a day, and 25 of them (1% of total) consumed a diet that contained less than 24% of total calories from carbohydrate.[46] Thus, to date, only a minority of subjects listed in the registry are low carbohydrate devotees; these people are more commonly consuming a low fat, high carbohydrate diet.

The low carbohydrate diet can have significant adverse effects.[42,43] Excess loss of water and sodium can lead to dehydration, so people on the plan need to drink plenty of fluids. Possible breakdown of protein and fat increases renal solute load, thus the diet should be used with caution in patients with renal dysfunction. Hyperuricemia leading to gout is another concern. The extreme ketogenic diet used for epilepsy has led to kidney stones, acidosis, and water soluble vitamin deficiencies, and the same adverse effects are theoretically possible with long term adherence to a low carbohydrate diet. In one study, adolescents using a very low calorie, low carbohydrate diet showed increases in calcium excretion and decreases in total bone mineral content, and this deserves further investigation.[47]

The effect of low carbohydrate diets on blood lipid levels seems to vary among individuals. Although it would be expected that people receiving a high percentage of their calories from fat might exhibit worsening of lipid profiles, this has not been uniformly reported.[43] Some studies in obese individuals have shown improvements in lipid profiles, perhaps related to the weight loss seen on the diets. On the other hand, worsening of the lipid profile has been reported in lean subjects following these diets. The number of subjects in these studies is limited, and duration of study is typically short, leaving this issue as another worthy of further investigation.

An interesting debate between leading proponents of two disparate diets occurred at the 2001 American College of Cardiology meeting.[48] Dr. Robert Atkins, champion of the high fat, low carbohydrate Atkins diet, squared off against Dr. Dean Ornish, the guiding force behind the Ornish plan, which promotes lifestyle changes and a very low fat diet. As might be expected, no clear winner of the debate emerged.

EXERCISE AS A MODALITY FOR WEIGHT LOSS AND WEIGHT MAINTENANCE

Since weight homeostasis depends on both energy intake and energy expenditure, increasing physical activity could be useful for the overweight and obese patient. The AHA states that "exercise should be considered one of the highest priorities of a weight management program."[49]

The NHLBI guidelines reviewed the effect of physical activity on weight loss and weight maintenance.[4] The guidelines concluded that aerobic exercise results in modest weight loss in overweight and obese persons independent of dietary caloric reduction. The studies also showed that diet-only groups achieved more weight loss than exercise-only groups. Cross-sectional and longitudinal studies said that exercise helps with long-term maintenance of body weight and in preventing weight gain with age. A limited number of studies looked at the effect of physical activity on waist circumference; it was concluded that physical activity modestly reduces abdominal fat in overweight and obese patients.

In general, studies used for NHLBI guidelines concluded that a combination of a reduced calorie diet and an increase in physical activity produced greater weight losses than either of the modalities alone.[4] The combination therapy also resulted in greater reductions in waist circumference.

BEHAVIORAL THERAPY IN WEIGHT MANAGEMENT

The NHLBI guidelines define behavior therapy as "those strategies, based on learning principles such as reinforcement, that provide tools for overcoming barriers to compliance with dietary therapy and/or increased physical therapy."[4] The literature reviewed indicated that behavior therapy provides benefit in short term (up to 1 year) weight loss efforts when used in combination with other approaches. However, at 3 to 5 years, no additional benefit was seen in patients who received behavioral therapy during the first year, perhaps due to infrequent practice as time goes on.

Various behavioral therapies are recommended by the NHLBI guidelines, including self-monitoring of eating habits and physical activity, stress management, stimulus control, and social support.[4] No one strategy emerges as clearly superior. Intense multimodal strategies utilizing several of the above methods appear to work best.

PHARMACOTHERAPY OF OBESITY

Many people find it difficult to achieve and maintain a desirable body weight. Drug therapy may be helpful for some people. The NHLBI and NAASO, Shape Up America, and the American Obesity Association all recommend reserving drug therapy for those with a BMI of 30 kg/m^2 or greater without comorbidities and those with a BMI of 27 kg/m^2 or greater with comorbidities such as hypertension, dyslipidemia, coronary heart disease, type 2 diabetes, or sleep apnea.[4,8,50] These guidelines are also used by the American Pharmaceutical Association in its drug treatment protocol for weight management.[51]

All of these organizations stress that pharmacotherapy should not be used alone for weight control. However, it may be effective in the context of a comprehensive weight management program, which also includes a sensible diet, physical activity, and behavioral modification. The NHLBI and NAASO guidelines suggest that pharmacotherapy may be considered if at least 6 months of a regimen including a low calorie diet, increased physical activity, and behavior therapy has not resulted in weight loss of 1 pound per week.[8] These guidelines also emphasize that pharmacotherapy should not be used for cosmetic weight loss, but rather to decrease medical risk.

Some medications for the treatment of obesity have been misused, with disastrous results. Thyroid extract used for obesity in the late 1800s led to hyperthyroidism with the attendant problems of that condition.[52,53] History has been known to repeat itself in the realm of obesity treatment: the Food and Drug Administration (FDA) recently pulled some dietary supplements containing the thyroid extract triiodothyroacetic acid (TRIAC or tiratricol) from the market due to risk of myocardial infarction and stroke.[54] Dinitrophenol, a compound that uncouples oxidative phosphorylation, was used in the early 1900s to help with weight control, and neuropathies and cataracts were some of the adverse side effects.[52]

Amphetamines were discovered to have appetite suppressant properties as early as the 1930s. They fell into disfavor in the late 1960s when experts realized people could become addicted, and as a result amphetamines were classified as controlled substances by the Drug Enforcement Administration (DEA).[52,53] Use of digitalis and diuretics as weight loss adjuvants led to several deaths, but diuretics continue to be included in dietary supplements marketed as weight control agents.[52]

Aminorex was a serotonergic appetite suppressant available in Europe in the early 1970s and was associated with cases of primary pulmonary hypertension.[52] Use of the non-FDA approved combination of phentermine and fenfluramine (two drugs approved for use alone in the early 1970s) in the 1990s led to the wild popularity of this regimen. Some people who received the drugs suffered from cardiac valvular abnormalities and primary pulmonary hypertension, so fenfluramine and dexfenfluramine were withdrawn from the market in 1997. These agents were serotonergic agents similar to aminorex.[55]

Phenylpropanolamine, a centrally acting adrenergic agent available in the United States for many years as a nonprescription weight control agent, was withdrawn in 2000. Although serious adverse effects of this agent had been reported for many years, it took a large multicenter case control study to finally move the FDA to request removal of this product from the market.[56]

A recent analysis of the 1998 BRFSS led to the estimate that about 2.5% of U.S. adults (4.0% of women and 0.9% of men) used prescription weight loss medications during the period 1996 to 1998.[57] Of people with a BMI greater than 30 kg/m², 10.2% of women and 3.1% of men reported use. About 1/4 of them had a BMI less than 27 kg/m², making them ineligible for such therapy according to authoritative guidelines. Pill use was highest in women in the 25 to 44 age group. Highest usage of the medications for men was in the 35 to 64 age group.

Agents for the treatment of obesity can be divided into several broad categories.[58] Centrally acting adrenergic agents and the adrenergic plus serotonergic agent sibutramine decrease appetite or increase satiety through modulation of neurotransmitters. Thermogenic agents contribute to weight loss by increasing diet-induced thermogenesis, or by increasing energy expenditure through heat production in the body. Digestive inhibitors act directly on the gastrointestinal tract. The gene products are experimental agents that are involved in the hormonal regulation of eating.

Of the commercially available prescription agents, only orlistat and sibutramine have FDA approval for long-term use (defined as therapy for greater than 3 months at a time). These two drugs may be continued as long as they are effective and the adverse effects are manageable.[8]

Because obesity is a chronic disease, short-term use of pharmacotherapy is not helpful. NHLBI guidelines recommend that these drugs should only be used in the context of a long-term treatment strategy. With sibutramine, if initial weight loss on a standard starting dosage is less than expected in the context of good adherence to the overall treatment regimen, the dosage may need to be increased. If maximum dosages of the drugs are ineffective

Classification of Agents for Treatment of Obesity

Appetite suppressants / satiety enhancers
    Centrally acting adrenergic
        Benzphetamine (Didrex)*
        Diethylpropion (Tenuate)**
        Mazindol (Mazanor, Sanorex)**
        Phendimetrazine (various)*
        Phentermine (various)**
    Serotonergic
        Selective serotonin reuptake inhibitors
    Adrenergic plus serotonergic
        Sibutramine (Meridia)**
Agents increasing energy expenditure (thermogenic agents)
    Adrenergic
        Ephedra alkaloids
        Ephedrine plus caffeine
        β-3 agonists (investigational)
Digestive inhibitors
    Lipase inhibitor
        Orlistat (Xenical)
    Fat substitutes
        Olestra
    Cholesterol inhibitors
        Plant stanols (Benecol)
        Plant sterols (Take Control)
Gene products
    Leptin analogs (investigational)
    Neuropeptide Y antagonists (investigational)

* DEA controlled substance category III
** DEA controlled substance category IV

after a period of several weeks, discontinuation of treatment should be considered.[4]

Sibutramine

Sibutramine (Meridia) is an inhibitor of serotonin and norepinephrine reuptake; it is also a weak inhibitor of dopamine reuptake.[59] The effects on serotonin and norepinephrine are important for sibutramine's satiety effect; the drug is sometimes referred to as a serotonin-norepinephrine reuptake inhibitor. The drug was initially developed as an antidepressant, but when its effects on depression proved disappointing, research efforts shifted.[60] Sibutramine was approved for treatment of obesity in late 1997, just months after the removal of fenfluramine and dexfenfluramine from the market.

Two of the metabolites of sibutramine, as well as the parent compound, are active.[59] Metabolism occurs mainly by CYP3A4 in the liver.[59] Long half-lives of the active metabolites allow for dosing once a day.[59] Taking the drug with food alters its peak concentration and time to achieve this peak, but does not alter the area under the concentration curve. Therefore, the drug can be taken either with or without food.[59]

Sibutramine is supplied in 5, 10, and 15 mg capsules. Recommended starting dosage is 10 mg once daily. The manufacturer suggests that the dosage should be conservative in elderly patients, due to higher frequency of decreased hepatic, renal, or cardiac function and concomitant disease and drug therapy. The manufacturer also cautions that the drug should not be used in patients with severe renal impairment, and that sibutramine safety and efficacy in children under 16 years of age are unknown.

Two methods are widely used to report efficacy in weight loss trials. Some studies report results as the percentage of patients losing at least some percentage of initial body weight, such as 5%, 10%, or 15%. Other studies report mean weight reduction in kilograms or pounds compared to baseline.

Studies of people taking 10 to 15 mg per day of sibutramine for 6 months to 1 year have typically shown weight loss between about 5 and 7 kg (10 to 15 pounds).[61-64] The number of those losing at least 5% of baseline weight varied between about 50% and 65%. Between 15% and 35% of the group lost at least 10% of baseline weight. People lost the most weight in the first 6 months of therapy, and continued drug therapy helped to maintain weight loss through 12 and 24 months compared to placebo in studies of longer duration.[63,64] In the Sibutramine Trial of Obesity Reduction and Maintenance, a multicenter European study in which patients received sibutramine for up to 2 years, drug dosage was increased to 20 mg during the maintenance phase (after 6 months) if weight regain occurred.[64]

Most of the clinical trials showing weight loss with sibutramine include diet and behavioral therapy in addition to drug therapy. Thus the results seen in these trials may be more dramatic than in general clinical practice, where the patient will typically not be receiving the same intensity of follow-up.

A recent study emphasizes this.[65] In a 1-year trial of sibutramine, the drug was prescribed to a group of obese women along with recommendations for exercise (working up to four to five sessions per week of 30 to 40 minutes per session) and dietary restriction (1200 to 1500 kcal per day). In a second group, the drug was prescribed in combination with a group lifestyle modification program (weekly group meetings with a psychologist). A third group received the drug and a combined treatment of the group lifestyle modification program, plus a 1000 kcal per day diet for the first 4 months. This was followed by instructions to consume 1200 to 1500 kcal per day for the remainder of the study.

Weight loss at month 12 in the three groups was 4.1, 10.8, and 16.5% of initial body weight, respectively, emphasizing that use of the drug alone (as is probably often the case in actual use outside a clinical trial setting) is not as effective as when it is combined with lifestyle modification and diet. Maximal weight loss was seen at 6 months in all three groups (5.8%, 11.0%, and 17.7%, respectively). These represented mean losses of 5.6, 11.4, and 17.9 kg, respectively; the losses in the latter two groups are larger than those seen in many of the previously published clinical studies with this drug.

This study also showed that women who lost more weight in the first month of the study continued to lose more weight at months 2, 4, 6, and 12, compared to counterparts who lost less weight initially. Patients had very unrealistic weight loss expectations; at the beginning of the study, they expected, on average, to lose 25% of their initial body weight in a year, even though the researchers repeatedly told them to anticipate a 5% to 15% weight loss. The authors of this study emphasize the importance of patients keeping food records; the more food records patients kept during the first 4 months of the study, the greater their weight loss over the short and long term.

Study design will influence interpretation of results, and must be considered before findings are extrapolated to the general population. For example, in a study by Apfelbaum et al., treatment with sibutramine 10 mg daily plus a low calorie diet for 12 months resulted in a weight loss of about 14 kg, compared to a 9 kg weight loss in patients on a low calorie diet given placebo.[63] However, the weight losses in both groups of this study included approximately an 8 kg weight loss achieved during a 1 month lead in period, where patients received a very low calorie diet prior to placement in sibutramine or placebo groups.

Another important consideration is that the percentage of patients completing the longer term trials was sometimes about 50%. The data are typically recorded for the last observation carried forward (LOCF) for the various patients. Data from later in these studies represent smaller numbers of patients (i.e., those who stuck with the rigors of the diet and drug therapy) than data from earlier in the study. Again, this must be taken into account when trying to extrapolate the results of the clinical trials to general populations.

Several clinical trials have investigated the effects of weight loss and sibutramine therapy on serum lipid levels. The product information for Meridia gives data for a combined analysis of 11 placebo-controlled studies ranging in duration from 12 to 52 weeks.[59] This analysis showed that in patients losing at least 5% of body weight, serum triglycerides declined on average about 15% in patients receiving placebo and 17% in patients receiving sibutramine. Total cholesterol declined about 6% in these same placebo patients and 6% in patients receiving sibutramine.

Low-density lipoprotein (LDL) cholesterol dropped about 6% in weight losing placebo patients and about 5% in weight losing sibutramine patients. In other words, the changes in these lipid levels seemed to be associated with weight loss rather than with the drug. On the other hand, HDL cholesterol rose about 1% in weight losing placebo patients and about 5% for weight losing sibutramine patients. The manufacturer does not claim statistical significance for this latter finding, but it is intriguing and deserves further investigation. A recent abstract from an NAASO meeting also indicated that sibutramine may have beneficial effects on HDL cholesterol over that seen with weight loss alone.[66]

Sibutramine is classified by the DEA as a Class IV controlled substance. At least two studies have examined the abuse potential of the medication. In the first of these studies, slightly supratherapeutic dosages of sibutramine (20 and 30 mg) produced stimulation and euphoria similar to placebo. The subjects were recreational stimulant users, and they rated perceived street value of sibutramine and session enjoyment as low.[67] In the second study, polydrug abusers given a high dose of sibutramine (75 mg) experienced anxiety and confusion and stated that they would rather give up their study pay than retake the drug.[68] These studies would indicate that the abuse potential of the drug is low.

Since sibutramine is a serotonergic agent (like fenfluramine and dexfenfluramine), there is some concern about its potential for cardiac valvular damage. Bach et al., studied 210 obese type 2 diabetic patients receiving sibutramine or placebo for an average of 7.6 months (range 14 to 487 days).[69] The prevalence of left-sided valve dysfunction as evidenced by echocardiogram was similar in both groups. Post-marketing surveillance studies should continue to monitor for this devastating side effect.

Other adverse events associated with sibutramine are increased blood pressure and heart rate. With weight loss, one would expect to see a decline in blood pressure and indeed this may be seen in some patients receiving sibutramine. However, a significant number of patients receiving the drug will actually have increases in blood pressure. The product information states that 0.4% of patients enrolled in pre-marketing studies were discontinued from the studies because of hypertension, compared to 0.4% in control groups; 0.4% of sibutramine patients were discontinued secondary to tachycardia compared to 0.1% of control patients.[59] Although the mean increase in blood pressure in these trials was only 1 to 3 mm Hg and the mean increase in pulse rate 4 to 5 beats per minute compared to placebo, a number of patients experienced significant problems.[59]

Results from two studies presented in the product information defined outliers as patients who had increases in systolic blood pressure above baseline of at least 15 mm Hg, increases in diastolic blood pressure of at least 10 mm Hg, or increases in pulse rate of at least 10 beats per minute for three consecutive visits.[59] Compared to placebo, patients treated with sibutramine 10 mg daily were more likely to be outliers in terms of systolic blood pressure (12% vs. 9%), diastolic blood pressure (15% vs. 7%), and pulse (28% vs. 12%).[59] The statistical significance of these findings is not presented, nor is the number of patients on which these data are based.

Despite the possibility of increased blood pressure associated with sibutramine use, the drug has been studied in patients with a history of hypertension.[70] Patients who control hypertension with a calcium channel blocker (with or without a thiazide diuretic) were given either sibutramine or placebo for a year. The mean increase in diastolic blood pressure in sibutramine-treated hypertensives in this study was 2 mm Hg, and the mean increase in pulse rate was about five beats per minute. Sibutramine was discontinued in about 5% of patients due to hypertension.

Weight loss over a year in patients receiving sibutramine in this study was modest (mean of 4.4 kg or 4.7% of baseline body weight). This may be because these patients received minimal behavioral intervention. The authors concluded that sibutramine could be used in most people with controlled hypertension if close monitoring is employed. An added benefit of sibutramine demonstrated in this study was a decrease in serum uric acid levels beyond the decrease seen with equivalent weight loss alone.

Other common adverse reactions of sibutramine include dry mouth, insomnia, constipation, headache, and (ironically) increased appetite.[59] The manufacturer's product information indicates several contraindications for the drug.[59] Sibutramine is not recommended for patients receiving monoamine oxidase inhibitors because of concerns regarding the development of a hypertensive crisis with concomitant use. People who are hypersensitive to the drug or who have anorexia nervosa or severe renal or hepatic dysfunction should avoid the drug.

Patients taking other centrally acting appetite suppressants and those with a history of coronary artery disease, congestive heart failure, arrhythmias, or stroke should avoid the drug. Special caution should be taken when using sibutramine in patients with narrow-angle glaucoma or a history of seizures.[59] The drug has not been studied in children less than 16 years of age, and is not recommended for women who are pregnant or lactating.[59] There is some concern regarding the concomitant use of sibutramine with other serotonergic agents, including the selective serotonin reuptake inhibitors, due to the potential development of serotonin syndrome.[59]

Orlistat

The second medication approved by the FDA for long-term use in the treatment of obesity is orlistat (also known as tetrahydrolipstatin). This drug is a digestive inhibitor which binds reversibly to gastric and pancreatic lipases in the gastrointestinal tract lumen, making them unavailable to hydrolyze dietary triglycerides into absorbable free fatty acids and monoglycerides.[71] At the recommended dosage of 120 mg three times a day before meals, the drug inhibits dietary fat absorption by about 30%. Increasing the dosage above the recommended level does not appreciably increase the percentage of fat absorption inhibition.[72] If the patient skips a meal or anticipates ingestion of a meal containing no fat, the dose should be withheld. The drug itself is minimally absorbed.[73] Orlistat is supplied as 120 mg capsules.

Weight loss with orlistat tends to be more modest than with sibutramine. The product information outlines five placebo-controlled studies lasting 1 year in which more than 3000 patients received orlistat.[74] Mean weight loss after 1 year was 6.1 kg in the intent to treat population (i.e., all patients were followed until the end of the study regardless of whether they withdrew from the treatment). Of patients completing a year of orlistat, 57% lost at least 5% of initial body weight.

Again, caution is advised in interpreting the results of these studies when trying to extrapolate to general clinical practice. One must be careful to look at intent to treat results as well as LOCF results, since significant numbers of patients dropped out of the studies. In addition, a placebo lead-in period was included in some of these studies, during which people lost additional weight. One reviewer observed that treatment groups in these trials may have become unblinded due to the gastrointestinal side effects of orlistat.[75]

Two-year efficacy data from the studies mentioned above are also given in the product information.[74] Of patients completing 2 years of orlistat therapy, 40% lost more than 5% of initial body weight. The relative weight loss advantage between orlistat and placebo was the same after 2 years as it had been after a year.

In a multicenter European study, patients received either orlistat 120 mg three times a day or placebo for 1 year in combination with a hypocaloric diet (600 kcal per day deficit).[76] At the end of 1 year, patients were reassigned to either orlistat or placebo and prescribed a weight maintenance diet. During the 2nd year, patients who continued on orlistat regained on average only half as much weight as patients switched to placebo. Similarly, patients switched from placebo to orlistat for the second year lost 0.9 kg during this year, whereas patients remaining on placebo regained 2.5 kg.

A recently published 2-year study explored the efficacy of orlistat in a primary care setting where limited dietary and behavioral counseling were provided.[77] This study again used the 4-week lead-in period, with a reduced calorie diet before randomization to orlistat or placebo groups. Patients were initially counseled by a primary care physician regarding the diet prior to the lead-in period; dietitians and psychologists were not used at any stage of the study. Patients were instructed to stay on this diet for the first year after randomization.

Seventy-two percent of the patients completing the lead-in period who were randomized to orlistat 120 mg three times a day completed the first year of the study. The prescribed caloric intake was increased slightly for patients who were still losing weight at the end of the first year, as the goal of the second year was aimed more at weight maintenance. During the second year, patients viewed behavior modification videos and were given weight management and diet pamphlets four times each. Fifty-six percent of patients in the orlistat 120 mg three times a day group completed the second year of study.

At 1 year, patients receiving orlistat 120 mg three times a day had lost about 7.9 kg (2.5 kg of which was lost during the lead-in period) compared to about 4.1 kg (2.7 kg in the lead-in period) in placebo-treated patients. At the end of 2 years, some weight regain had occurred, with the orlistat patients remaining about 5 kg below baseline weight and the placebo group remaining about 1.7 kg below baseline weight. The authors concluded that orlistat is effective as an adjunct to diet, even in primary care settings.

One study tested whether orlistat might be useful for weight maintenance after conventional dieting.[78] Obese subjects who had lost at least 8% of their baseline body weight during a 6-month lead-in period (utilizing a 1000 kcal per day deficit diet) were assigned to receive varying dosages of orlistat or placebo for a year, in combination with a maintenance diet. Subjects treated with orlistat 120 mg three times a day regained less weight than those treated with placebo. Similar results on prevention of weight gain were seen in a second study, in which patients were given orlistat plus a hypocaloric diet for a year, followed by orlistat plus a weight maintenance diet for a second year.[79]

Orlistat also has potential for weight reduction and subsequent improvement of glycemic control and reduction of cardiovascular risk factors, particularly in type 2 diabetic patients. In fact, Hoffman La-Roche, Inc., the product manufacturer of Xenical, submitted a supplemental application to the FDA in March 2001 for a new indication: to improve glycemic control when used as an adjunct to other antidiabetic treatments in overweight or obese patients with type 2 diabetes.[80]

In a 1-year, multicenter, double-blind study of type II diabetic patients on sulfonylurea medications, subjects received either orlistat 120 mg three times a day or placebo along with a mildly hypocaloric diet.[81] Although differences in weight lost over the year were modest (6.2 +/- 0.45% vs. 4.3 +/- 0.49% of initial weight in the two groups, respectively, expressed as mean +/- standard error of the mean), over twice as many patients receiving orlistat lost at least 5% of initial body weight (49% vs. 23%).

One review of orlistat pointed out that results like these on mean initial weight loss appear to be similar, without much variation.[75] However, if standard errors of the mean are converted to standard deviations, it becomes obvious that the response to therapy with orlistat and diet is quite variable. In this study, orlistat-treated patients had significantly larger decreases in hemoglobin A_{1C} levels and fasting plasma glucose levels. They were also able to decrease their doses of sulfonylurea.

Data from three double-blind placebo-controlled trials explored the role of orlistat and dietary intervention on glucose tolerance and deteriorating diabetes status.[82] The mean length of follow-up was 582 days. Orlistat-treated patients lost more weight, and fewer with impaired glucose tolerance at baseline progressed to a diagnosis of diabetes, compared to control patients (3.0% vs. 7.6%). Additionally, in patients with impaired glucose tolerance at baseline, glucose levels were closer to normal in orlistat-treated patients (71.6%) than in placebo-treated patients (49.1%).

Pooled data from five studies quoted in the product information for Xenical showed a 6.7 pmol/L decrease in fasting insulin levels in orlistat-treated patients, compared to a 5.2 pmol/L increase in placebo-controlled patients.[74] No claims of statistical significance are made for these data, and this finding has not been consistent in all studies.[81,83]

Many studies have looked at the effect of orlistat-associated weight loss on blood lipid levels.[76,78,81,83] These studies have typically shown greater reductions in total cholesterol and LDL cholesterol with orlistat treatment than in patients receiving placebo. In these studies the orlistat-treated groups experienced greater weight loss, which could explain some but probably not all of the more favorable lipid profile.[76,81] The product information for Xenical shows similar results from pooled data from five studies, although the statistical analysis is not presented.[74]

There is some concern about the effect of orlistat on fat-soluble vitamin status, since absorption of these nutrients might decrease with decreased fat absorption induced by the drug. Data included in the product information indicate that the incidence of low vitamin A levels in the blood on two or more consecutive visits in nonsupplemented patients with normal baseline values was 2.2% in orlistat-treated patients and 1.0% in placebo-treated patients.[74] Similar values for vitamin D, vitamin E, and beta carotene were 12% versus 6.6%, 5.8% versus 1%, and 6.1% versus 1.7%, respectively.

Based on these results, the manufacturer recommends that patients receiving orlistat take a multivitamin supplement that contains fat-soluble vitamins.[74] The supplement should be separated by at least 2 hours from dosages of orlistat.

One editorialist has raised the concern that osteopenia and osteoporosis not correlated with low vitamin D concentrations have been documented in patients with pancreatic insufficiency and steatorrhea.[84] Long-term orlistat users should be aware of their calcium balance, and bone mineral density measurements are necessary for those who are peri- and postmenopausal and thus at risk for osteoporosis.

The pharmacist will recognize the concern about possible interaction between orlistat and warfarin through effects on the absorption of fat-soluble vitamin K. A normal volunteer study showed that orlistat in normal dosage did not significantly change the pharmacokinetics or pharmacodynamics of a single 30-mg dose of warfarin.[85] However, vitamin K levels tended to decline with orlistat use.[74] Although vitamin A, vitamin E, and beta carotene serum levels were measured in several of the clinical trials, vitamin K levels were not reported.[76,78,83] Therefore, it is necessary to monitor the international normalized ratio very closely in patients on concomitant orlistat and warfarin.

Another theoretical concern regarding the use of orlistat is the potential for an increased rate of colon cancer, secondary to increased exposure of the colon to triglycerides. However, short term data indicate that increased colonic cell turnover and increased bile acid concentrations do not occur with orlistat therapy.[86]

In premarketing clinical trials, an increased incidence of breast cancer was seen in patients treated with orlistat compared to placebo-treated controls.[87] Retrospective analysis and subsequent data indicate that this finding was an artifact, and that the drug is not associated with an increased risk of breast cancer.[87]

As might be expected from its mechanism of action of decreasing fat absorption, orlistat is associated with gastrointestinal side effects. Listed in the product information are oily spotting, flatus with discharge, fecal urgency, fatty or oily stool, oily evacuation, increased defecation, and fecal incontinence.[74] Since the gastrointestinal events increase with increasing dietary fat, it is recommended that fat be distributed fairly evenly between the three main meals of a day.

The literature states that side effects usually occur within 3 months of initiating therapy.[74] About half of these incidences lasted for less than 1 week, with the majority lasting for no more than 4 weeks. The manufacturer goes on to say that 8.8% of orlistat-treated patients (compared to 5.0% of placebo-treated patients) discontinued treatment secondary to adverse effects.[74]

The use of orlistat is contraindicated in people with chronic malabsorption syndromes and hypersensitivity to the drug.[74] Patients with cholestasis should not receive the medication, since it may theoretically impair gallbladder motility and predispose them to gallstone formation, a problem which is also associated with significant weight loss. The manufacturer warns that orlistat should be used with caution in patients with hyperoxaluria or a history of calcium oxalate nephrolithiasis, as the drug can induce increased levels of urinary oxalate. Orlistat is classified as a Pregnancy Category B drug, so its use for pregnant or lactating women has not been studied.

Significant drug interactions with orlistat have been limited (excepting vitamin K and warfarin), perhaps because of the drug's limited absorption. That is, the interactions would be expected as a consequence of impaired absorption of other drugs rather than effects on metabolism. Case reports of reductions in cyclosporine levels in orlistat patients have led the manufacturer to recommend that the drugs not be coadministered.[74,88] Since the interaction is presumably due to decreases in cyclosporine absorption, the two agents should be separated by at least 2 hours if administered concomitantly.[74]

Little data exist regarding combination therapy with sibutramine and orlistat. In a recent study of obese women, an 11.6% loss of body weight was achieved during a year of treatment with sibutramine and lifestyle modification.[89] This was followed by randomization for 16 more weeks of either sibutramine plus orlistat or sibutramine plus placebo. No difference between groups was seen in the final 16 weeks, with the combination drug therapy group gaining an average of 0.1 kg and the sibutramine alone group gaining 0.5 kg. A problem in this study may have been that patients knew which group they were assigned to, due to the gastrointestinal side effects of orlistat.

Other Weight Loss Agents

Other digestive inhibitors include olestra and plant stanols and sterols. Olestra (Olean) is a nondigestible, nonabsorbable fat substitute made by combining sucrose and methyl esters of fatty acids.[90] It has been incorporated into certain snack foods, such as chips and crackers. Consumption of foods containing olestra may decrease total fat and saturated fat in the diet of some people, which would be the desired effect.[91] As with orlistat, there is concern that consumption of substantial amounts of olestra may result in malabsorption of fat soluble vitamins. Thus, foods containing this fat substitute are supplemented with vitamins A, D, E, and K.[90] Other lesser-known fat substitutes which are carbohydrate- or protein-based include carbohydrate-based polymers such as maltodextrin and microparticulated egg white and milk protein such as Simplesse.[92]

Plant stanols and sterols have recently been introduced into the American food industry in the form of margarines and salad dressings. Trade names of products containing these products include Benecol and Take Control. They decrease the absorption of cholesterol from the gastrointestinal tract, thus lowering serum cholesterol concentrations.[93] A 2 g amount of these substances found in an average daily portion (three servings) results in a reduction in serum LDL cholesterol of about 10% to 15%.[93] These products are currently quite expensive compared to their more conventional counterparts.

Adrenergic agents approved by the FDA for short-term treatment of obesity include benzphetamine (Didrex), diethylpropion (Tenuate), mazindol (Mazanor, Sanorex), phendimetrazine (various), and phentermine (various). One approach would be to use one of these agents for a period of time, discontinue the therapy, and then restart it when weight regain begins. Another approach has been to use one of these agents on an "on-off" schedule. For example, one study showed that using phentermine for 4 weeks followed by a 4-week hiatus resulted in weight loss as effective as when the drug was used continuously.[94]

This approach was also used by the researchers who performed the landmark studies with the fenfluramine-phentermine combination.[95] From weeks 34 to 104 of this 2-year study, some patients were cycled on and off the anorectics, with the end-of-year holidays and spring targeted as times to have subjects on active drugs. A 2-week taper-off period was employed when patients went off drug therapy. The intermittent groups did almost as well as the continuous therapy groups in terms of weight lost at the end of the study, but the intermittent group had more problems adhering to diet and with appetite control during the periods off the drugs. The intermittent groups also complained of more side effects, and more of these patients dropped out of the study compared to patients treated continuously. The authors of this study concluded that continuous therapy was superior to intermittent therapy.

Selective serotonin reuptake inhibitors such as fluoxetine have been investigated as weight loss agents since some patients do lose weight when initiated on this class of drugs. None of these agents is currently approved by the FDA for this use. Patients receiving fluoxetine have been shown to have decreases in caloric intake with no decrease in frequency of eating, suggesting that the primary mechanism of weight loss with these agents may be to induce satiety rather than to decrease appetite.[96]

Studies with fluoxetine have shown that although weight loss may occur during the first 6 months of therapy, after 6 months weight regain is frequent.[53] Since the effect of fluoxetine on satiety begins within 4 to 6 days of starting therapy, one author has suggested that the drug might be useful for short periods when overeating is anticipated, such as holidays or vacations.[96] Data to specifically support this hypothesis have not yet been published.

A plethora of nonprescription medications and dietary supplements have been marketed for use in weight control programs. Until recently, the nonprescription adrenergic agent phenylpropanolamine was listed by the FDA

Selected Dietary Supplements Included in Weight Loss Products

- ❏ L-carnitine
- ❏ Cayenne
- ❏ Chromium
- ❏ Corn silk
- ❏ Couchgrass
- ❏ Cranberry
- ❏ *Garcinia cambogia*
- ❏ Ginger
- ❏ Ginseng
- ❏ Guarana
- ❏ Juniper berry
- ❏ Ma huang
- ❏ Parsley
- ❏ Purple willow
- ❏ Uva ursi

as a Category I (safe and effective) agent for weight control. The potential for central nervous system (CNS) toxicities (such as nervousness, insomnia, and headache) and cardiovascular system toxicities (such as hypertension and stroke) with phenylpropanolamine use have long been recognized.

A study late in 2000 showed a 17-fold increase in hemorrhagic strokes in women who had taken phenylpropanolamine. This publication led to a request to the manufacturers by the FDA to remove products containing this medication from the market.[56] Controversy continues as to whether this action was truly justified given the available evidence, but it is unlikely to be reversed.[97] This ingredient removal affects not only the weight loss market, but also the common cold products market and the veterinary market. Phenylpropanolamine has been commonly used to treat urinary incontinence in cats and dogs.[97]

Some dietary supplements in popular weight loss products include ma huang, hydroxycitric acid, and chromium. Limited data exist to support whether they actually promote weight loss. In addition, safety and efficacy data are lacking concerning the many combinations of these ingredients found in commercially available products.

Dietary supplements containing ephedra alkaloids, such as ma huang, have also been associated with severe CNS and cardiovascular side effects.[98] The ephedra alkaloids include ephedrine, pseudoephedrine, and norpseudoephedrine.[99] The FDA has been attempting to pass rules restricting single serving amounts and daily consumption guidelines of ephedra since 1997.[100]

This effort has been complicated by criticism from another governmental agency, the General Accounting Office (GAO).[101] The GAO claimed that the FDA failed to establish a scientific basis for its regulations on ephedra, questioning the reliability of the MedWatch reports upon which the regulations were partially based. The Dietary Supplement Health and Education Act of 1994, which minimizes the ability of the FDA to regulate dietary supplements, further complicates this issue. Ironically, with manufacturer withdrawal of phenylpropanolamine from the marketplace, some manufacturers are promoting ephedrine-containing products in their place for weight loss.[97]

Another dietary supplement promoted as an antiobesity agent is hydroxycitric acid, the active compound in the herbal product *Garcinia cambogia*. This ingredient inhibits the enzyme adenosine triphosphate-citrate and could theoretically reduce fat mass by inhibiting lipogenesis.[102] This agent was studied in a 12-week randomized, double-blind, placebo-controlled trial.[102] The study failed to show significantly greater weight or fat mass loss in the *Garcinia* group.

Some experts criticized this study because, for the drug to effectively inhibit lipogenesis, it needs to be administered with a carbohydrate-rich diet.[103,104] Also, the energy restricted diet utilized did not allow evaluation of hydroxycitric acid's ability to decrease food intake.[104] Another limitation of this study should be taken into account when performing or interpreting clinical studies with all dietary supplements: since these agents are very loosely regulated, studies should measure blood levels of the active ingredient, when this is known, to make sure that the product utilized has acceptable bioavailability.[104]

Chromium, particularly as the picolinate salt, is another dietary supplement promoted for weight loss. Chromium has long been recognized as a component of the so-called glucose tolerance factor, and is considered a cofactor in lipid and carbohydrate metabolism.[99] Picolinic acid forms a stable complex with chromium, resulting in good bioavailability.[99] Dietary intake of chromium in humans may be suboptimal; a person's response to chromium depends on chromium status as well as type of diet consumed.[105] Limited data would support that chromium supplementation may increase lean body mass and decrease body fat in some individuals, if given in adequate dosages for sufficient lengths of time.[105]

Other agents with potential in the treatment of obesity include the thermogenic β-3 agonists and the gene products leptin and neuropeptide Y antagonists. The β-3 receptor enhances thermogenesis in brown adipose tissue in animal models.[106] β-3 receptor agonists also improve insulin sensitivity and blood lipid levels, indicating promise for treatment of patients with diabetes.[58] Some of the failure to produce an effective β-3 agonist for weight control in humans may relate to differences between rodent and human receptors, which differ by 10% to 20% in their amino acid sequences.[106] Some researchers have proposed that brown adipose tissue is a relatively unimportant site for thermogenesis in humans.[58] Although brown fat is abundant in human neonates, it is greatly reduced in adults.[106] Poor bioavailability has also been a problem with some of the compounds tested.

Leptin is a hormone synthesized in adipose tissue which circulates in the serum.[107,108] It binds to receptors in the hypothalamus, altering expression of several neuropeptides that regulate energy intake and expenditure.[107] One of these neuropeptides is neuropeptide Y; leptin downregulates neuropeptide

Y, resulting in reduced appetite.[107] Administration of leptin to leptin-deficient obese mice results in weight loss. Although a few leptin-deficient obese people have been identified, circulating leptin levels are actually elevated in most of them, indicating that obesity in humans may typically represent a disease of leptin resistance.[107] Although it remains to be seen whether leptin or its analogues will play a therapeutic role in the treatment of obesity, the study of this hormone is helping to increase knowledge of energy homeostasis.

SURGICAL TREATMENT OF OBESITY

The most successful technique for long-term treatment of morbid obesity is surgery. Patients whose BMI exceeds 40 are potential candidates for bariatric surgery. Patients with BMIs of 35 to 40 who also have high-risk comorbid conditions such as life-threatening cardiopulmonary problems or severe diabetes mellitus are also considered surgical candidates.

Details of surgical procedures are beyond the scope of this discussion, but can be found in other references.[109-111] The reader is also referred to other references for descriptions of liposuction and its potential side effects.[112,113] Matarasso, et al., state that the purpose of liposuction is more to "achieve greater harmony in body proportions rather than to produce weight loss or a change in body or clothing size."[112]

ECONOMIC IMPACT OF OVERWEIGHT AND OBESITY

The economic impact of overweight and obesity is substantial, but specific estimation of costs is difficult for several reasons.[114] Disparate definitions of overweight and obesity exist, in a variety of studies and from different countries. Estimates of cost are influenced by the selection of which obesity-associated diseases to include. As well, it is hard to determine how much of the cost of treating a disease is associated with obesity. Mortality rates should be taken into account when making estimates, since obese people tend to have higher mortality rates.

Published studies from around the world indicate that obesity-related treatments represent between 2% and 7% of the total health expenditure in industrialized countries. Studies from the United States usually show estimates toward the higher end of this range.[114]

A study from a health maintenance organization in the United States reported a correlation between health costs and BMI.[115] Costs were about 25% higher for individuals with a BMI of 30 to 34.9 compared to those with a BMI of 20 to 24.9. Costs were 44% higher for those with a BMI of 35 or more.

In the year 2000, the Internal Revenue Service of the United States revised policies to allow tax relief to some individuals who pay out-of-pocket for weight loss programs.[116] These policies were liberalized in 2002. The American Obesity Association, which has lobbied for these Internal Revenue Service policy changes, now states that "obesity is medically accepted to be a disease in its own right" and that "Uncompensated amounts paid by individuals for participation in a weight-loss program as treatment for a specific disease or diseases (including obesity) diagnosed by a physician are expenses for medical care that are deductible."

CONCLUSIONS

Achievement and/or maintenance of a healthy weight is a life-long struggle for many people. Various strategies, including regular exercise programs, dietary discretion, and other behavioral modifications may be helpful. For those who are obese, or those who are significantly overweight with comorbid conditions who have failed with other measures, pharmacotherapy may be an option.

At this time, though, no "magic bullet" exists which makes weight loss or weight maintenance easy. The prescription agents indicated for long term use are expensive. Even people who can afford them may be disappointed with their own results, especially if they are not motivated to combine the drugs with exercise and diet. Bariatric surgery may be a viable option for some morbidly obese patients. But for most, the "secret" to weight maintenance consists of a healthy diet, a regular fitness plan, and the discipline to make good habits a part of everyday life.

REFERENCES

1. BRFSS Prevalence Data Gender Grouping. (2000). Available from: http://apps.nccd.cdc.gov/brfss/sex.asp?cat=WC&yr=2000&qkey=4386&state=US. Accessed June 12, 2002.
2. Partnership for Healthy Weight Management. (2001). Available from: http://www.consumer.gov/weightloss/. Accessed June 13, 2002.
3. National Task Force on the Prevention and Treatment of Obesity. Overweight, obesity, and health risk. *Arch Intern Med.* 2000;160:898-904.
4. National Heart, Lung, and Blood Institute of the National Institutes of Health. Clinical guidelines on the identification, evaluation, and treatment of overweight and obesity in adults: the evidence report (1998). Available from: http://www.nhlbi.nih.gov/guidelines/obesity/ob_gdlns.pdf. Accessed June 13, 2002.
5. Strawbridge WJ, Wallhagen MI, Shema SJ. New NHLBI clinical guidelines for obesity and overweight: will they promote health? *Am J Public Health.* 2000;90:340-3.
6. Eckel RH, Krauss RM. American Heart Association call to action: obesity as a major risk factor for coronary heart disease. *Circulation.* 1998;97:2099-100.
7. World Health Organization. Obesity epidemic puts millions at risk from related diseases. (1997). Available from: http://www.who.int/archives/inf-pr-1997/en/pr97-46.html. Accessed June 13, 2002.
8. National Heart, Lung, and Blood Institute of the National Institutes of Health and North American Association for the Study of Obesity. The practical guide: identification, evaluation, and treatment of overweight and obesity in adults. (2000). Available from: http://www.nhlbi.nih.gov/guidelines/obesity/prctgd_c.pdf. Accessed June 13, 2002.
9. World Health Organization. Controlling the global obesity epidemic. (2001). Available from: http://www.who.int/nut/obs.htm. Accessed June 13, 2002.
10. Mokdad AH, Serdula MK, Dietz WH, et al. The spread of the obesity epidemic in the United States, 1991-1998. *JAMA.* 1999;282:1519-22.
11. Centers for Disease Control. Update: prevalence of overweight among children, adolescents, and adults. United States, 1988-1994. *MMWR Morb Mortal Wkly Rep.* 1997;46:199-202.
12. Centers for Disease Control. Physical activity trends: United States, 1990-1998. *MMWR Morb Mortal Wkly Rep.* 2001;50:166-9.
13. Wilding J. Science, medicine, and the future: obesity treatment. *Br Med J.* 1997;315:997-1000.

14. Centers for Disease Control. Prevalence of overweight among children and adolescents: United States, 1999. (2001). Available from: http://www.cdc.gov/nchs/products/pubs/pubd/hestats/over99fig1.htm. Accessed June 14, 2002.

15. North American Association for the Study of Obesity. Frequent dieting among youth may increase future obesity risk. (2000). Available from: http://www.naaso.org/newsflash/dieting.htm. Accessed June 13, 2002.

16. Bray GA. Obesity: a time bomb to be defused. *Lancet*. 1998;352:160-1.

17. Allison DB, Fontaine KR, Manson JE, et al. Annual deaths attributable to obesity in the United States. *JAMA*. 1999;282:1530-8.

18. Manson JE, Willett WC, Stampfer JM, et al. Body weight and mortality among women. *N Engl J Med*. 1995;333:677-85.

19. Brown CD, Higgins M, Donato KA, et al. Body mass index and the prevalence of hypertension and dyslipidemia. *Obes Res*. 2000;8:605-19.

20. Shekelle RB, Shyrock AM, Paul O, et al. Diet, serum cholesterol, and death from coronary heart disease: The Western Electric study. *N Engl J Med*. 1981;304:65-70.

21. Reeder BA, Angel A, Ledoux M, et al. Obesity and its relation to cardiovascular disease risk factors in Canadian adults: Canadian Heart Health Surveys Research Group. *CMAJ*. 1992;146:2009-19.

22. Colditz GA, Willett WC, Rotnitzky A, et al. Weight gain as a risk factor for clinical diabetes mellitus in women. *Ann Intern Med*. 1995;122:481-6.

23. Ford ES, Williamson DF, Liu S. Weight change and diabetes incidence: findings from a national cohort of US adults. *Am J Epidemiol*. 1997;146:214-22.

24. Chan JM, Rimm EB, Colditz GA, et al. Obesity, fat distribution, and weight gain as risk factors for clinical diabetes in men. *Diabetes Care*. 1994;17:961-9.

25. Syngal S, Coakley EH, Willett WC, et al. Long term weight patterns and risk for cholescystectomy in women. *Ann Intern Med*. 1999;130:471-7.

26. Douketis JD. The long-term effectiveness of weight reduction interventions in patients with obesity: a critical review of the literature. *Journal of Clinical Outcomes Management*. 2000;7(5):31-44.

27. National Research Council. *Recommended Dietary Allowances*. 10th ed. Washington, DC: National Academy Press; 1989.

28. Pi-Sunyer FX. Obesity. In: Shils ME, Olson JA, Shike M, et al., eds. *Modern Nutrition in Health and Disease*. 9th ed. Baltimore: Williams & Wilkins; 1999.

29. Hill JO, Peters JC. Environmental contributions to the obesity epidemic. *Science*. 1998;280:1371-4.

30. Womble LG, Wang SS, Wadden TA. Behavioral treatment of obesity. *TEN The Economics of Neurosciences*. 2000;2(8):53-8.

31. American Dietetic Association. Weight management: position of ADA. *J Am Diet Assoc*. 1997;97:71-4.

32. American Dietetic Association. Position of The American Dietetic Association: very-low-calorie weight loss diets. *J Am Diet Assoc*. 1990;90:722-6.

33. Howard AN. The historical development of very low calorie diets. *Int J Obesity*. 1989;13(suppl 2);1-9.

34. Rossner S. Intermittent vs. continuous VLCD therapy in obesity treatment. *Int J Obesity*. 1998;22:190-2.

35. Bray GA, Popkin BM. Dietary fat intake does affect obesity! *Am J Clin Nutr*. 1998;68:1157-73.

36. Willett WC. Is dietary fat a major determinant of body fat? *Am J Clin Nutr*. 1998;67:556S-62S.

37. Willett WC. Dietary fat and obesity: an unconvincing relation. *Am J Clin Nutr*. 1998;68:1149-50.

38. Seedily JC. Dietary fat and obesity: an epidemiologic perspective. *Am J Clin Nutr*. 1998;67:546S-50S.

39. United States Department of Agriculture. Dietary Guidelines for Americans. (2000). Available from: http://www.health.gov/dietaryguidelines/dga2000/document/frontcover.htm. Accessed June 14, 2002.

40. United States Department of Agriculture. Food Guide Pyramid. (2000). Available from: http://www.pueblo.gsa.gov/cic_text/food/food-pyramid/main.htm. Accessed June 14, 2002.

41. Rolls BJ, Miller DL. Is the low-fat message giving people a license to eat more? *J Am Coll Nutr*. 1997;16:535-43.

42. Allara L. The return of the high-protein, low-carbohydrate diet: weighing the risks. *Nutr Clin Pract*. 2000;15:26-9.

43. Westman EC. A review of very low carbohydrate diets for weight loss. *Journal of Clinical Outcomes Management*. 1999;6(7):36-40.

44. Official Atkins Website. (2001). Available from: http://www.atkinsdiet.com. Accessed June 14, 2002.

45. National Weight Control Registry. (2001). Available from: http://www.uchsc.edu/nutrition/nwcr.htm. Accessed June 14, 2002.

46. North American Association for the Study of Obesity. New research examines effectiveness and weight loss maintenance of the low carbohydrate diet. (2001). Available from: http://www.naaso.org/newsflash/atkins.htm. Accessed June 14, 2002.

47. Willi SM, Oexmann MJ, Wright NM, et al. The effects of a high-protein, low-fat, ketogenic diet on adolescents with morbid obesity: body composition, blood chemistries, and sleep abnormalities. *Pediatrics.* 1998;101:61-7.

48. American College of Cardiology. Sessions highlight importance – and controversies – of heart-healthy diets. (2001) Available from: http://www.acc.org/media/session%5Finfo/newsconf/acc2001/2001index.htm#tuesday. Accessed June 14, 2002.

49. American Heart Association. Guidelines for weight management programs for healthy adults. (1994). Available from: http://216.185.112.5/presenter.jhtml?identifier=1226. Accessed June 14, 2002.

50. Shape Up America and American Obesity Association. Guidance for treatment of adult obesity. (1998). Available from: http://secure.cartsvr.net/catalogs/catalog.asp?prodid=1348864&showprevnext =1. Accessed June 14, 2002.

51. APhA Comprehensive Weight Management Protocol Panel. APhA Drug Treatment Protocols: comprehensive weight management in adults. *J Am Pharm Assoc.* 2001;41:25-31.

52. Apovian CM. Antiobesity drugs: should they be used in the treatment of obesity? *Nutr Clin Pract.* 1998;13:251-6.

53. Hensrud DH. Pharmacotherapy of obesity. *Med Clin North Am.* 2000;84:441-62.

54. Office of Public Affairs, Food and Drug Administration. FDA warns against consuming dietary supplements containing tiratricol. (2000). Available from: http://www.fda.gov/bbs/topics/ANSWERS/ANS01057.html. Accessed June 14, 2002.

55. Connolly HM, Crary JL, McGoon MD, et al. Valvular heart disease associated with fenfluramine-phentermine. *N Engl J Med.* 1997;337:581-8.

56. Kernan WN, Viscoli CM, Brass LM, et al. Phenylpropanolamine and the risk for hemorrhagic stroke. *N Engl J Med.* 2000;343:1826-32.

57. Khan LK, Serdula MK, Bowman BA, et al. Use of prescription weight loss pills among U.S. adults in 1996-1998. *Ann Intern Med.* 2001;134:282-6.

58. Cerulli J, Lomaestro BM, Malone M. Update on the pharmacotherapy of obesity. *Ann Pharmacother.* 1998;32:88-102.

59. Meridia [package insert]. Mt. Olive, NJ: Knoll Pharmaceutical Company; 2000.

60. Luque CA, Rey JA. Sibutramine: a serotonin-norepinephrine reuptake-inhibitor for the treatment of obesity. *Ann Pharmacother.* 1999;33:968-78.

61. Bray GA, Ryan DH, Gordon D, et al. A double-blind randomized placebo-controlled trial of sibutramine. *Obes Res.* 1996;4:263-70.

62. Bray GA, Blackburn GL, Ferguson JM, et al. Sibutramine produces dose-related weight loss. *Obes Res.* 1999;7:189-98.

63. Apfelbaum M, Vague P, Ziegler O, et al. Long-term maintenance of weight loss after a very-low-calorie diet: a randomized blinded trial of the efficacy and tolerability of sibutramine. *Am J Med.* 1999;106:179-84.

64. James WPT, Astrup A, Finer N, et al. Effect of sibutramine on weight maintenance after weight loss: a randomised trial. *Lancet.* 2000;356:2119-25.

65. Wadden TA, Berkowitz RI, Sarwer DB, et al. Benefits of lifestyle modification in the pharmacologic treatment of obesity. *Arch Intern Med.* 2001;161:218-27.

66. Anonymous. Weight loss drug aids heart health. *US Pharmacist.* 2001;26(1):10.

67. Cole JO, Levin A, Beake B, et al. Sibutramine: a new weight loss agent without evidence of the abuse potential associated with amphetamines. *J Clin Psychopharmacol.* 1998;18:231-6.

68. Schuh LM, Schuster CR, Hopper JA, et al. Abuse liability assessment of sibutramine, a novel weight control agent. *Psychopharmacology (Berl).* 2000;147:339-46.

69. Bach DS, Rissanen AM, Mendel CM, et al. Absence of cardiac valve dysfunction in obese patients treated with sibutramine. *Obes Res.* 1999;7:363-9.

70. McMahon FG, Fujioka K, Singh BN, et al. Efficacy and safety of sibutramine in obese white and African American patients with hypertension: a one-year, double-blind, placebo-controlled, multicenter trial. *Arch Intern Med.* 2000;160:2185-91.

71. Hadvary P, Sidler W, Meister W, et al. The lipase inhibitor tetrahydrolipstatin binds covalently to the putative active site serine of pancreatic lipase. *J Biol Chem.* 1991;266:2021-7.

72. Hauptman JB, Jeunet FS, Hartman D. Initial studies in humans with the novel gastrointestinal lipase inhibitor Ro 18-0647 (tetrahydrolipstatin). *Am J Clin Nutr.* 1992;55:309-13S.

73. Zhi J, Melia AT, Eggers H, et al. Review of limited systemic absorption of orlistat, a lipase inhibitor, in healthy human volunteers. *J Clin Pharmacol.* 1995;35:1103-8.

74. Xenical [package insert]. Nutley, NJ: Roche Laboratories Inc; 1999.

75. Heck AM, Yanovski JA, Calis KA. Orlistat, a new lipase inhibitor for the management of obesity. *Pharmacotherapy.* 2000;20:270-9.

76. Sjostrom L, Rissanen A, Andersen T, et al. Randomised placebo-controlled trial of orlistat for weight loss and prevention of weight regain in obese patients. *Lancet.* 1998;352:167-73.

77. Hauptman J, Lucas C, Boldrin MN, et al. Orlistat in the long-term treatment of obesity in primary care settings. *Arch Fam Med.* 2000;9:160-7.

78. Hill JO, Hauptman J, Anderson JW, et al. Orlistat, a lipase inhibitor, for weight maintenance after conventional dieting: a one year study. *Am J Clin Nutr.* 1999;69:1108-16.

79. Rossner S, Sjostrom L, Noack R, et al. Weight loss, weight maintenance, and improved cardiovascular risk factors after two years treatment with orlistat for obesity. *Obes Res.* 2000;8:49-61.

80. Anonymous. Roche seeks new indication for Xenical for treatment of type 2 diabetes. (2001 Mar 22). Available from: http://www.rocheusa.com/newsroom/current/2001/pr2001032201.html. Accessed June 14, 2002.

81. Hollander PA, Elbein SC, Hirsch IB, et al. Role of orlistat in the treatment of obese patients with type 2 diabetes: a one year randomized double-blind study. *Diabetes Care.* 1998;21:1288-94.

82. Heymsfield SB, Segal KR, Hauptman J, et al. Effects of weight loss with orlistat on glucose tolerance and progression to type 2 diabetes in obese adults. *Arch Intern Med.* 2000;160:1321-6.

83. Davidson MH, Hauptman J, DiGirolamo M, et al. Weight control and risk factor reduction in obese subjects treated for two years with orlistat: a randomized controlled trial. *JAMA.* 1999;281:235-42.

84. Halstad CH. Is blockade of pancreatic lipase the answer? *Am J Clin Nutr.* 1999;69:1059-60.

85. Zhi J, Melia AT, Guerciolini R, et al. The effect of orlistat on the pharmacokinetics and pharmacodynamics of warfarin in healthy volunteers. *J Clin Pharmacol.* 1996;36:659-66.

86. Sjostrom L, Rissanen A, Golay A. Orlistat and weight loss: author's reply. *Lancet.* 1998;352:1474.

87. Food and Drug Administration. Meeting 69, NDA 20-766, Xenical (Orlistat tetrahydroliastatin [sic]). (1998 Mar 13). Available from: http://www.fda.gov/ohrms/dockets/ac/98/transcpt/3393t2.rtf. Accessed June 14, 2002.

88. Colman E, Fossler M. Reduction in blood cyclosporine concentrations by orlistat. *N Engl J Med.* 2000;13:1141-2.

89. Wadden TA, Berkowitz RL, Womble LG, et al. Effects of sibutramine plus orlistat in obese women following one year of treatment by sibutramine alone: a placebo-controlled trial. *Obes Res.* 2000;8:431-7.

90. Lawson KD, Middleton SJ, Hassall CD. Olestra, a nonabsorbed, noncaloric replacement for dietary fat: a review. *Drug Metab Rev.* 1997;29:651-703.

91. Patterson RE, Kristal AR, Peters JC, et al. Changes in diet, weight, and serum lipid levels associated with olestra consumption. *Arch Intern Med.* 2000;160:2600-4.

92. Warshaw H, Franz M, Powers MA, et al. Fat replacers: their use in foods and role in diabetes medical nutrition therapy. *Diabetes Care.* 1996;19:1294-301.

93. Law M. Plant sterol and stanol margarines and health. *Br Med J.* 2000;320:861-4.

94. Munro JF, MacCuish AC, Wilson EM et al. Comparison of continuous and intermittent anorectic therapy in obesity. *Br Med J.* 1968;1:352-4.

95. Weintraub M, Sundaresan PR, Schuster B, et al. Long-term weight control study. II: weeks 34 to 104. *Clin Pharmacol Ther.* 1992;51:595-601.

96. Greeno CG, Wing RR. A double-blind, placebo-controlled trial of the effect of fluoxetine on dietary intake in overweight women with and without binge-eating disorder. *Am J Clin Nutr.* 1996;64:267-73.

97. Otto A. Was it really necessary to take PPA off the market? *Pharmacy Today.* 2001;7(3):1-2.

98. Haller CA, Benowitz NL. Adverse cardiovascular and central nervous system events associated with dietary supplements containing ephedra alkaloids. *N Engl J Med.* 2000;343:1833-8.

99. Doering PL. Overweight and obesity. In: *Handbook of Nonprescription Drugs.* 12th ed. Washington, DC: American Pharmaceutical Association; 2000:465-80.

100. Food and Drug Administration: Dietary Supplements Containing Ephedrine Alkaloids; Proposed Rule. Federal Register 1997. Available from: http://www.cfsan.fda.gov/~lrd/fr97064a.html. Accessed June 14, 2002.

101. Blumenthal M. GAO criticizes Food and Drug Administration's (FDA) proposed regulations on ephedrine-containing dietary supplements: report notes lack of science in FDA process. *HerbalGram.* 1999;47:34-7.

102. Heymsfield SB, Allison DB, Vasselli JR, et al. Garcinia cambogia (hydroxycitric acid) as a potential antiobesity agent: a randomized controlled trial. *JAMA.* 1998;280:1596-600.

103. Badmaev V, Majeed M, Conte AA. Garcinia cambogia for weight loss. *JAMA.* 1999;282:233-4.

104. Schaller JL. Garcinia cambogia for weight loss. *JAMA.* 1999;282:234.

105. Anderson RA. Effects of chromium on body composition and weight loss. *Nutr Rev.* 1998;56:266-70.

106. Lowell BB, Flier JS. Brown adipose tissue, β3-adrenergic receptors, and obesity. *Annu Rev Med.* 1997;48:307-16.

107. Mantzoros CS. The role of leptin in human obesity and disease: a review of the current evidence. *Ann Intern Med.* 1999;130:671-80.

108. Rosenbaum M, Leibel RL, Hirsch J. Obesity. *N Engl J Med.* 1997;337:396-406.
109. National Institutes of Health, Consensus statement. *Gastrointestinal surgery for severe obesity.* 1991;9(1):1-20.
110. Mun EC, Blackburn GL, Matthews JB. Current status of medical and surgical therapy for obesity. *Gastroenterology.* 2001;120:669-81.
111. Shikora SA. Surgical treatment for severe obesity: the state-of-the-art for the new millennium. *Nutr Clin Pract.* 2000;15:13-22.
112. Matarasso A, Hutchinson OHZ. Liposuction. *JAMA.* 2001;285:266-8.
113. Rao RB, Ely SF, Hoffman RS. Deaths related to liposuction. *N Engl J Med.* 1999;340:1471-5.
114. Kortt MA. Obesity cost-of-illness studies: an international perspective. *TEN The Economics of Neuroscience.* August 2000;2:59-62.
115. Quesenberry CP Jr, Caan B, Jacobson A. Obesity, health services use, and health care costs among members of a health maintenance organization. *Arch Intern Med.* 1998;158:466-72.
116. American Obesity Association. IRS figures weight loss programs into tax deductible medical expenses. Available from: http://www.obesity.org/subs/tax/taxguide.shtml. Accessed June 14, 2002.

CHAPTER 9

DIET AND DISEASE

Melvin Baron, Lisa Nicholson

Diet exerts a strong influence over medical illness. A healthy diet can prevent or delay the development of a chronic illness, while a poor diet may be one of many risk factors that hasten its progression. Yet diet tends to be underappreciated as a factor in disease prevention and outcomes.

Atherosclerosis is a classic example of this medical phenomenon: a high-fat diet increases the risk, while a low-fat, high-fiber diet lowers serum lipids and may actually reverse plaque buildup in the arteries. Some conditions, such as certain types of anemia, can even be cured by diet. For other diseases, diet is an effective treatment. In the progression from chronic renal disease to renal failure, dietary management prevents further symptoms and reduces complications.

Eating habits include both the behaviors involved in eating and the actual foods consumed. Both are key considerations when evaluating a patient's diet and the role it may play in an illness. Dietary interventions, to be successful, must begin with assessing what patients eat as well as when and why they eat what they do. A patient may know what diet is best for a medical condition, but be unable to, or simply choose not to, follow that diet. Factors such as socioeconomic status, access to healthy foods, cultural beliefs, and personal values can have a profound influence.

Medical nutrition therapy is the application of dietary interventions to the treatment of a medical illness or condition. It has several components, consisting first of the assessment of nutritional status, followed by diet, counseling, and specialized nutrition therapy. Often medical nutrition therapy involves educating patients, breaking down their barriers to change, and guiding them toward more desirable eating habits. Examples of conditions that can be managed with medical nutrition therapy include hypertension, hyperlipidemia, type 2 diabetes mellitus, osteoporosis, and obesity.

All of these chronic medical conditions may respond to nutritional intervention; for some, however, pharmacotherapy will also be necessary. Therefore, an initial risk stratification by the clinical team is desirable. Nutritional and pharmacological therapy will be used sequentially or concurrently in many patients, and the intensity of pharmacotherapy depends on the patient's disease risk

341

classification, the speed with which control is needed, and the risk of experiencing drug-related adverse events. In low-risk individuals, diet and lifestyle changes may be tried initially, but for patients who do not succeed or respond to such changes, drugs may be prescribed. Patients who have trouble changing their nutritional and lifestyle habits may eventually need more intense pharmacotherapy to control their symptoms than would otherwise be required. For some patients, the possibility of avoiding uncomfortable and expensive multiple drug regimens may be a motivating factor to make lifestyle changes.

This chapter broadly reviews several chronic diseases or medical conditions, including type 2 diabetes mellitus, cardiovascular disease (e.g., coronary heart disease, hypertension, stroke, and atherosclerosis), renal disease, anemia, osteoporosis, cancer, dental health, and eating disorders. Nutritional care approaches are recommended for each. Also included for each disease or condition is a set of questions that can be used by pharmacists to gauge patients' medical and nutritional status, as well as their understanding and self-management of their conditions.

Providing optimal care to patients requires more than one concerned pharmacist, however. It takes physicians, pharmacists, dietitians, and other members of the health care team working together. When weighing therapeutic options, the best approach is to conduct a thorough individualized assessment of the potential benefits and risks of each potential treatment. This is only achieved through a coordinated multidisciplinary effort.[1]

DIABETES MELLITUS

Diabetes mellitus is a group of metabolic diseases characterized by a defect in insulin secretion, insulin action, or both. Insulin, a hormone produced by the beta cells of the pancreas, is necessary for the metabolism of carbohydrate, protein, and fat. When the body is unable to utilize carbohydrates effectively, the result is high blood glucose levels, or hyperglycemia, which can lead to serious short-term and long-term complications.

Some of the short-term consequences of insufficient blood glucose control include glycosuria, water and electrolyte loss, ketoacidosis, and coma. Long-term risks include neuropathy, retinopathy, nephropathy, generalized degenerative changes in large and small blood vessels, and increased susceptibility to infection. These gradual tissue changes may lead to debilitating complications such as limb ischemia and amputation, vision loss, and kidney failure. In addition, diabetes is associated with a very high risk of heart disease. All of this explains why good control of diabetes mellitus is so important. In fact, most people with diabetes are able to sufficiently control their condition to prevent or minimize serious complications.

Diabetes affects an estimated 16 million Americans. More than 10 million people have been diagnosed, and an estimated 5.4 million people have undiagnosed forms of the disease. The risk of diabetes increases with age and also is higher in certain ethnic groups in the United States, including Hispanics, Native Americans, African Americans, Asian Americans, and Pacific Islanders. The prevalence is slightly higher in women than in men.[2]

The American Diabetes Association (ADA), the National Institute of Diabetes and Digestive and Kidney Diseases, and the Centers for Disease Control and Prevention adopted new diagnostic criteria for diabetes in 1997. The routine diagnostic test is now the fasting plasma glucose test rather than the oral glucose tolerance test. A confirmed fasting plasma glucose value of greater than or equal to 126 mg/dL is the diagnostic threshold. When diabetes symptoms are present, a confirmed nonfasting plasma glucose value of greater than or equal to 200 mg/dL indicates a diagnosis of diabetes.

The same group of organizations reached a consensus to eliminate the terms "insulin-dependent diabetes mellitus" (IDDM) and "non-insulin dependent diabetes mellitus" (NIDDM). These have been replaced by the terms "type 1" and "type 2" diabetes, respectively.[3]

Diabetes treatments include medical nutrition therapy, exercise, blood glucose monitoring, and, frequently, medications (i.e., exogenous insulin or drugs that increase insulin secretion or action). Dietary self-management is the cornerstone of disease treatment, but a great deal of patient education and training are required to master blood sugar monitoring and proper dietary balance. The goal of treatment is to normalize blood glucose levels to prevent or delay complications, while minimizing weight gain and hypoglycemia. Morbidity and mortality can be reduced by early treatment and good metabolic control. See page 348 for counseling tips.

Type 1 Diabetes

Type 1 diabetes is characterized by destruction of the insulin-producing beta cells located in the pancreas. The cause is not well known, but appears to relate to an autoimmune process set in motion early in life by a "trigger" mechanism, such as a virus, allergy, environment toxin, or stressful lifestyle. It may take months or years to develop, or type 1 diabetes may also have a sudden onset, when pancreatic trauma or disease damages or destroys the beta cells. In either case, the symptoms of type 1 diabetes become noticeable at a fairly advanced stage, when around 70% of the beta cells have been destroyed. Most individuals progress to absolute insulin deficiency (i.e., when the body produces no insulin), and exogenous insulin will be needed to prevent ketoacidosis and death.

Type 1 diabetes accounts for 5% to 10% of all diagnosed cases of diabetes.[2] Although it may occur at any age, most cases are diagnosed in people younger than 30 years of age, with a peak incidence between the ages of 10 and 12 years in girls and 12 and 14 years in boys. For this reason, type 1 diabetes used to be referred to as "juvenile onset" diabetes.

Type 2 Diabetes

Type 2 diabetes is characterized by insulin resistance (i.e., its diminished effectiveness in lowering blood sugar levels) and relative, rather than absolute, insulin deficiency. The insulin concentration may be normal, depressed, or elevated, but it is inadequate to overcome the decreased tissue sensitivity and responsiveness associated with the insulin resistance. The cause of type

2 diabetes may relate to a variety of factors ranging from deficiencies in the amount or function of insulin receptors (possibly due to a genetic susceptibility, a virus, or another trauma), to "lifestyle" triggers such as obesity, lack of exercise, age, and chronic stress. Insulin secretion and function decline with age, and insulin resistance increases with age. The prevalence of diabetes is almost 10% for Americans over the age of 60.

Patients with type 2 diabetes are not prone to developing ketoacidosis except during times of severe stress. Therefore, most of them do not require exogenous insulin for survival. However, approximately 40% of them will eventually require exogenous insulin for adequate blood glucose control. Insulin may also be required for control during periods of stress-induced hyperglycemia.[4]

Type 2 diabetes accounts for 90% to 95% of all diagnosed cases. Approximately 80% of patients are obese or have a history of obesity at the time of diagnosis; however, type 2 diabetes can occur in nonobese people as well, especially in the elderly.[4] Along with advancing age, obesity, and physical inactivity, additional risk factors include a family history of diabetes, a prior history of gestational diabetes, impaired glucose homeostasis, and ethnicity.[2]

Nutritional Care of Diabetes

Nutritional therapy is an essential component in managing type 1 and type 2 diabetes. The primary goal is to help patients improve their metabolic control by modifying their eating and exercise habits. Specifically, medical nutrition therapy helps patients to:[5]

- Maintain near-normal blood glucose levels.
- Control serum lipids.
- Improve dietary and lifestyle habits.
- Prevent future complications.

Patients can achieve most of these goals by following the Dietary Guidelines for Americans.[6] The following recommendations are of particular importance to patients with diabetes:

- Choose a diet that is low in saturated fat and cholesterol and moderate in total fat.
- Consume a variety of grains daily, especially whole grains.
- Eat a variety of fruits and vegetables daily.
- Pick beverages and foods that help to moderate your intake of sugars.
- If you drink alcoholic beverages, do so in moderation.
- Be physically active each day.

Carbohydrate Intake

In the past, diabetic patients were advised to reduce their intake of carbohydrate-rich foods, especially those containing simple sugars. Under current recommendations, all individuals, including those with diabetes, are advised to consume at least 55% of their daily calories from carbohydrates. Complex carbohydrates (e.g., whole grain foods, fruits, and vegetables) are emphasized as the best choices because they contain more dietary fiber and nutrients than refined or simple carbohydrates. However, the glycemic response of carbohydrates cannot always be predicted by their molecular structure (i.e., starch versus sugar). Research has shown that starches can have the same glycemic response as sucrose and a higher glycemic response than fruits or milk.[5] There is ongoing research into the glycemic effect of complex carbohydrates and simple sugars.

Fat Intake

Diabetic patients are at high risk of developing cardiovascular disease. As a result, they need to minimize their dietary fat intake, especially the saturated fats found in animal foods. This will improve the blood lipid profile and help protect against vascular disease. In addition, a high-fat diet has been shown to increase insulin resistance.

Protein Intake

Diabetic individuals with normal kidney function should eat a moderate amount of protein, typically comprising around 10% to 15% of their total daily calories. Some patients with kidney disease may need to modify their protein intake downward from this level, while others might need to increase protein intake, depending on the nature and extent of their kidney damage.

Meal Planning and Timing

Preventing weight gain is a critical priority for people with diabetes. Consistency in food intake, as well as an individualized meal plan, improves glycemic control and weight management. Unfortunately, adherence to meal plans can be the most challenging aspect of diabetes care.[4] Therefore, to facilitate achievement of these objectives, the ADA emphasizes the importance of individualized nutritional management. In other words, the diet must meet the nutritional, emotional, and cultural needs of the diabetic patient.

Day-to-day consistency in the timing and the amount of food is also important, particularly for patients receiving conventional insulin therapy (i.e., one or two injections per day, as opposed to an insulin pump). Patients should synchronize meals and snacks with the action of their insulin, monitor their blood glucose levels, and when necessary, adjust insulin dosage to the amount of food eaten. Intensive insulin therapy (i.e., three or more injections per day) or the use of an insulin infusion pump gives the patient greater flexibility to choose when and what to eat. Aggressive management of blood glucose has been shown to prevent or delay the progression of retinopathy, microalbuminuria, and neuropathy in patients with type 1 diabetes. In general, this management approach consists of monitoring blood glucose levels and administering insulin with greater frequency compared with conventional control.[7]

Diet and Exercise

For people with type 2 diabetes, diet and exercise are the key components of managing their disease. Moderate weight loss, regardless of initial body weight, has been shown to reduce hyperglycemia, insulin resistance, dyslipidemia, and hypertension.[5] Even small amounts of weight loss (i.e., under 10 lbs) can improve diabetes control. However, this is a very difficult undertaking for many people, and most do not succeed in losing pounds and maintaining a lower body weight. Diabetic individuals may be more effective at maintaining a metabolically healthy weight if they are encouraged to focus on the "total picture" of diabetes self-management—controlling their blood glucose, eating a balanced diet, and increasing daily physical activity—rather than simply on losing weight.

Synchronizing Medications with Meals

When blood glucose levels cannot be adequately controlled by diet and exercise alone, medications are added. Some medications, including sulfonylurea drugs, biguanides (such as metformin), and alpha glucosidase inhibitors (such as acarbose), are sensitive to dietary composition or timing of meals. Acarbose slows gastrointestinal absorption of carbohydrates by inhibiting the production of enzymes that hydrolyze glucosides. Both the side effects and the efficacy of the drug are linked to the carbohydrate content of the diet.[4] Metformin functions as an "insulin sensitizer" by decreasing hepatic glucose production and improving glucose uptake in muscle, and may be less well absorbed when taken with meals. Sulfonylurea agents increase insulin secretion, and vary with regard to whether or not they should be taken with meals. These and other drug-nutrient interactions for selected type 2 diabetes medications are summarized in Table 9-1.

CARDIOVASCULAR DISEASE

Cardiovascular disease (CVD) is the name given to a broad disease syndrome relating to the heart and the blood vessels or the circulation. It is manifested in a number of chronic or episodic conditions, including coronary heart disease, hypertension, stroke, peripheral artery disease, and atherosclerosis. Many of these conditions are life threatening. Often they occur in combination. See page 356 for patient counseling tips.

Atherosclerosis

Atherosclerosis is the major underlying cause of many forms of CVD, including the most lethal of these, coronary heart disease (see sidebar on page 350). It is a slow, progressive disease that begins in childhood and takes decades to advance.

TABLE 9-1 Drug and Nutrient Interactions in Diabetes Mellitus

Drug	With Food	Empty Stomach	Comments	Nutritional Interactions
Glyburide	X			May deplete coenzyme Q_{10}.
Glipizide		X	Take 30 min before meal to increase effectiveness.	
Glimepiride	X			
Acarbose	X		Take with the first bite of each main meal.	May decrease serum Ca and vitamin B_6 levels.
Miglitol	X		Take with the first bite of meal.	
Metformin	X		Food decreases and delays absorption.	Decreases serum vitamin B_{12} levels in 7% of patients.
Repaglinide		X	Take from 30 minutes before meal to immediately before meal.	
Rosiglitazone			Take with or without meals.	
Pioglitazone			Take with or without meals.	

Source: References 8 and 9.

The root cause of atherosclerosis is structural and compositional changes in the innermost intimal layer of the large arteries. Due to these changes, lipid deposits and other materials build up along the intima, or arterial wall. These deposits are referred to as arterial plaque, or atheroma.

Currently, atherosclerosis is understood as both an inflammatory and a proliferative response to arterial wall injuries,[10] with plaque forming in response to the damaged endothelium. Risk factors leading to injury may include hypercholesterolemia, oxidized low-density lipoprotein, hypertension, cigarette smoking, diabetes, obesity, elevated homocysteine, and diets high in cholesterol and saturated fat.

There is a direct relationship between total blood cholesterol (TC) and the incidence of CHD and its associated mortality. In addition, epidemiologic studies have shown that populations consuming diets high in saturated fat, such as in the United States, have higher blood cholesterol levels and greater CHD risk than elsewhere. However, the good news is that the progression of atherosclerosis can be slowed or halted and coronary heart disease can be considerably reversed through lifestyle modification.[1]

Low-density lipoprotein cholesterol (LDL-C), sometimes referred to as "bad" cholesterol, is the main culprit and the primary transporter of cholesterol in the blood. LDL-C can be oxidized and taken up by endothelial cells and macrophages in the arterial wall, leading to the first stages of atherosclerosis. Levels of LDL-C are highly correlated with TC and CHD risk.

High-density lipoprotein cholesterol (HDL-C), or "good" cholesterol, is engaged in reverse transport, or removal of LDL-C from the blood. High

Educating Patients About Diabetes: Questions Pharmacists Should Ask

Q. How long ago were you diagnosed with diabetes?

(This information helps you to determine the patient's risk of complications based on number of years since diagnosis.)

Q. Do you have any other health problem, such as kidney disease, heart disease, high blood pressure, vision problems, pain in your hands or feet, or increased frequency of colds?

(Patients should report other health problems, especially sudden changes in symptoms, to their physicians.)

Q. Do you know how to measure your blood sugar? How often do you measure your blood sugar? Do you keep a record of results to show your physician?

(Keeping frequent and accurate blood glucose records will help the physician determine the most appropriate timing, spacing, and type of insulin for them.)

Q. Do you know what blood sugar levels you are trying to achieve at different times of day (i.e., morning, after meals, and before bedtime)? Which numbers indicate that your blood sugar is too high or too low?

(Explain the importance of keeping blood sugar levels within a safe range, and encourage patients to talk with their physicians if they cannot identify these numbers. Describe how the timing of meals and medications, poor fluid intake, changes in injection site, exercise changes, stress, illness, and use of other medications can affect blood sugar control.)

Q. What do you do if you have low blood sugar numbers?

(Explain that low blood sugar can occur when a meal is skipped or after exercise. Encourage patients to keep juice or glucose tablets with them for such occasions. Make sure patients on insulin understand the potential risk of using too much insulin without food to balance the dose.)

Q. Do you measure ketones in your urine? Do you know the symptoms of ketoacidosis?

(High ketone levels, high blood sugar, thirst, and frequent urination are the first symptoms of ketoacidosis. Symptoms progress to nausea, vomiting, and confusion. If these symptoms appear, patients should warn someone that they may be going into diabetic shock and should seek medical treatment immediately. Diabetic ketoacidosis can result in coma and death. See note on the following page about MedicAlert bracelet.)

Q. How many injections of insulin do you use daily? Which types do you use? What combinations have worked best for you? Do you vary your injection sites?

(Do the type of insulin and number of injections seem appropriate for this patient?)

Q. How are you storing your insulin?

(Remind the patient to store insulin in the refrigerator and to follow any other recommendations made by the manufacturer.)

Q. Have you talked with your physician or a dietitian recently about your diet? Do you know how to plan your meals using the dietary exchange lists?

(Refer the patient to the ADA or the American Dietetic Association to learn about meal planning and exchange lists. Advise patients to review their dietary plan regularly with their physicians, diabetes educators, or dietitians.)

Q. Have you been gaining or losing weight?

(Unintended weight gain or loss may indicate a problem with their disease management. Advise patients to check with their physician because changes in weight may require adjustments in medication.)

Q. What other medications, vitamins, or herbs do you take?

(Is the patient taking dietary supplements or other medications that influence diabetic control?)

Q. Do you wear a MedicAlert bracelet or other identification that shows you have diabetes?

(Recommend that the patient obtain a bracelet and provide the phone number for MedicAlert.)

levels of HDL-C are associated with reduced risk of atherosclerosis, and the ratio between TC and HDL-C can also be used to predict the risk of coronary events. A high risk of CHD is associated with a TC:HDL-C ratio of 5.6 or greater in women and 6.4 or greater in men. Therefore, a TC:HDL-C ratio of 6 in women or 7 in men is considered the target for starting intervention.

Cholesterol Screening and Treatment Guidelines

Guidelines for preventing and treating atherosclerosis are coordinated on a national level through the National Cholesterol Education Program (NCEP) of the National Heart, Lung, and Blood Institute. New clinical guidelines for cholesterol testing and management were published by the NCEP in 2001,

The Real Killer: Coronary Heart Disease

Coronary heart disease (CHD) is the most deadly of all cardiovascular diseases. Also known as coronary artery disease or ischemic heart disease, it is caused by obstructions in the network of blood vessels surrounding and serving the heart, leading to a chronic or abrupt halt in blood flow that can damage the myocardium (heart muscle tissue). When the damage is sudden (such as when plaque ruptures along the arterial wall and blocks the passage of blood through the artery), the result is a heart attack, or acute myocardial infarction. The primary underlying cause is atherosclerosis.

One in nine women and one in six men have coronary heart disease by the age of 65 years. Myocardial infarction is the leading cause of death in American men and women, and is responsible for half of all deaths from cardiovascular causes in the United States. Mortality from heart disease increases with age in all races.

and are contained in the *Third Report of the Expert Panel on Detection, Evaluation, and Treatment of High Blood Cholesterol in Adults* (Adult Treatment Panel III, or ATP III guidelines).[11]

As a starting point, NCEP recommends that all people age 20 and older obtain a fasting lipoprotein profile (consisting of TC, LDL-C, HDL-C, and triglyceride measurements) at least once every 5 years. The ATP III risk classification system is described in the sidebar on page 351. Patients at increased risk of developing CHD are those with high TC and LDL-C, and those with low HDL-C, according to the ATP III guidelines. Interventions are based on a stepped-care approach and focus on the use of CHD risk status to guide the intensity of therapy and to pinpoint the cholesterol-lowering goals (e.g., the target serum cholesterol levels).

The recommended treatment for atherosclerosis and elevated risk of CHD consists of monitoring cholesterol levels, instituting lifestyle interventions (i.e., diets that progressively reduce saturated fat and cholesterol, combined with weight reduction, physical activity, and smoking cessation), and prescribing medications. Interventions will be more intensive in patients who have an increased risk of developing CHD than for those at lower risk.

Treatment decisions concerning dietary requirements, the frequency of cholesterol measurement, and the need for medication are determined by cholesterol measurements combined with the individual's CHD risk profile (i.e., the presence and number of multiple CHD risk factors). Numerous factors besides serum cholesterol determine CHD risk, including the presence of CHD, diabetes, hypertension, or low HDL-C; cigarette smoking; family history of premature CHD; and age (with the risk increasing at 45 years and above in men and 55 years and above in women).

Additional risk assessments may be conducted in people who appear to have an elevated risk of atherosclerosis and CHD, and these results also may contribute to the treatment plan. An example would be arterial imaging,

The NCEP Adult Treatment Panel III Classification of LDL, Total, and HDL Cholesterol Levels

Total Cholesterol (TC)

Less than 200 mg/dL (5.20 mmol/L)	Desirable
200 to 239 mg/dL (5.20–6.15 mmol/L)	Borderline high
240 mg/dL (>6.20 mmol/L) and above	High

Low-Density Lipoprotein Cholesterol (LDL-C)

Less than 100 mg/dL (<2.58 mmol/L)	Optimal
100 to 129 mg/dL (2.58–3.35 mmol/L)	Near or above optimal
130 to 159 mg/dL (3.35–4.10 mmol/L)	Borderline high
160 to 189 mg/dL (4.15–4.88 mmol/L)	High
190 mg/dL (4.90 mmol/L) and above	Very high

High-Density Lipoprotein Cholesterol (HDL-C)

Less than 40 mg/dL (1.03 mmol/L)	Low
60 mg/dL (1.55 mmol/L) or above	High

Source: Reference 11.

where the degree of change in vessel stenosis may be used to make treatment decisions.

Diet has long been recognized as the cornerstone to lowering blood cholesterol. The NCEP's ATP III guidelines recognize this, and recommend dietary therapy as the first approach. Aggressive therapy is recommended for people with preexisting CHD or at least two CHD risk factors. Dietary management is the first step in treatment, and medications are recommended only if nutritional intervention fails to reduce LDL-C levels below 100 mg/dL (2.58 mmol/L) in patients with CHD, or below 130 mg/dL (3.35 mmol/L) in patients with two or more CHD risk factors.

When pharmacotherapy is required, the availability of new and more effective cholesterol-lowering drugs, including a new generation of statin agents, can be expected to improve compliance with medications. However, drug therapy does not eliminate the need for continued nutrition intervention in people at risk for CHD.[11]

It is important to note that a number of other medications, in addition to cholesterol-lowering agents, are commonly prescribed for patients with extremely high cholesterol or existing CHD. Table 9-2 describes the drug-nutrient interactions for many of these cardiovascular medications.

Hypertension

High blood pressure in adults, or hypertension, is defined as a systolic pressure of 140 mm Hg or higher and/or a diastolic pressure of 90 mm Hg or higher on two or more separate visits. It affects an estimated 50 million

TABLE 9-2 Drug–Nutrient Interactions for Cardiovascular Medications

Drug	With Food	Empty Stomach	Food Interactions/Effects on Nutrients
Atenolol			May be taken without regard to meals; may deplete coenzyme Q_{10}.
Labetalol	X		Food may increase bioavailability; may deplete coenzyme Q_{10}.
Metoprolol	X		Food enhances bioavailability; may deplete coenzyme Q_{10}.
Nadolol			May be taken without regard to meals; may deplete coenzyme Q_{10}.
Furosemide		X	Food decreases bioavailability; may deplete Ca, Mg, K, Zn, and thiamin.
Triamterene/HCTZ			May deplete K, Ca, and folic acid.
Hydrochlorothiazide			May deplete Mg, K, Na, and Zn.
Spironolactone		X	May interact with food; may deplete Ca and folic acid.
Captopril		X	Administer one hour before meals; may deplete Zn; use caution with K.
Verapamil	X		Sustained release; should be given with food.
Isosorbide mononitrate			Do not drink alcohol.
Isosorbide dinitrate			Do not drink alcohol.
Digoxin			Patient must maintain normal serum K, Mg, and Ca levels to avoid toxicity.
Nitroglycerin			Do not drink alcohol.
Nitroquick			Do not drink alcohol.
Hydralazine	X		Taking with food will result in higher plasma levels; may deplete vitamin B_6.
Terazosin			Do not drink alcohol; use caution with valerian and kava kava.
Prazosin			Do not drink alcohol; use caution with valerian and kava kava.
Warfarin			Patient must maintain constant intake of vitamin K (green leafy vegetables); avoid ginkgo and high doses of vitamin E.
Pentoxifylline	X		

Source: Reference 8.

Americans, or about one in every four adults. However, only an estimated two-thirds of adults with hypertension are properly diagnosed. The remaining one-third of individuals have undiagnosed hypertension.[13]

Lifestyle modifications are recognized as the first steps in preventing and treating high blood pressure.[1] The Joint National Committee on Detection, Evaluation, and Treatment of High Blood Pressure has issued Step 1 and Step 2 recommendations. Step 1 therapy consists of lifestyle modification alone, including weight reduction, exercise, increased dietary potassium, and elimination of alcohol consumption. Step 2 continues lifestyle modification and introduces pharmacological treatment, and is initiated when there is an inadequate response to Step 1.

Weight reduction and dietary modifications can be effective early steps for reducing blood pressure for many people. In one study of patients with high-normal diastolic blood pressure (DBP), moderate sodium restriction lowered diastolic pressure by 0.9 mm Hg and weight reduction lowered diastolic pressure by over twice that amount, or 2.3 mm Hg.[1] Pooled data from several randomized clinical trials reinforce these findings, and show that DBP reductions of 2.6 mm Hg can be attained in most patients in response to moderate sodium restriction.

Results obtained with various types of lifestyle modification have been compared among themselves and with that of drug therapy. Decreases in DBP totaling 8.6 mm Hg can be achieved with a combination of lifestyle changes (i.e., weight loss, dietary sodium reduction, decreased alcohol intake, and increased physical activity), and this is compared with decreases averaging 12.3 mm Hg for all drug treatments.[1] Weight loss of approximately 10 kg has been shown to reduce blood pressure without sodium restriction, and with or without concomitant pharmacotherapy.[1] Therefore, evidence suggests that improved blood pressure control can be achieved with current levels of pharmacotherapy when weight loss occurs. When additional steps are taken to restrict sodium and increase dietary potassium intake, it may be possible to reduce levels of medication for hypertension.[1]

Stroke

Stroke is the acute onset of a focal or global neurologic deficit lasting more than 24 hours, attributable to diseases of the intra- or extra-cranial neurovasculature. Severe strokes may be preceded by transient ischemic attacks (TIAs).

Stroke is the third most common cause of death in the United States, accounting for 150,000 deaths annually. Advanced age is the most significant risk factor; however, among modifiable risk factors, hypertension and smoking rank highest. Other risk factors for stroke are CVD, including CHD, atherosclerosis, and atrial fibrillation; diabetes; and oral contraceptive use, particularly by female smokers.

Eighty-five percent of strokes are incited by a thromboembolic event, for which atherosclerosis is a key risk factor. Embolic stroke occurs when a blood clot or plaque travels to the brain from another part of the body and blocks a brain artery. Thrombotic stroke occurs when a local cholesterol plaque ruptures and lodges in an already narrowed brain artery, and resulting platelet aggregation blocks blood flow.

Nutritional Care of Cardiovascular Disease

The NCEP diet modifications have traditionally been aimed at lowering blood cholesterol levels to reduce risk of atherosclerosis and CHD. The long-standing and primary goal has been to lower LDL-C levels by lowering total fat, saturated fat, and cholesterol in the diet, and by adjusting energy intake to achieve appropriate body weight.

ATP III has taken a somewhat different approach and now recommends a complete lifestyle approach to reducing CHD risk. The guidelines refer to

NCEP ATP III Therapeutic Lifestyle Changes (TLC) Dietary Guidelines

Nutrient	Recommended Amount
Saturated fat[a]	Less than 7% of total calories
Polyunsaturated fat	Up to 10% of total calories
Monounsaturated fat	Up to 20% of total calories
Total fat	25% to 35% of total calories
Cholesterol	Less than 200 mg/day
Carbohydrate[b]	50% to 60% of total calories
Fiber	20 to 30 g/day
Protein	Approximately 15% of total calories
Total calories[c]	Balance energy intake and expenditure to maintain desirable body weight and prevent weight gain

a. *Trans* fatty acids are another category that elevates LDL-C and should be kept at a low intake.
b. Carbohydrates should be derived predominantly from foods rich in complex carbohydrates, including grains, especially whole grains, fruits, and vegetables.
c. Daily energy expenditure should include at least moderate physical activity, i.e., enough to expend approximately 200 kcal/day.

Source: Reference 11.

this approach as "Therapeutic Lifestyle Changes" (TLC),[11] and it now replaces the previous NCEP Step I and Step II diets. The new TLC dietary guidelines are summarized in the sidebar above.

The initial step in TLC is to reduce saturated fat and cholesterol intake and to increase physical activity. After 6 weeks, the LDL-C response should be evaluated. If the LDL-C target has not been achieved, the next step is to reinforce the need to reduce intake of saturated fat and cholesterol, and to boost soluble fiber intake. Consideration should be given to adding plant stanols/sterols to the diet, with these latter supplements now available in medical margarines. Once again, it will be necessary to reassess serum cholesterol levels to determine the response to these dietary changes. If the LDL-C goal is still unmet and progress has not reached appropriate levels, weight management and physical activity should be intensified and drug therapy may be considered.

Numerous dietary factors interact to affect serum lipids, atherogenesis, and CHD risk. Many dietary substances have been investigated: not only fat and cholesterol quantity and quality, but also the role of fiber, antioxidants, and other dietary components.

High fat diets increase postprandial lipidemia and chylomicron remnants (i.e., the least dense of the plasma lipoproteins that transport cholesterol in the blood), both of which are associated with increased risk of CHD. In general, saturated fatty acids are the worst offenders. When substituted for carbohydrate or other fatty acids, they tend to elevate blood cholesterol in all lipoprotein fractions. Consuming fish and fish oils rich in omega-3 fatty acids tend to reverse this process, and has been associated with decreased platelet aggregation and reduced risk of stroke.[14]

The amount of total fat in the diet is related to obesity, which affects many of the major risk factors for atherosclerosis. Individuals with baseline high-fat diets, simply by losing weight, may find their TC has been reduced by as much as 25%. A meta-analysis of 2244 dietary intervention studies has estimated that a change from the typical American diet to the NCEP Step I diet would result in average TC and LDL-C reductions of 5%.[1]

Dietary cholesterol also raises TC and LDL-C, but to a lesser extent than saturated fat. Cholesterol responsiveness varies widely among individuals. Some people are hyporesponders (i.e., their plasma cholesterol level does not increase after dietary cholesterol challenge), while others are hyperresponders (i.e., serum cholesterol levels respond to a cholesterol challenge more strongly than expected).

Dietary factors that reduce circulating serum cholesterol are also important. Soluble fibers such as pectins, gums, mucilages, algal polysaccharides, and some hemicelluloses serve to lower serum TC and LDL-C. These substances are found in legumes, oats, fruits, and psyllium. Insoluble fibers, such as cellulose and lignin, have no effect on serum cholesterol levels. The recommended fiber intake is 25–30 g per day for adults, and 6–10 g should be from soluble fiber. This level can be achieved with the recommended five or more servings of fruits and/or vegetables per day and six or more servings of grains, as long as whole grains and high fiber cereals are chosen.

Dietary factors can inhibit the oxidation of circulating cholesterol, which reduces cholesterol buildup in plaque. Two dietary factors that affect oxidation are the amount of oxidizable substrates and the amount of antioxidants available to protect the lipoprotein molecule. For example, when the diet is high in polyunsaturated fatty acids the lipoprotein molecule has many easily oxidized elements. But when antioxidants such as vitamins C and E are available, the lipoprotein molecule has protection against oxidation. Epidemiologic studies support this finding and suggest that antioxidant vitamins reduce CVD; however, randomized trials have not consistently supported this concept. Evidence is strongest for the role of vitamin E in cholesterol protection; one of vitamin E's major functions is to prevent oxidation of polyunsaturated fatty acids in the cell membrane. Other antioxidants, such as the carotenoids, may have a greater protective effect later in the process of atherosclerosis than they do in the earliest stages of plaque development.

Most types of CVD respond well to dietary intervention; however, primary prevention remains the cornerstone for managing stroke. This can be accomplished in part by dietary means, along with other lifestyle behaviors. Once stroke has occurred, however, dietary reduction of cholesterol, fat, and salt are of questionable benefit. Malnutrition is predictive of a poor outcome in stroke management, and therefore efforts at that point are directed toward maintaining nutritional status. In addition, often a stroke will introduce physical or neurologic deficiencies that make eating difficult and tend to limit

Educating Patients About Cardiovascular Disease: Questions Pharmacists Should Ask

Q. Has your physician told you that you have heart disease? What type of heart disease do you have and how long have you had it?

(Determine which types of cardiovascular disease the individual has; encourage patients to see their physicians regularly to discuss symptoms and any problems they have complying with treatment or medications).

Q. What symptoms are you experiencing? How often do you experience these symptoms and have they changed recently?

(Determine whether patient is having serious symptoms. A change in symptoms may indicate a worsening of the condition. Patients experiencing serious or new symptoms should be encouraged to talk with a physician as soon as possible).

Q. Are you currently taking any prescription or over-the-counter (OTC) drugs? Which ones?

(Determine whether patients are taking drugs that do not seem appropriate for the condition they described, or are taking drugs that interact with each other's effectiveness or tolerability.)

Q. Are you taking vitamins, minerals, herbal products, or any other type of dietary supplements? Which ones, and why do you take them?

(Is the patient taking any drugs or supplements that may interfere with their treatment, cause side effects, or interact with other prescription medications? Advise patients to discontinue any supplements that are contraindicated due to their existing medications or disease. Explain to patients that even OTC drugs or supplements should not be taken without their physician's knowledge or approval.)

Q. Has your physician or dietitian given you a special diet? How well do you follow those instructions?

(Diet and lifestyle changes can be extremely successful at improving risk factors and preventing or delaying the progression of cardiovascular disease. Therefore, you should reinforce dietary instructions provided by the dietitian or physician. Finally, re-emphasize the importance of losing weight or maintaining a healthy body weight; reducing levels of total fat and saturated fat in the diet; increasing the intake of fruits, vegetables, and whole grains; and exercising regularly in a manner that is appropriate for the patient's cardiovascular condition.)

Q. Do you know the sources of cholesterol and saturated fat in your diet?

(Cholesterol is found only in animal foods. Decreasing the consumption of meat, cheese, and other animal foods reduces dietary cholesterol. Saturated fats usually come from animal foods and are always solid at room temperature. They are contained in meats, milk products, butter, and vegetable shortenings. Liquid fats, such as cooking oils, are typically unsaturated fats.)

Q. Do you have high blood cholesterol levels? Have you tried increasing your intake of soluble fiber foods, or perhaps trying a fiber-rich dietary supplement, such as Metamucil, to help decrease your cholesterol?

(Soluble fiber inhibits absorption of cholesterol from the intestinal tract and thus reduces serum cholesterol levels. Dietary sources of soluble fiber include legumes, oatmeal and oat bran, berries, and some other fruits. Patients should check with their physicians before trying OTC fiber products.)

dietary choices. Patients who are admitted to the hospital after a stroke and who have problems chewing or swallowing may require nutritional support, at least temporarily, until regular eating can be resumed.

RENAL DISEASE

Renal disease has many presentations, including nephrotic syndrome, nephritic syndrome, acute renal failure, tubular defects, renal stones, and end stage renal disease. These different types are a consequence of the portion of the nephron most affected. Treatment approaches and objectives of medical nutrition therapy will vary accordingly. See page 362 for counseling tips.

Nephrotic Syndrome

Nephrotic syndrome, or nephrosis, stems from loss of the glomerular barrier to protein, resulting in increased permeability of the glomerular capillary membranes. This clinical state is characterized by massive edema, proteinuria, hypoalbuminemia, hypercholesterolemia, hypercoagulability, and abnormal bone metabolism. The etiology may be unknown, or related to glomerulonephritis, diabetic glomerulosclerosis, systemic lupus erythematosus, amyloidosis, renal vein thrombosis, or hypersensitivity to various toxic agents.

Nephritic Syndrome

Nephritic syndrome is characterized by inflammation of the capillary loops of the glomerulus. It can be caused by a streptococcal infection, by primary kidney disease, or as a complication of systemic lupus erythematosus. Nephritic syndrome often has a sudden onset and may resolve quickly and proceed to recovery, or may result in chronic nephrotic syndrome or end stage renal disease. Blood in the urine is a symptom of the capillary inflammation, and nephritic syndrome may be accompanied by hypertension and mild loss of renal function.

Acute Renal Failure

Acute renal failure is characterized by a sudden reduction in glomerular filtration rate and a change in the kidneys' ability to excrete the daily load of wastes. It occurs in previously healthy kidneys and may be identified by a sudden reduction in urine output. Duration varies from a few days to several weeks. The long-term outcome is determined by the extent of destruction to renal tissue.

The cause of acute renal failure may be inadequate renal perfusion, diseases within the renal parenchyma, or obstruction. Typically patients develop this condition as a complication of sustained shock due to an overwhelming infection, severe trauma, surgical accident, or cardiogenic shock. Hemodialysis is used to reduce the acidosis, correct the uremia, and control hyperkalemia with the disease. Acute renal failure can sometimes be short-lived and require no particular nutritional intervention as long as attention is paid to diagnosing and correcting the prerenal and obstructive causes. Recovery is characterized first by an increase in urine output and later by the return of waste elimination.

End Stage Renal Disease

End stage renal disease (ESRD) is characterized by the kidney's lasting inability to excrete waste products, maintain fluid and electrolyte balance, and produce hormones. ESRD can result from a variety of kidney diseases and chronic illnesses, and 90% of patients have chronic diabetes mellitus, glomerulonephritis, or hypertension. As renal failure slowly progresses, a point is reached at which the level of circulating waste products leads to symptoms of uremia. ESRD requires either transplantation or dialysis treatment. If transplantation is anticipated it is important to maintain optimal nutritional status.

Hemodialysis and Peritoneal Dialysis

Dialysis, or artificial filtration of waste products from the blood, can be accomplished in one of two ways. The most common method is hemodialysis, in which blood passes through the semipermeable membrane of an artificial kidney. Hemodialysis requires permanent access to the bloodstream through a surgically created fistula. Waste products and electrolytes move by osmosis from the blood into the dialysate and are removed. Dietary protein needs increase to about 1 to 1.2 g/kg body weight to make up for losses through the dialysate.[15]

Peritoneal dialysis makes use of the semipermeable membrane of the peritoneum. A catheter is surgically implanted in the abdomen and into the peritoneal cavity. Dialysate containing a high-dextrose concentration is instilled into the peritoneum, where diffusion carries waste products from the blood through the peritoneal membrane and into the dialysate. Peritoneal dialysis is a less efficient method of removing waste products from the blood, and patients with peritoneal dialysis have higher protein needs (1.2–1.5 g/kg) because of greater protein losses.[15]

Nutritional Care of Renal Disease

Nephrotic Syndrome

Medical nutrition therapy for nephrosis is principally aimed at managing symptoms of edema, hypoalbuminemia, and hyperlipidemia; decreasing the risk of progression to renal failure; and maintaining nutritional stores. The diet should provide sufficient protein and energy to maintain positive nitrogen balance and produce an increase in plasma albumin concentration, leading to resolution of the edema. Historically, patients with nephrotic syndrome received diets high in protein (up to 1.5 g/kg) to increase serum albumin; however, a high protein diet also leads to increased urinary losses. Research has shown that a reduction of protein intake to as low as 0.8 mg/kg can decrease proteinuria without adversely affecting serum albumin.[15] For optimal protein utilization, the use of high quality proteins is recommended.

Edema is the most obvious clinical symptom of nephrosis, and indicates a state of total body sodium overload. However, attempts to limit sodium intake more than modestly and to eliminate large amounts of extra sodium with diuretics can result in marked hypotension, exacerbation of the coagulopathy, and deterioration of renal function. Control of edema in nephrotic syndrome should therefore entail only moderate sodium restriction (of approximately 3 g per day), and must rely to some extent on elastic full-length support hose, which create pressure to return blood from the lower body to the heart and brain. Because of the associated risk of atherosclerosis with nephrotic syndrome, lipid-lowering agents may be prescribed.

Acute Renal Failure

During acute renal failure, physiological stresses that increase protein needs, such as infection or tissue destruction, may be concurrent with the uremia, metabolic acidosis, and fluid and electrolyte imbalances. Nutritional care of this condition is therefore complicated because protein and calorie needs must be balanced with the treatment of acidosis and excessive nitrogenous waste. The key nutrients to monitor are protein, calories, sodium, and potassium. Adequate calories and carbohydrates are needed to prevent the breakdown of protein for energy.

The preferred treatment is parenteral administration of glucose, lipids, and a mixture of essential and nonessential amino acids. Protein needs are influenced by the underlying cause of renal failure and the presence of other conditions. A high-calorie, low-protein diet may be used in cases where dialysis and hemofiltration are unavailable. In addition to the usual high-calorie foods

Dietary Counseling for Renal Patients: Expected Outcomes

After undergoing dietary counseling, renal patients should be able to:

- ❏ Identify high-protein foods and other nutrients as appropriate.
- ❏ Choose foods and amounts according to the meal plan.
- ❏ Eat meals and snacks according to the meal plan.
- ❏ Accurately read food labels.
- ❏ Modify recipes as needed.
- ❏ Use appropriate cooking methods.
- ❏ Avoid or limit alcohol.
- ❏ Select appropriately from restaurant menus.
- ❏ Verbalize potential food/drug interactions.
- ❏ Verbalize importance of regular exercise and smoking cessation.

Source: Reference 16.

such as refined sweets and fats, special high-calorie, low-protein, low-electrolyte formulas are available to augment the diet. Fluid and electrolyte intake should balance the net output. All fluid above the daily calculated water loss should be replaced with a balanced salt solution.

Potassium balance and excretion are disrupted during renal failure. Potassium intake needs to be individualized according to serum levels. The primary mechanism of potassium removal is dialysis. Control of serum potassium levels between dialysis administrations relies mainly on intravenous infusions of glucose, insulin, and bicarbonate, all of which serve to drive potassium into the cells. Exchange resins such as Kayexalate, which exchange K^+ for Na^+ in the gastrointestinal tract, can be used to treat high potassium concentrations, but the treatment is unpleasant. Hyperkalemia, commonly associated with cyclosporine therapy, warrants dietary potassium restriction, although this is usually only temporary.

ESRD

The goals of nutritional management in ESRD are:

1. To prevent nutrient deficiency and maintain good nutritional status and, in the case of children, growth, through adequate protein, calorie, vitamin, and mineral intake.
2. To control edema and electrolyte imbalance by controlling sodium, potassium, and fluid intake.
3. To prevent or retard the development of renal osteodystrophy by controlling calcium, phosphorus, and vitamin D intake.
4. To enable the patient to eat a palatable, attractive diet that fits his or her lifestyle as closely as possible.

The desired outcomes for renal patient counseling are listed in the sidebar above.

Kidney Transplant

Nutritional care of the adult patient who has received a transplanted kidney is directed primarily towards the metabolic effects of the immuno-suppressive therapy. Long-term medications that are typically used include steroids, cyclosporine, azathioprine, and mycophenolate mofetil. Cortico-steroids are associated with accelerated protein catabolism, hyperlipidemia, sodium retention, weight gain, glucose intolerance, and inhibition of normal calcium, phosphorus, and vitamin D metabolism.[8]

ANEMIA

Anemia is a condition characterized by alterations in the number and/or size of red blood cells. Because red blood cells transport oxygen from the lungs to the tissues, a reduction in their size or number results in a limited capacity to oxygenate the tissues. The clinical symptoms include lethargy, weakness, poor concentration, shortness of breath after minor exertion, pale complexion, increased susceptibility to colds and infection, and mild depression. In advanced stages of anemia, the fingernails also become thin and flat, the tongue becomes smooth and waxy, and stomach disorders develop.

Anemias are typically caused by a lack of nutrients required for normal erythrocyte synthesis, principally iron, vitamin B_{12}, and folic acid. In addition, anemia can result from severe blood loss following an accident or surgery; low-grade, chronic internal bleeding; long-term dietary deficiencies (e.g., deficiencies of iron, vitamin B_{12}, folic acid, vitamin B_6, vitamin C, vitamin E, protein, or copper); impaired absorption or metabolism of nutrients; and negative drug-nutrient interactions involving these nutrients.

Classification of anemia is based on red blood cell size and appearance, and hemoglobin content. The red blood cells may be macrocytic (large), normocytic (normal in size), microcytic (small), hypochromic (pale in color), or normochromic (normal in color). See page 366 for counseling tips.

Megaloblastic Anemia

Megaloblastic anemia is characterized by the presence of large, immature, abnormal red blood cell progenitors in the bone marrow. Vitamin B_{12} and folic acid are essential to the synthesis of nucleoproteins and deficiencies of these vitamins are responsible for 95% of cases of megaloblastic anemia. Resulting hematologic changes are the same for both deficiencies; however, the folic acid deficiency is the first to appear.

Folic acid deficiency anemia is associated with tropical sprue (i.e., a primary intestinal malabsorption associated with enteric infection and nutritional deficiency). It can affect pregnant women, and occurs in infants born to mothers with folic acid deficiency. Chronically deficient diets, faulty absorption and utilization of folic acid, and increased requirements due to growth are the most frequent causes. Because alcohol interferes with the

Educating Patients About Renal Disease: Questions Pharmacists Should Ask

Q. What type of kidney disease do you have? How long have you had this condition and have you experienced any changes in symptoms recently?

(Determine the patient's status and likelihood of complications. Changes in symptoms should be reported to the physician treating the disease.)

Q. Are you on dialysis treatment? What type of dialysis? How are you managing between dialysis treatments?

(Fluid and dietary restrictions are necessary for patients on dialysis. Review the food and liquid aspects of disease management and determine whether the patient is having difficulty complying with the restrictions.)

Q. Do you keep track of your fluid intake each day?

(Ask patients whether they experience fluid buildup, swelling, or weight gain between dialysis sessions. Explain that extra fluid affects their blood pressure and makes their heart work harder. Encourage patients to comply with fluid restrictions and offer tips to help them do so, such as drinking from smaller cups and freezing juice in ice cube trays to eat like popsicles.)

Q. Have you noticed changes in how much water you are retaining? Is there swelling around your ankles? Elsewhere?

(Explain that edema should be monitored, and worsening of edema may indicate poor management of the disease.)

Q. Have you noticed any change in your urine, such as the presence of blood?

(Changes in urine volume or color and the presence of blood in the urine can indicate changes in the disease condition. If so, the patient should report this to the physician. Changes in medication and treatment may be needed.)

Q. What prescription and OTC medications are you taking?

(Determine whether there might be interactions between these medications, or whether any of the prescription or OTC drugs might produce side effects or interfere with disease treatment. Potential interactions should be explained to patients and they should be advised to check with their physicians or pharmacists before taking any OTC drugs or products.)

Q. Do you take multivitamins? Did your physician prescribe them?

(Vitamins and minerals may be missing from the diet due to dietary restrictions, and patients may benefit from a supplement. However, regular supplements purchased off the shelf may contain harmful levels of nutrients. Ask whether their physician has prescribed a special vitamin and mineral supplement, such as Nephrocaps.)

Q. What are your current eating habits? Are you following a specific eating plan?

(Ask about the amount of protein, salt, potassium, and phosphorus the patient is consuming. Explain that the patient may need to increase or decrease certain foods, depending on the renal condition. Foods rich in high-quality protein include meat, fish, poultry, eggs, and milk products. Foods high in sodium include table salt, soups, pretzels and chips, cheeses, cured meats, and processed foods. Foods high in potassium include bananas, dried fruits, kiwis, some salt substitutes, and many fruits and vegetables. Foods high in phosphorus include milk and cheese, meats, dried beans, peas, and nuts.)

folate enterohepatic cycle, most alcoholics have a negative folate balance and the majority are folate deficient.

Administration of folic acid will correct megaloblastosis due to either folate or vitamin B_{12} deficiency. However, folic acid administration can mask the neurologic damage of vitamin B_{12} deficiency and permit the nerve damage to progress to the point of irreversibility.

Pernicious Anemia

Pernicious anemia is a macrocytic, megaloblastic anemia caused by a deficiency of vitamin B_{12} secondary to lack of intrinsic factor. Intrinsic factor is a glycoprotein secreted by the parietal cells of the gastric mucosa and is necessary for the absorption of dietary vitamin B_{12}. Pernicious anemia affects not only the blood, but also the gastrointestinal tract and the peripheral and central nervous systems.

Microcytic Anemia

Microcytic anemia is the last stage of iron deficiency and represents the end of a long period of iron deprivation. The condition is characterized by microcytic erythrocytes (i.e., mean corpuscular volume of 80 cu micrometer or less) and lower circulating hemoglobin concentration.

Iron deficiency is the most common nutrient deficiency in the world. It affects work capacity by reducing blood hemoglobin concentration, thereby decreasing the transport and utilization of oxygen. Iron deficiency in pregnant women is associated with a greater likelihood of low birth weight infants. In infants and young children, iron deficiency adversely affects mental development and behavior.

In the United States, iron deficiency is most common in children age 1–2 years (9%) and females age 12–49 years (9% to 11%).[17] This reflects increased iron needs due to rapid growth in children and menstrual blood losses in women. The many possible causes of iron deficiency anemia are listed in the sidebar on the following page.

> ## Causes of Iron Deficiency Anemia
>
> ❑ Inadequate dietary intake of iron.
> ❑ Poor iron absorption resulting from
>   —Diarrhea
>   —Achlorhydria
>   —Intestinal disease
>   —Atrophic gastritis
>   —Partial or total gastrectomy
>   —Drug interference (antacids, cholestyramine, cimetidine, pancreatin, ranitidine, and tetracycline).
> ❑ Inadequate utilization secondary to chronic gastrointestinal disturbances.
> ❑ Increased iron requirement for growth of blood volume, which occurs during infancy, adolescence, pregnancy, and lactation.
> ❑ Increased iron loss due to excessive menstrual bleeding.
> ❑ Increased iron loss due to hemorrhage or injuries.
> ❑ Chronic blood loss from a bleeding ulcer, bleeding hemorrhoids, esophageal varices, regional enteritis, ulcerative colitis, parasites, or malignant disease.
> ❑ Defective release of iron from iron stores into the plasma.
> ❑ Defective iron utilization due to chronic inflammation.
>
> Source: Reference 4.

Nutritional Care of Anemia

Megaloblastic Anemia

Megaloblastic anemia is usually caused by a deficiency of vitamin B_{12} or folic acid, both of which are essential to the synthesis of nucleoproteins. Normal body folate stores are depleted after 2–4 months of a diet deficient in folic acid, whereas vitamin B_{12} stores are depleted only after several years of inadequate intake. Deficiencies in vitamin B_{12} intake may result from a diet that lacks animal foods and microorganisms, which are the sole sources of vitamin B_{12} in the diet. This eating pattern may be seen with strict vegetarians and with some fad diets.

Diseases that affect the intestinal tract and may affect nutrient absorption, such as tropical sprue and celiac disease, are additional risk factors for megaloblastic anemia. People with chronic alcoholism are also at risk due to poor intake, disruption of the folate enterohepatic cycle by alcohol, and gastrointestinal problems.

A dose of 1 mg of folic acid, taken orally every day for 2 to 3 weeks, will replenish folate stores. When folic acid deficiency is complicated by alcoholism or other conditions that suppress hematopoiesis, increase folate requirements, or decrease absorption, therapy should begin at a dosage of 500 to 1000 mcg per day. Symptoms may improve long before blood values are within normal limits. Rich dietary sources of folate include oranges, orange juice, meats, legumes, soybeans, fruits, vegetables, and fortified cereals.

A deficiency of either vitamin B_{12} or folic acid causes serum homocysteine levels to rise. Abnormally high serum homocysteine levels are associated with heart attacks, clotting strokes, and peripheral vein occlusions. High homocysteine levels are usually treated with vitamin B_6 in infants and children, with folic acid in women of childbearing age, and with oral vitamin B_{12} in the elderly. In elderly patients, the absorption of vitamin B_{12} declines because of gastric atrophy.

Pernicious Anemia

A high-protein diet (1.5 g/kg of body weight) is recommended for patients with pernicious anemia because it is desirable for liver function and for blood regeneration. Because green leafy vegetables contain both iron and folic acid, the diet should contain increased amounts of these foods. Animal source protein is of high biological value and contains heme iron, the most bioavailable form of iron. Liver is a good food choice because it contains iron, vitamin B_{12}, folic acid, and other important nutrients. Food sources of vitamin B_{12} include organ meats, fish, and other meats and dairy products. Vitamin B_{12} treatments include subcutaneous or intramuscular injections of vitamin B_{12}. A nasal gel is also available.

Iron Deficiency Anemia

If the patient has been diagnosed with iron deficiency anemia, attention should be given to the amount of absorbable iron in the diet. Liver, kidney, beef, egg yolk, dried fruits, dried peas and beans, nuts, green leafy vegetables, molasses, whole-grain breads and cereals, and fortified cereals are among the foods highest in iron. If the diet contains mostly non-heme iron from plant foods, beverages or foods rich in vitamin C (citrus fruits and juices, berries) should be included at each meal. Vitamin C can enhance the absorption of iron. Drinking coffee and tea with meals should be discouraged because these beverages can decrease iron absorption.[18]

Repletion of iron stores, not merely alleviation of anemia symptoms, should be the goal of treatment of iron deficiency anemia. Treatment usually involves oral administration of inorganic ferrous iron. Ferrous sulfate is the most widely used preparation. Gastrointestinal side effects of iron supplements include nausea, epigastric discomfort and distention, heartburn, diarrhea, or constipation. Increasing the dose slowly over a few days can minimize the side effects. The dosage can be divided and taken throughout the day to increase iron absorption and decrease side effects.

OSTEOPOROSIS

Osteoporosis, or porous bone, is a disease characterized by low bone mass and structural deterioration of bone tissue. The specific skeletal site cannot withstand ordinary strains, leading to bone fragility and increased

---

Educating Patients About Anemia: Questions Pharmacists Should Ask

Q. Did a qualified medical professional say you have anemia? Was the diagnosis confirmed by blood test? What type of anemia do you have?

(If the patient has been diagnosed, follow up with appropriate dietary or pharmacological goals. If not, ask additional questions to determine what symptoms the patient is experiencing.)

Q. Did your doctor mention iron deficiency anemia?

(Determine whether the patient is taking iron supplements, and which type. Explain the different types of iron and the best way to take the product.)

Q. Did your doctor mention pernicious anemia or vitamin B_{12}?

(Was the patient given advice about vitamin B_{12} or folic acid therapy? If patients have pernicious anemia, advise them not to take folic acid, as it may mask vitamin B_{12} deficiency. Vitamin B_{12} may be given as a supplement, an injection, or as a nasal gel. The physiological function of the patient's gastrointestinal tract will determine the mode of administration.)

Q. Are you taking prescription or OTC drugs for any medical condition?

(Is the patient taking medications that might promote anemia by interfering with iron, folic acid, or vitamin B_{12} metabolism, or by promoting gastrointestinal bleeding?)

---

susceptibility to fractures of the hip, spine, and wrist. Primary osteoporosis occurs in both genders and at all ages but most often strikes postmenopausal women. Secondary osteoporosis is a result of medications or other diseases, including genetic disorders, hypogonadal states, endocrine disorders, gastrointestinal diseases, connective tissue disease, nutritional deficiencies, renal disease, and alcoholism. Glucocorticoid use is the most common form of drug-related osteoporosis and long-term administration for disorders such as rheumatoid arthritis and pulmonary disease is associated with a high rate of fracture.

Osteoporosis or osteopenia (low bone mass) affects 28 million Americans. Ten million people already have osteoporosis and 18 million have osteopenia, placing them at increased risk for this disease. It is estimated that one out of every two women and one out of eight men over the age of 50 years will have an osteoporosis-related fracture in their lifetime.[19]

Osteoporosis is irreversible. It may be prevented by maximizing peak bone mass during the first 2 to 3 decades of life. There is strong evidence that adequate calcium intake and physical activity early in life contributes to higher peak bone mass. Exercise during the later years, in the presence of

TABLE 9-3 Drug and Nutrient Interactions in Bone Disease

Drug	With Food	Empty Stomach	Food Interactions/Effects on Nutrients
Alendronate		X	Must be taken 30 minutes before the first food, beverage, or medication of the day, with plain water only.
Risedronate		X	Must be taken 30 minutes before the first food, beverage, or medication of the day, with plain water only.
Raloxifene			May be taken without regard to meals.

Source: Reference 8.

adequate calcium and vitamin D intake, probably has a modest effect on slowing the decline in bone mineral density (BMD).

Estrogen replacement therapy (ERT) is an established approach for osteoporosis prevention and treatment. There are now several medications that prevent bone loss, strengthen bones, or inhibit fractures in menopausal women. Table 9-3 summarizes the drug–nutrient interactions for these drugs. Optimal treatment of osteoporosis requires that calcium and vitamin D intake meet the recommended levels. See page 370 for counseling tips.

Nutritional Care of Osteoporosis

The most important determinant of skeletal health is the bone mass accumulated early in life. The goal for practitioners is to maximize bone mass early in adulthood and to minimize bone loss later in life. This involves regular physical activity; adequate estrogen status in women; optimal intakes of calcium, vitamin D, and magnesium; limited intakes of dietary protein, sodium, and alcohol; and avoidance of smoking.

The nutrients or food components that are linked to bone health include calcium, vitamin D, magnesium, sodium, protein, caffeine, phosphorus, fluoride, and phytoestrogens for women. Other nutrients may affect bone, such as vitamin K, vitamin C, vitamin A, manganese, copper, iron, zinc, and fatty acids; however, there is insufficient evidence to make recommendations for these nutrients.

Calcium is a fundamental nutrient for maximizing peak bone mass and preventing or treating osteoporosis. Currently, there are two sets of recommendations for dietary calcium: the Institute of Medicine's Dietary Reference Intakes (published in 1997) and the recommendations of a National Institutes of Health Consensus Development Panel on Optimal Calcium Intakes (published in 1994).[20,21] Both sets of recommendations are shown in Table 9-4. Although they may differ by several hundred milligrams of calcium for a particular age or gender group, both sets are notably higher than the previous recommended dietary allowances (RDA). They are also considerably higher than the typical daily calcium intake of all women and for most men.[22]

TABLE 9-4   Recommended Calcium Intakes Throughout the Life Cycle (mg/day)

Institute of Medicine (1997)		National Institutes of Health (1994)	
Birth to 6 months	210	Birth to 6 months	400
6 months to 1 year	270	6 months to 1 year	600
1 to 3 years	500	1 to 10 years	800–1200
4 to 8 years	800	11 to 24 years	1200–1500
9 to 13 years	1300	25 to 50 years (women and men)	1000
14 to 18 years	1300	51 to 64 years (women on ERT and men)	1000
19 to 30 years	1000	65 years or older	1500
31 to 50 years	1000	Pregnant or lactating women	1200–1500
51 to 70 years	1200		
70 years or older	1200		
Pregnant or lactating			
14 to 18 years	1300		
19 to 50 years	1000		

Source: References 20 and 21.

Eating low-fat dairy products is the most desirable way to meet calcium goals. It is much more difficult to meet the recommended calcium intake when dairy products are eliminated from the diet. Other sources of calcium include tofu, sardines and other fish eaten with the bones, and green leafy vegetables. However, the calcium in spinach and some leafy vegetables has low bioavailability. Calcium-fortified beverages and calcium supplements are recommended for patients who cannot get enough calcium from their foods.

Vitamin D is a major determinant of intestinal calcium absorption and it is required for normal bone metabolism. Consumption of vitamin D-fortified dairy products tends to decrease after childhood, and vitamin D intake may not be adequate to support optimal calcium absorption in adolescents and adults. Vitamin D deficiency occurs in older adults, particularly in frail elderly people living in northern climates. The new Dietary Reference Intake for vitamin D increases from 400 IU to 600 IU per day in people over age 70.[20]

Magnesium deficiency disrupts the normal regulation of calcium, vitamin D, and parathyroid hormone. As such, magnesium deficiency may be an important risk factor for osteoporosis, particularly in postmenopausal women.

High intakes of dietary sodium, protein, and caffeine increase the loss of calcium in the urine; however, as long as dietary calcium is adequate, the impact is generally minimal. For every 500 mg increase in dietary sodium, there is an additional loss of 10 mg urinary calcium. For every 50 g increase in dietary protein, there is an additional loss of 60 mg urinary calcium. Although the current medical literature regarding the effects of sodium and protein on bone health is sparse, moderate intakes are advised. In addition to sodium and protein, caffeine increases urinary calcium loss and decreases intestinal calcium absorption, shifting calcium balance in the negative direction. The effect of caffeine becomes most pronounced when dietary calcium is inadequate.

Dietary phosphorus intakes are generally higher than recommended and have been increasing over the last several decades. Some researchers suggest that the combination of high phosphate and low calcium in the diet may increase bone resorption and/or decrease bone formation. However, other researchers conclude that the typical range of phosphorus intake has little effect on bone health.

Isoflavones, coumestans, and lignans are phytoestrogens that, because of their structure, act as estrogen agonists or antagonists. Isoflavones are found in soybeans and they may have protective effects on the bones. Animal studies show promising results, but the role of phytoestrogens in protecting against bone loss in postmenopausal women is unclear.

Early studies of fluoride treatment for osteoporosis have been disappointing because of the narrow therapeutic window and side effects of fluoride. However, recent studies using sustained-release sodium fluoride in combination with calcium citrate demonstrate improved bone mass and reduced spinal fractures.[23] Currently, this medication is not approved for osteoporosis treatment.

Physical activity is essential for bone health. Although the type, frequency, duration, and intensity of exercise affect the outcome, exercise intervention generally increases BMD by 1% to 5% in premenopausal and postmenopausal women. In addition, physical activity may improve muscle strength, balance, coordination, and flexibility, all of which may forestall a fractured bone from a fall.

CANCER

Cancer is a group of diseases characterized by uncontrolled growth and spread of abnormal cells. The root of the problem is damage to their deoxyribonucleic acid (DNA) that interferes with mechanisms that normally regulate the growth and spread of cells. This damage leading to cancer can be caused by external factors (chemicals, radiation, and viruses) or internal factors (hormones, immune conditions, and inherited mutations), and the causative factors may act together or in sequence to initiate and promote carcinogenesis. Ten or more years may pass between carcinogen exposure or mutations and detectable cancer. Surgery, radiation, chemotherapy, hormones, and immunotherapy are used to treat cancer. However, cancer is still the second leading cause of death in the United States.

Nutrition addresses both the causes and the consequences of cancer. Poor nutrition may be related to the etiology of cancer, and existing cancer may affect nutritional status. In addition, many cancer therapies have side effects that affect nutritional intake and status.

Carcinogenesis is a multistage process often described in three progressive stages: initiation, promotion, and tumor progression. Nutrition and cancer relationships may differ according to the stage and type of cancer. A dietary factor that is protective against the initiation of abnormal cells may no longer be protective in the later stages of promotion or progression. This may be one

Educating Patients About Bone Health: Questions Pharmacists Should Ask

Q. Did your doctor diagnose you with osteoporosis? How long have you had this condition?

(Determine how long the patient has had osteoporosis in order to gauge the progression or state of the disease.)

Q. Were you given any dietary advice or medications for your condition?

(Encourage patients to comply with their medication regimens and to follow diet, exercise, and other lifestyle advice. Doing so can delay bone loss and the complications of excess bone loss.)

Q. Do you eat dairy products? How many servings each day? Do you use a vitamin and mineral supplement?

(Assess the patient's eating habits for adequate calcium intake. It may be appropriate to recommend that the patient take a calcium supplement in addition to a multivitamin, multimineral supplement that contains vitamin D.)

Q. Are you being treated for any other medical condition? Are you taking other medications?

(Decide if the patient is at risk for bone loss due to diseases or medications that promote bone loss or interfere with nutrients essential for bone health. If so, recommend that the patient consult their physician about BMD testing.)

Q. I see you have a bone fracture. Have you ever had your BMD tested?

(Determine if the patient has had BMD testing. Adults with vertebral, rib, hip, or distal forearm fractures should be evaluated for osteoporosis and given appropriate therapy. Those patients most likely to have osteoporosis are females of Caucasian or Asian race who have slight body build and are older (i.e., postmenopausal). Recommend that these patients, especially, consult their physicians about BMD testing.)

Q. Are you having any difficulty performing your regular activities?

(Is osteoporosis affecting the patient's quality of life? Elderly patients can be referred to the local agency on aging for assistance such as transportation services or home health care.)

explanation for the results of the Beta Carotene and Retinol Efficacy Trial, in which the use of beta carotene supplements was associated with increased risk of lung cancer in a sample of long-term smokers.[24] Nutrition may be involved at all stages of carcinogen metabolism, cellular and host defenses, cell differentiation, and tumor growth. See page 374 for counseling tips.

American Cancer Society Guidelines on Diet, Nutrition, and Cancer Prevention

❑ Choose most of the foods you eat from plant sources.
❑ Eat five or more servings of fruits and vegetables each day.
❑ Eat other foods from plant sources, such as breads, cereals, grain products, rice, pasta, or beans several times each day.
❑ Limit your intake of high-fat foods, particularly from animal sources.
❑ Choose foods low in fat.
❑ Limit consumption of meats, especially high-fat meats.
❑ Be physically active: achieve and maintain a healthy weight.
❑ Be at least moderately active for 30 minutes or more on most days of the week.
❑ Stay within your healthy weight range.
❑ Limit consumption of alcoholic beverages, if you drink at all.

Source: Reference 25.

Nutritional Care of Cancer

It is estimated that about one-third of the 500,000 cancer deaths that occur in the United States each year may be associated with dietary factors. Another third is due to cigarette smoking. Therefore, among the large majority of Americans who do not smoke cigarettes, dietary choices and physical activity become the most important modifiable determinants of cancer risk.

Although genetics is a factor in the development of cancer, cancer cannot be explained by heredity alone. Behavioral factors such as cigarette smoking, dietary choices, and physical activity modify the risk of cancer at all stages. The introduction of healthful diet and exercise practices at any time from childhood to old age can promote health and reduce cancer risk.[25]

The Cancer Prevention Diet

The goal of cancer chemoprevention is to reverse carcinogenesis in the premalignant phase, reverse precancerous lesions, prevent disease in populations at high risk for recurrent or new disease, and reduce the incidence of specific tumors in the general population. Green tea, various carotenoids, vitamin C, vitamin E, selenium, and folic acid are all being investigated for their chemopreventive potential. The American Cancer Society recommends choosing most foods from plant sources, especially cruciferous vegetables like broccoli and cauliflower, and limiting high-fat foods, especially those from animal sources. The American Cancer Society guidelines for nutritional chemoprevention are in the sidebar above.

TABLE 9-5   How Cancer Treatment Can Affect Nutrition and Eating[26]

Cancer Treatment	Effects on Eating	Potential Side Effects
Surgery	May slow digestion. May lessen the ability of the mouth, throat, and stomach to work properly.	After surgery, some patients may not be able to eat normally and may require nutrition support.
Radiation Therapy	May also damage healthy cells.	Treatment of head, neck, or breast may cause dry mouth, sore mouth or throat, dental problems, difficulty swallowing, and change in food tastes. Treatment of stomach may cause nausea, diarrhea, vomiting, bloating, cramps.
Chemotherapy	May affect the digestive system and decrease the desire to eat.	May cause nausea, vomiting, loss of appetite, sore mouth or throat, diarrhea, constipation, weight gain or loss, change in taste of foods.
Immunotherapy	Can affect the desire or the ability to eat.	May cause nausea, vomiting, sore or dry mouth, severe weight loss, diarrhea, change in taste of food, muscle aches, fatigue, or fever.
Hormonal Therapy	Can increase appetite and change the way the body handles fluids.	May cause changes in appetite, fluid retention.

Source: Reference 26.

The Nutritional Impact of Disease

Cachexia is one of the most severe side effects of cancer. Cachexia is a syndrome of progressive anorexia, weight loss, debility, anemia, and abnormalities in protein, fat, and carbohydrate metabolism.

Recent research has focused on the role of the cytokines to explain metabolic changes and wasting in the individual with cancer. A number of pharmacological agents are being investigated for managing the anorexia-cachexia syndrome including thalidomide, corticosteroids, progestational agents, and recombinant human growth hormone.

Dietary Changes to Accommodate Cancer Therapy

Cells that normally grow and divide rapidly, such as the epithelial cells in the mouth and digestive tract, are most likely to be affected by cancer therapies. Cell damage produces the unpleasant side effects that cause eating problems. Table 9-5 shows some of the gustatory, digestive, and nutritional consequences that may result from cancer treatment.

Many cancer patients lose weight during their treatment. This is partly due to the effects of the cancer itself, but also to the nausea, vomiting, and appetite changes that occur as a result of treatment. Many of the side effects can be controlled with new drugs, so pharmacotherapy should be used in conjunction with dietary management. However, the emotional toll of dealing with cancer can also affect eating habits and body weight.

Additional calories and protein can be added to the diet from commercial meal replacements, such as drinks or shakes, or from supplemental products that can be added to any food or beverage. These supplements are high in protein and calories and have extra vitamins and minerals.

On some cancer treatments, patients may gain weight. If this occurs, patients should be advised to notify their physician to determine what is causing the weight gain. If the weight gain is due to edema, then diuretics or a reduced sodium diet may be indicated. Breast cancer patients with a primary diagnosis of cancer tend to fall into this category, where over half of them actually gain rather than lose weight during treatment.

Patients should be advised to try to eat meals and snacks with sufficient protein and calories to maintain energy, prevent body tissues from breaking down, and rebuild the tissues that cancer treatment may harm. Many patients find their appetite is better in the morning, and if this is the case, they might consider eating their main meal early in the day and have liquid meal replacements later on, when they are less interested in eating. It is a good thing to encourage patients by telling them that they may feel more like eating in a few days, and should not worry about 1 or 2 days with no appetite. If lack of appetite is a persistent problem, they should notify their physicians.

Combined with a loss of appetite, there may be other problems, such as mouth sores or a tender mouth, or difficulty chewing or swallowing. Here are some dietary tips to improve nutritional intake:

- Patients should be advised to eat frequent small meals throughout the day, rather than fewer large ones.
- Beverages are often easier to tolerate than solid foods.
- Softer, cool, or frozen foods, such as yogurt, milkshakes, or popsicles are often the easiest to eat.
- Limiting fluid intake during meals may preserve appetite and help patients consume more food and more calories.
- Foods should be cooked until tender or even pureed before eating, because soft foods are easier to chew and swallow.
- Foods or liquids that can irritate the mouth should be avoided (e.g., acid, spicy or salty foods; rough, coarse or dry foods; and commercial mouthwashes that contain alcohol).

Another side effect of cancer treatment may be a changed sense of taste or smell during the illness or treatment. Foods, especially meat or other high-protein foods, can begin to have a bitter or metallic taste. Many foods will have less taste. Using strong seasoning often increases the interest in food. Alternate sources of protein, such as legumes, may be preferred over meat. Dental problems also can change the way foods taste. For most people, changes in taste and smell go away when their cancer treatment is finished.

Educating Patients About Cancer: Questions Pharmacists Should Ask

Q. Did a physician diagnose you with cancer? Do you think you might have cancer? Why?

(Has the patient been diagnosed with cancer, and what kind? If the patient has noticed something abnormal, such as a lump or growth, unusual discharges or blood in the stool, and symptoms of pain or fatigue, he or she should be encouraged to see their doctor.)

Q. What type of treatment are you getting for your cancer?

(What current and previous treatments has the patient received?)

Q. How long have you been in treatment? Are you noticing any changes in your symptoms or side effects?

(Symptoms may continue even though the patient is receiving treatment; however, patients should report any new or changed symptoms to their doctors. Side effects that were not present at the beginning of radiation or chemotherapy may emerge after a period of time [such as radiation burns or increased fatigue after a prolonged period of ongoing treatment]. Reassure the patient that this is normal.)

Q. Does your treatment cause you to lose your appetite?

(Some treatments can cause loss of appetite, difficulty eating, or nausea. Patients should talk with their physicians or dietitians for tips on how to eat a healthy diet in spite of loss of appetite or nausea. Antiemetics may be used to control nausea.)

Q. Are you taking prescription or OTC drugs for any other condition?

(Interactions may occur between the cancer drugs, and also OTC drugs may produce side effects or interfere with cancer treatment. These potential interactions should be explained. Patients must be advised to check with their physicians or pharmacists before taking any OTC drugs or products.)

Q. Are you using any complementary or alternative medical treatments for your cancer?

(Patients can learn more about alternative cancer therapies from the National Center for Complementary and Alternative Medicine[27] and the Office of Cancer Complementary and Alternative Medicine,[28] but they should be advised to discuss different treatment options with their physicians. All members of the treatment team should know what alternative therapies the patient is currently using.)

DENTAL HEALTH

Diet and nutrition are involved in tooth development, gingival and oral tissue health, bone strength, and the prevention and management of oral diseases. Specific foods may affect tooth condition, and overall diet may affect oral health. Infant feeding practices affect tooth development. In addition, oral health may influence dietary intake.[4] See page 377 for counseling tips.

Dental Caries

Dental caries are caused by the bacterial production of acid resulting from fermentation of carbohydrates in the mouth. This leads to demineralization of tooth enamel and destruction of the tooth structure. Caries are a major cause of tooth loss in the United States. Caries can occur if four factors are present: a susceptible host or tooth surface; microorganisms in the dental plaque; fermentable carbohydrate in the diet; and adequate time in the mouth for bacteria to metabolize the carbohydrate, produce acids, and cause a drop in salivary pH.

Fermentable carbohydrates are found in grains, starches, fruits and fruit juices, sodas, dairy products, and sugars. Dried fruits are especially cariogenic. Xylitol, a five-carbon sugar alcohol, is anticariogenic. Noncarbohydrate sweeteners are cariostatic, meaning they do not contribute to tooth decay.

Chewing promotes saliva production. The flow of saliva clears food from around the teeth and buffers the acid produced by bacteria. Saliva is supersaturated with calcium and phosphorus. Fluoride is the most effective anti-caries agent, and if fluoride is present in the saliva, these minerals are deposited in the erosion resistant form of fluorapatite.

Although saliva is protective, saliva production can decrease as a result of radiation therapy to the head and neck or with the use of some medications. Medications that reduce salivary flow include anti-anxiety agents, anticonvulsants, antidepressants, antihistamines, antihypertensives, diuretics, narcotics, and sedatives.[29]

Periodontal Disease

Periodontal disease is an oral infectious disease characterized by inflammation and destruction of the attachment apparatus of the teeth, including the ligamentous attachment of the tooth to the surrounding alveolar bone. Gingivitis, an early form of periodontal disease, is an inflammation and infection of the gums.

Nutrition is a minor part of the etiology or control of periodontal disease; however, nutrient deficiencies can compromise the associated inflammatory response and wound healing. Malnutrition can alter the volume or the protective properties of saliva. Changes in gum and tooth structure or loss of teeth can affect the ability to chew foods properly and may cause the patient to avoid many foods.

Caries Prevention Guidelines

❑ Brush at least twice daily, preferably after meals.
❑ Rinse mouth after meals and snacks when brushing is not possible.
❑ Chew sugarless gum for 15 to 20 minutes after meals and snacks.
❑ Floss twice daily.
❑ Use fluoridated toothpastes.
❑ Pair cariogenic foods with cariostatic foods.
❑ Snack on cariostatic and anticariogenic foods, such as cheese, nuts, popcorn, and vegetables.
❑ Limit between-meal eating and drinking of fermentable carbohydrates.

Source: Reference 4.

Plaque is the sticky colorless mass of microorganisms, salivary proteins, and polysaccharides that adheres to teeth and gums. In time the plaque combines with calcium and hardens to form calculus. In this state plaque becomes a local irritant to the gums and is a significant factor in the development of periodontal disease. Plaque in the gingival sulcus produces toxins that destroy tissues and permit loosening of the teeth. Healthy epithelial tissue prevents the penetration of bacterial endotoxins into subgingival tissue. Deficiencies of vitamin C, folate, and zinc increase the permeability of the gingival barrier and increase susceptibility to periodontal disease.

Nutritional Care to Promote Dental Health

The major components of a preventive dental regimen include nutrition counseling, fluoride therapy, use of sealants, and control of cariogenic bacteria. The primary factors to consider in determining the cariogenic or anticariogenic properties of food are as follows:

- The form of the food (i.e., liquid, solid, sticky, or long lasting).
- Frequency of consumption of sugar and other fermentable carbohydrates.
- Nutrient composition.
- Sequence of food intake.
- Combinations of foods consumed.

The form and consistency of a food influence its cariogenic potential because of the duration of exposure (retention time). Liquids are rapidly cleared from the mouth and have low adherence capabilities. Solid foods such as crackers, chips, and cookies can stick between the teeth. Chewy foods stimulate saliva production and have a lower adherence potential than solid, sticky foods, such as pretzels or potato chips. Starchy foods have longer duration when stuck between the teeth, because salivary amylase hydrolyzes the starch into simple sugars.

Educating Patients About Dental Health: Questions Pharmacists Should Ask

Q. Do you wear dentures? Are you having any trouble with them?

(Poor fitting dentures may cause patients to change their eating habits, and this could lead to weight loss or nutrient deficiencies.)

Q. How often do you brush your teeth? How often do you floss your teeth?

(Emphasize the importance of brushing the teeth after meals or at least before bedtime. Daily brushing and flossing reduce cavities and decrease the plaque build-up that leads to periodontal disease.)

Q. Are you taking any medicines that dry out your mouth?

(Determine whether any of the patient's medications might decrease saliva production. When saliva production is low, the risk of caries and plaque increases. Recommend that the patient drink water frequently and if necessary, use artificial saliva products.)

Q. Have you noticed soreness around your gums? Have you noticed bleeding when you brush your teeth?

(These may be signs of dental disease and the patient should see a dentist for proper care.)

Caries prevention focuses on a balanced diet, modification of the sources and quantities of fermentable carbohydrates, and the integration of oral hygiene practices into individual lifestyles. Patients using oral rinses or gels should not eat or drink for 30 minutes after using the product. Patients who are taking sodium fluoride should not take it with milk. Brushing, rinsing the mouth with water, or chewing sugarless gum for 15 to 20 minutes should follow meals and snacks. Additional guidelines for preventing dental caries are shown in the sidebar on page 376.

Periodontal Disease

Diet and nutrition also have a distinct bearing on development of periodontal disease. Diet contributes to plaque build-up in the gingival crevices between teeth. Food that is retained around the teeth is metabolized by oral bacteria and contributes to plaque accumulation. Therefore, the same guidelines for caries prevention are useful in prevention of periodontal disease.

EATING DISORDERS

Eating disorders, while considered to be psychiatric disorders, are notable for their nutrition-related aspects. Both anorexia nervosa and bulimia nervosa concern issues such as food intake and related behaviors, body image, and weight regulation, all of which need to be resolved for a patient to fully recover. In many ways, successful treatment amounts to resolving the entire nutritional lifestyle. A medical nutrition therapy approach to lifestyle change is therefore appropriate for these illnesses. However, treatment needs to deal with the psychological and nutritional aspects of eating disorders throughout the recovery period.

The clinical features of anorexia and bulimia vary, but the American Psychiatric Association's *Diagnostic and Statistical Manual of Mental Disorders* (DSM-IV) lists the criteria that are used to establish these diagnoses (see sidebars on pages 379 and 380).[30] DSM IV criteria have also been established for Eating Disorders Not Otherwise Specified (EDNOS) and Binge Eating Disorder.

The primary symptoms of anorexia and bulimia are preoccupation with weight and excessive self-evaluation of weight and shape. Among women, the lifetime prevalence of anorexia nervosa is 0.5% to 3.7%. The lifetime prevalence of bulimia is 1.1% to 4.2%. Far more women than men suffer from these disorders, and the male-to-female prevalence ratio ranges from 1:6 to 1:10. See page 385 for patient counseling tips.

Anorexia Nervosa

Anorexia nervosa (AN) is characterized by the refusal to maintain body weight at or above a minimally normal weight for age and height. A disturbance in the way in which one's body weight or shape is experienced by the self, the undue influence of body weight or shape on self-evaluation, or denial of the seriousness of the current low body weight are diagnostic criteria for AN. Many patients with the disorder look emaciated, but are convinced they are overweight and remain intensely fearful of gaining weight.

This disease usually begins in young people around the time of puberty. It is related to a person's poor self-image, which is also a symptom of this disorder. Patients suffering from this disorder believe that their body weight, shape, and size is directly related to how good they feel about themselves and their worth as a human being. Patients often deny the seriousness of their condition and cannot objectively evaluate their own weight. They may adhere to strict exercise routines to keep off weight. Loss of monthly menstrual periods is typical in women with the disorder. Men with anorexia often become impotent.

Treatment Approaches

The treatment of this disorder is notoriously difficult. Many patients see no problem with their body weight. They may come for treatment as unwilling and uncooperative participants, brought in by family, friends, or another concerned professional. All clinical team members who treat patients with eating disorders need to be cooperative and supportive of the patient's efforts throughout treatment.

DSM-IV Criteria for Anorexia Nervosa

CRITERIA DESCRIPTION:

❑ Refusal to maintain body weight at or above a minimally normal weight for age and height (i.e., weight loss leading to maintenance of body weight less than 85% of that expected or failure to make expected weight gain during period of growth, leading to body weight less than 85% of that expected).

❑ Intense fear of gaining weight or becoming fat, even though underweight.

❑ Disturbance in the way in which one's body weight or shape is experienced, undue influence of body weight or shape on self-evaluation, or denial of the seriousness of the current low body weight.

❑ In postmenarcheal females, amenorrhea defined as the absence of at least three consecutive menstrual cycles. (A woman is considered to have amenorrhea if her periods occur only following hormone administration, e.g., estrogen.)

TYPES:

Restricting Type

❑ During the current episode of anorexia nervosa, the person has not regularly engaged in binge-eating or purging behavior (i.e., self-induced vomiting or the misuse of laxatives, diuretics, or enemas).

Binge-Eating/Purging Type

❑ During the current episode of anorexia nervosa, the person has regularly engaged in binge-eating or purging behavior (i.e., self-induced vomiting or the misuse of laxatives, diuretics, or enemas).

Source: Reference 30.

The goals of treatment for anorexia nervosa are to restore patients to a healthy weight, treat the physical complications, enhance the patient's motivation to cooperate with treatment, and provide education about healthy nutrition and eating habits. Other goals of treatment include correcting maladaptive thoughts, attitudes, and feelings related to the eating disorder; treating associated psychiatric conditions; enlisting family support; and attempting to prevent relapse. Medication should be considered in the treatment of anorexia, but should not be the sole or primary treatment.

If the patient is not in immediate crisis or suffering from medical complications from the disorder, individual psychotherapy is usually a good starting point for treatment. Cognitive-oriented therapies, focusing on issues of self-image and self-evaluation, are likely to be the most beneficial to the

DSM-IV Criteria for Bulimia Nervosa

CRITERIA DESCRIPTION:

❑ Recurrent episodes of binge eating, as characterized by the following:
   —Eating within a discrete period of time (i.e., any 2-hour period) an amount of food that is definitely larger than most people would eat during a similar period of time and under similar circumstances.
   —A sense of lack of control over eating during the episode (i.e., a feeling that one cannot stop eating or control what or how much one is eating).
❑ Recurrent inappropriate compensatory behavior to prevent weight gain, such as self-induced vomiting; misuse of laxatives, diuretics, enemas, or other medications; fasting; or excessive exercise.
❑ Frequency of binge eating and inappropriate compensatory behaviors both occurring, on average, at least twice a week for 3 months.
❑ Self-evaluation unduly influenced by body shape and weight.
❑ Disturbance not occurring exclusively during episodes of anorexia nervosa.

TYPES:

Purging Type

❑ During the current episode of bulimia nervosa, the person has regularly engaged in self-induced vomiting or the misuse of laxatives, diuretics, or enemas.

Nonpurging Type

❑ During the current episode of bulimia nervosa, the person has used other inappropriate compensatory behaviors, such as fasting or excessive exercise, but has not regularly engaged in self-induced vomiting or the misuse of laxatives, diuretics, or enemas.

Source: Reference 30.

patient. Some medications can be extremely helpful in treating patients with AN. Compliance should be carefully monitored, however, because patients may induce vomiting, which decreases effectiveness of the medication. Antidepressants are the usual drug treatment and may speed up the recovery process. Chlorpromazine may be beneficial for patients suffering from severe obsessions and increased anxiety and agitation.

The prognosis for recovery from an eating disorder is increased if patients do not binge or purge and if they have had the disorder for less than 6 months. A good support system is essential to quick recovery. The percentage of patients with AN who fully recover is modest, however. Although some improve over time, many continue to suffer from a distorted body image, disordered eating habits, and psychiatric difficulties.

Self-help support groups are an especially powerful and effective means of ensuring long-term treatment compliance and minimizing risk of relapse. Many such groups have established themselves within communities for the purpose of helping patients with this disorder share their common experiences and feelings. Patients find they can bounce ideas off of one another, get objective feedback about body image, and gain increased social support.

Bulimia Nervosa

Bulimia nervosa (BN) is characterized by recurrent episodes of binge eating, occurring at least twice a month for a minimum of 3 months. After binging, many bulimic individuals use a variety of methods to "purge." For example, they induce vomiting, abuse laxatives or diuretics, take enemas, refuse to eat, or exercise obsessively. Some of them use a combination of all these forms of purging.

There are two major subtypes of disorders found within BN. The 'Purging Type' defines the person who regularly engages in self-induced vomiting or the misuse of laxatives, diuretics, or enemas. The 'Non-Purging Type' is characterized by the use of other inappropriate compensatory behaviors, such as fasting or excessive exercise, but has not regularly engaged in self-induced vomiting or the misuse of laxatives, diuretics, or enemas.

Because many individuals with bulimia "binge and purge" in secret, and maintain normal or above normal body weight, they can often successfully hide their problem from others for years. Many patients remain at normal body weight or above because of their frequent binges and purges, which can range from once or twice a week to several times a day. Dieting heavily between episodes of binging and purging is also common.

Eventually, half of those individuals who are diagnosed with anorexia will develop bulimia. As with anorexia, bulimia typically begins during adolescence. The condition is most prevalent in women but is also found in men. Many people with bulimia are ashamed of their behavior and do not seek help until they reach their 30s or 40s. By this time, their eating behavior is deeply ingrained and more difficult to change.

Treatment Approaches

Patients with BN require specific nutritional counseling and psychosocial intervention. Some medications can be extremely helpful in treating a person who suffers from bulimia. Antidepressants (such as imipramine, desipramine, or phenelzine) are often an effective component of initial treatment, particularly if the patient has significant symptoms of depression, anxiety, obsessions, or impulse disorders. Selective serotonin reuptake inhibitors (SSRIs) are considered the safest medication option in patients who appear to be at suicide risk. The SSRIs and other newer medications that affect neurotransmitters, such as dopamine or norepinephrine, generally have fewer side effects than other drug treatments. Phenytoin and carbamazepine may help to reduce the frequency of the binging behaviors. Compliance with medical therapy should be carefully monitored, especially since the patient may be vomiting or taking large amounts of laxatives, both of which can have an impact on drug use and effectiveness.

Many of the issues relevant to anorexia treatment are similar in BN treatment, including distorted self-esteem and self-perception. A complete medical examination is usually warranted to evaluate the patient's health and medical status. Underweight or overweight patients often suffer from medical complications, especially if they are using laxatives or vomiting as a method of controlling their overeating.

Therapy is most effective when it examines the causes of those behaviors, such as poor self-perception. If the patient is not in immediate crisis or suffering from medical complications from the disorder, individual psychotherapy is usually a good starting point for treatment. Cognitive-oriented therapies, focusing on issues of self-image and self-evaluation, are likely to be the most beneficial.

Little is known about the long-term prognosis of patients with untreated bulimia. In one long-term study of patients with bulimia who were treated in an intensive program, 60% had a good outcome 6 years after successful treatment.[31] The prognosis for recovery from an eating disorder is increased if the patient does not binge or purge and has had the disorder for less than 6 months. A good support system is essential to quick recovery.

The Female Athlete Triad

The female athlete triad refers to a problematic triad of disorders that are distinct yet interrelated. They are disordered eating, amenorrhea, and osteoporosis.

In the disease progression, eating disorders often lead to menstrual dysfunction and subsequent premature osteoporosis. Not only can amenorrheic patients develop osteoporosis in their teens and 20s, they may never regain their previous bone densities. The presence of one disorder of the triad in a young female patient should prompt evaluation for the other two. Female athletes who have irregular periods require further assessment, including questions about nutrition, disordered eating habits, training intensity, and life stressors.

Anorexia Athletica

This subclinical eating disorder is not included in the DSM-IV. It occurs when an athlete uses at least one unhealthy method to control weight, including fasting, vomiting, diet pills, laxatives, or diuretics. Body builders and wrestlers have reported chronic dieting, preoccupation with food, and binge eating to achieve low body weight for competitions. Treatment should include education about the consequences of anorexia, gradually increasing meals and snacks to an appropriate level, and rebuilding the body to an appropriate weight. Treatment goals would be to establish a normal eating pattern and decrease any unhealthy preoccupation with food and weight. Preventive education for athletes may also be useful. It should instruct on how to get adequate calories from wholesome nutrient-dense foods, how to select an iron-rich diet, and how to allow for flexibility in their eating plan.

Nutritional Care of Eating Disorders

For all types of eating disorders, the goals of medical nutrition therapy are to restore patients to a healthy weight, treat their physical complications, enhance their motivation to cooperate with treatment, and provide education about healthy nutrition and eating habits.

Anorexia Nervosa

The nutritional assessment of AN routinely includes a diet history as well as the assessment of biochemical, metabolic, and anthropometric indices of nutritional status. AN is associated with chronic inadequate energy consumption, with reported calorie intakes of generally less than 1000 calories per day.

Patients with AN often require hospitalization to begin the refeeding process. Regardless of whether the patient is seen in an inpatient facility or presents to an outpatient center in a severely emaciated state, basic nutritional needs must first be met. This is often done through an intravenous line, because the patient will refuse to eat.

Daily fluid intake and weight should be monitored. Patients should be watched for a few hours after each meal to ensure no vomiting occurs. During the course of refeeding, the number of calories needed to gain weight increases. The patient's diet should begin between 1500 and 2000 calories per day, and the caloric intake can be increased gradually as the patient makes treatment gains. Severely anorexic patients can be started on a liquid food supplement or IV line, if necessary. Delayed gastric emptying with complaints of abdominal distention and discomfort after eating are common in AN.

The importance of the patient's weight should not be overemphasized. Weight is only the symptom in this disorder of poor body image and self-esteem problems. Therefore, while these primary difficulties should be the focus of any treatment approach, weight gain can be used as an objective measure as to treatment progress.

Patients may express multiple food aversions, especially to dietary fat. Prolonged dietary fat restriction may be a risk factor for essential fatty acid deficiency. In addition, patients with AN may hold illogical food beliefs and food avoidance patterns. For some, the compulsiveness shows up in strange eating rituals or the refusal to eat in front of others. It is not uncommon for people with anorexia to collect recipes and prepare gourmet feasts for family and friends, but not partake in the meals themselves. Nutrition education can help patients confront illogical beliefs.

Bulimia Nervosa

BN is described as a state of dietary chaos characterized by periods of uncontrolled, poorly structured eating, often followed by a period of restrained food intake. Total energy consumption in BN patients is unpredictable due to variability in the energy content of a binge, residual energy after a purge, and the degree of restrained eating between binge episodes. Binge episodes have been reported as ranging between 1200 to 11,500 calories per episode.

The nutrition plan therefore is aimed at promoting controlled eating and structure. Body weight should be stabilized although typically the patient will want to lose weight. A balanced macronutrient intake should be encouraged in patients with BN. This should include sufficient carbohydrate to prevent craving and adequate protein and fat to promote satiety. Patients with bulimia may avoid carbohydrates between binge episodes. Indeed, even restrained eating of carbohydrates may decrease normal brain serotonin and actually trigger binge-eating episodes.

Binging, purging, and restrained intake often impair recognition of hunger and satiety cues in bulimic patients. Therefore the cessation of purging behavior, coupled with a reasonable daily distribution of calories at three meals and prescribed snacks, can be instrumental in strengthening these biologic cues.

CONCLUSION

Health professionals play an important role in helping patients manage the relationship between diet and disease. Eating behavior is complex, and may be influenced by multiple factors including culture, economics, beliefs, habits, knowledge, and health.

The foremost goal for all health professionals should be to assist patients by providing factual, appropriate information regarding what can and cannot be achieved through diet. Dietary misinformation is pervasive and consumers are confused and overwhelmed by the amount of conflicting dietary advice they hear.

The psychology of eating affects both the interest and the ability to make dietary changes. During times of illness, some individuals believe that diet is one aspect of their life that they can control and they accomplish major dietary changes. Other individuals may realize that dietary changes will improve their health, but the personal barriers to making those changes are greater than the perceived benefits. Compliance to dietary prescriptions varies greatly. Therefore, supportive motivation for dietary change should come from all members of the patient's health care team.

The foundation of the treatment plan is a healthy lifestyle. Pharmacotherapy should complement this lifestyle. Even with the addition of medication, individuals should continue to meet the Dietary Guidelines for Americans, exercise regularly, and maintain a metabolically healthy body weight.

New fields of research, such as nutrition programming, the influence of diet in autoimmune disease, and gene–nutrient interactions, will greatly enhance the understanding of diet–disease relationships in the future. In addition, new drug therapies are constantly expanding treatment options for clinicians. The

Educating Patients About Eating Disorders: Questions Pharmacists Should Ask

Q. Have your family or friends expressed concern that your weight is unusually low? What do you think of your weight?

(Determine if the patient appears to have an eating disorder. If the patient appears below normal weight but expresses concerns about being overweight, encourage the patient to seek professional treatment.)

Q. Have you lost weight recently on purpose?

(Find out if the patient was intentionally trying to lose weight and if they are still dieting. Current research suggests that dieting may actually precipitate binge eating in biologically predisposed individuals.)

Q. Are there times during the day when you cannot stop eating? Do you ever find yourself eating unusually large amounts of food in a short period of time? Do you ever feel extremely guilty or depressed afterward?

(Explain that these behaviors are typical of eating disorders. Suggest that the patient seek treatment for an eating disorder.)

Q. Has your physician talked to you about the use of medications?

(Is the patient taking any medications for the condition? A variety of medications may be helpful in treating and managing eating disorders.)

Q. Are you taking prescription or OTC drugs for any other condition?

(Are there possibly interactions between prescribed drugs, or could any OTC drugs be producing side effects or interfering with treatment? Explain any potential interactions to the patient and advise him or her to check with the physician or pharmacist before taking any OTC drug or product.)

Q. Have you considered joining a support group for your condition?

(Support groups are very useful in treating eating disorders. Social support is important, especially when the problem is intractable.)

Q. Do you feel uncomfortably full after eating? Have you tried any meal replacement beverages?

(It is normal for recovering anorexic patients to feel uncomfortably full after eating. Suggest that the patient try high-calorie liquids to provide calories and other nutrients without the bulkiness of food.)

wealth of new information and choices increase the importance of multidisciplinary teamwork in assessing patients' needs and increasing their health and satisfaction.

REFERENCES

1. Position of the American Dietetic Association: medical nutrition therapy and pharmacotherapy. *J Am Diet Assoc.* 1999;99:227-30.
2. National Institute of Diabetes and Digestive and Kidney Diseases. Diabetes statistics. Available at: http://www.niddk.nih.gov/health/diabetes/pubs/dmstats/dmstats.htm. Accessed August 3, 2001.
3. Report of the Expert Committee on the Diagnosis and Classification of Diabetes Mellitus. *Diabetes Care* 1997;20:1183-97.
4. Mahan LK, Escott-Stump S. *Krause's Food, Nutrition, & Diet Therapy.* 10th ed. Philadelphia: WB Saunders; 2000.
5. American Diabetes Association. Nutrition recommendations and principles for people with diabetes mellitus. *Diabetes Care.* 2001;24(suppl 1):S44-7.
6. *Nutrition and Your Health: Dietary Guidelines for Americans.* Washington, DC: US Department of Agriculture; 2000. Home and Garden Bulletin No. 232.
7. Epidemiology of Diabetes Interventions and Complications (EDIC). Design, implementation, and preliminary results of a long-term follow-up of the Diabetes Control and Complications Trial cohort. *Diabetes Care.* 1999;22:99-111.
8. *Drug Facts and Comparisons 2001 Pocket Version.* 5th ed. St. Louis, MO: Facts and Comparisons; 2000.
9. Jellin JM, ed. *Natural Medicines Comprehensive Database.* Stockton, CA: Therapeutic Research; 2001.
10. Griffin, BA. Lipoprotein atherogenicity: an overview of current mechanisms. *Proc Nutr Soc.* 1999;58:163-9.
11. Expert Panel on Detection, Evaluation, and Treatment of High Blood Cholesterol in Adults. Executive Summary of the Third Report of the National Cholesterol Education Program (NCEP) Expert Panel on Detection, Evaluation, and Treatment of High Blood Cholesterol in Adults (Adult Treatment Panel III). *JAMA.* 2001; 285:2486-97.
12. Pronsky ZM. *Food Medication Interactions.* 11th ed. Birchrunville, PA: Food-Medication Interactions; 2000.
13. American Heart Association. High blood pressure statistics. Available at: http://www.americanheart.org/hbp/phys_stats.html. Accessed August 3, 2001.
14. Hu FB, Manson JE, Willett WC. Types of dietary fat and risk of coronary heart disease: a critical review. *J Am Coll Nutr.* 2001;20:5-19.
15. Kopple J. Renal disorders and nutrition. In: Shils ME, Olson JA, Shike M, et al., eds. *Modern Nutrition in Health and Disease.* 9th ed. Philadelphia: Lippincott, Williams & Wilkins; 1999:1439-72.
16. Coulston AM, Michels FG, eds. *Medical Nutrition Therapy Across the Continuum of Care: Client Protocols.* 2nd ed. Chicago, IL: The American Dietetic Association; 1998.
17. Looker AC, Dallman PR, Carroll MD, et al. Prevalence of iron deficiency in the United States. *JAMA.* 1997;277:973-6.
18. Fairbanks VF. Iron in medicine and nutrition. In: Shils ME, Olson JA, Shike M, et al., eds. *Modern Nutrition in Health and Disease.* 9th ed. Philadelphia: Lippincott, Williams & Wilkins; 1999:193-221.
19. National Institute of Arthritis and Musculoskeletal and Skin Diseases. Osteoporosis: progress and promise. Available at: http://www.nih.gov/niams/healthinfo/opbkgr.htm. Accessed August 3, 2001.
20. Standing Committee on the Scientific Evaluation of Dietary Reference Intakes, Food and Nutrition Board, Institute of Medicine. *Dietary Reference Intakes for Calcium, Phosphorus, Magnesium, Vitamin D, and Fluoride.* Washington, DC: National Academy Press; 1997.
21. National Institutes of Health. Optimal Calcium Intake. NIH Consens Statement 1994 Jun 6-8; 12(4): 1-31. Available at: http://consensus.nih.gov/cons/097/097_statement.htm. Accessed August 3, 2001.
22. US Department of Agriculture, Agricultural Research Service. Results from USDA's 1994-96 Continuing Survey of Food Intakes by Individuals and 1994-96 Diet and Health Knowledge Survey: table set 10. Available at: http://www.barc.usda.gov/bhnrc/foodsurvey/pdf/Csfii3yr.pdf. Accessed August 3, 2001.
23. Pak CY, Sakhaee K, Adams-Huet B, et al. Treatment of postmenopausal osteoporosis with slow-release sodium fluoride: final report of a randomized controlled trial. *Ann Intern Med.* 1995;123:401-8.
24. Omenn GS, Goodman GE, Thornquist MD, et al. Risk factors for lung cancer and for intervention effects in CARET, the Beta-Carotene and Retinol Efficacy Trial. *J Natl Cancer Inst.* 1996;88:1550-9.
25. American Cancer Society. The importance of nutrition in cancer prevention. Available at: http://www2.cancer.org/prevention/NutritionandPrevention.cfm. Accessed August 3, 2001.
26. National Cancer Institute. *Eating Hints for Cancer Patients Before, During, and After Treatment.* Bethesda, MD: National Cancer Institute; 1997. National Institutes of Health (NIH) Pub No. 98-2079.

27. National Center for Complementary and Alternative Medicine. Complementary and alternative medicine fact sheets. Available at: http://nccam.nih.gov/fcp/factsheets/index.html. Accessed August 3, 2001.

28. National Cancer Institute. Office of Cancer Complementary & Alternative Medicine. Available at: http://www.cancer.gov/occam. Accessed August 3, 2001.

29. Depaola D, Faine MP, Palmer CA. Nutrition in relation to dental medicine. In: Shils ME, Olson JA, Shike M, et al., eds. *Modern Nutrition in Health and Disease.* 9th ed. Philadelphia: Lippincott, Williams & Wilkins; 1999:1099-124.

30. American Psychiatric Association. Practice guideline for the treatment of patients with eating disorders [revision]. *Am J Psychiatry.* 2000;157(suppl 1):1-39.

31. Fichter MM, Quadflieg N. Six-year course of bulimia nervosa. *Int J Eat Disord.* 1997;22:361-84.

Appendices

Ira Wolinsky and Dorothy J. Klimis-Zacas

APPENDIX I   Dietary Reference Intakes and Recommended Intakes for Vitamins from the Food and Nutrition Board, Institute of Medicine, National Academy of Sciences

Life Stage Group	Vitamin A (mcg/d)a	Vitamin C (mg/d)	Vitamin D (mcg/d)b,c	Vitamin E (mg/d)d	Vitamin K (mcg/d)	Thiamin (mg/d)	Riboflavin (mg/d)	Niacin (mg/d)e	Vitamin B6 (mg/d)	Folate (mcg/d)f	Vitamin B12 (mcg/d)	Pantothenic Acid (mg/d)	Biotin (mcg/d)	Choline (mg/d)g
Infants														
0-6 mo	400*	40*	5*	4*	2.0*	0.2*	0.3*	2*	0.1*	65*	0.4*	1.7*	5*	125*
7-12 mo	500*	50*	5*	5*	2.5*	0.3*	0.4*	4*	0.3*	80*	0.5*	1.8*	6*	150*
Children														
1-3 y	300	15	5*	6	30*	0.5	0.5	6	0.5	150	0.9	2*	8*	200*
4-8 y	400	25	5*	7	55*	0.6	0.6	8	0.6	200	1.2	3*	12*	250*
Males														
9-13 y	600	45	5*	11	60*	0.9	0.9	12	1.0	300	1.8	4*	20*	375*
14-18 y	900	75	5*	15	75*	1.2	1.3	16	1.3	400	2.4	5*	25*	550*
19-30 y	900	90	5*	15	120*	1.2	1.3	16	1.3	400	2.4	5*	30*	550*
31-50 y	900	90	5*	15	120*	1.2	1.3	16	1.3	400	2.4	5*	30*	550*
51-70 y	900	90	10*	15	120*	1.2	1.3	16	1.7	400	2.4h	5*	30*	550*
>70 y	900	90	15*	15	120*	1.2	1.3	16	1.7	400	2.4h	5*	30*	550*
Females														
9-13 y	600	45	5*	11	60*	0.9	0.9	12	1.0	300	1.8	4*	20*	375*
14-18 y	700	65	5*	15	75*	1.0	1.0	14	1.2	400i	2.4	5*	25*	400*
19-30 y	700	75	5*	15	90*	1.1	1.1	14	1.3	400i	2.4	5*	30*	425*
31-50 y	700	75	5*	15	90*	1.1	1.1	14	1.3	400i	2.4	5*	30*	425*
51-70 y	700	75	10*	15	90*	1.1	1.1	14	1.5	400	2.4h	5*	30*	425*
>70 y	700	75	15*	15	90*	1.1	1.1	14	1.5	400	2.4h	5*	30*	425*
Pregnancy														
≤18 y	750	80	5*	15	75*	1.4	1.4	18	1.9	600j	2.6	6*	30*	450*
19-30 y	770	85	5*	15	90*	1.4	1.4	18	1.9	600j	2.6	6*	30*	450*
31-50 y	770	85	5*	15	90*	1.4	1.4	18	1.9	600j	2.6	6*	30*	450*
Lactation														
≤18 y	1,200	115	5*	19	75*	1.4	1.6	17	2.0	500	2.8	7*	35*	550*
19-30 y	1,300	120	5*	19	90*	1.4	1.6	17	2.0	500	2.8	7*	35*	550*
31-50 y	1,300	120	5*	19	90*	1.4	1.6	17	2.0	500	2.8	7*	35*	550*

Note: This table presents Recommended Dietary Allowances (RDAs) in **bold type** and adequate intakes (AIs) in ordinary type followed by an asterisk (*).

RDAs and AIs may both be used as goals for individual intake. RDAs are set to meet the needs of almost all (97% to 98%) individuals in a group. For healthy breastfed infants, the AI is the mean intake. The AI for other life-stage and gender groups is believed to cover needs of all individuals in the group, but the lack of data or uncertainty in the data prevent being able to specify with confidence the percentage of individuals covered by this intake.

a   As retinal activity equivalents (RAEs). 1 RAE=1 mcg retinal, 12 mcg beta carotene, 24 mcg alpha carotene, or 24 mcg beta cryptoxanthin in foods. To calculate RAEs from REs of provitamin A carotenoids in foods, divide the REs by 2. For preformed vitamin A in foods or supplements and for provitamin A carotenoids in supplements, 1 RE = 1 RAE.

b   Cholecalciferol. 1 mcg cholecalciferol = 40 IU vitamin D.

c   In the absence of adequate exposure to sunlight.

d   As α-tocopherol. α-tocopherol includes RRR-α-tocopherol, the only form of α-tocopherol that occurs naturally in foods, and the 2R-stereoisomeric forms of α-tocopherol (RRR-, RSR-, and RSS-α-tocopherol) that occur in fortified foods and supplements. It does not include the 2S-stereoisomeric forms of α-tocopherol (SRR-, SSR-, SRS-, and SSS-α-tocopherol) also found in fortified foods and supplements.

e   As niacin equivalents (NE). 1 mg of niacin = 60 mg of tryptophan; 0-6 months = preformed niacin (not NE).

f   As dietary folate equivalents (DFE). 1 DFE =1 mcg food folate = 0.6 mcg of folic acid from fortified food or as a supplement consumed with food = 0.5 mcg of a supplement taken on an empty stomach.

g   Although AIs have been set for choline there are few data to assess whether dietary supply of choline is needed at all stages of the life style, and it may be that the choline requirement can be met by endogenous synthesis at some of these stages.

h   Because 10% to 30% of people may malabsorb food-bound B_{12}, it is advisable for those older than age 50 to meet their RDA mainly by consuming foods fortified with B_{12} or a supplement containing B_{12}.

i   In view of evidence linking folate intake with neural tube defects in the fetus, it is recommended that all women capable of becoming pregnant consume 400 mcg of fortified foods in addition to intake of food folate from a varied diet.

j   It is assumed that women will continue consuming 400 mcg from supplements or fortified food until their pregnancy and they enter prenatal care, which ordinarily occurs after the end of the periconceptual period—the critical time for formation of the neural tube.

Source: Reference 5, Appendix 5.

Reprinted with permission: Trumbo P, Yates AA, Schlicker S, et al. Dietary reference intakes: vitamin A, vitamin K, arsenic, boron, chromium, copper, iodine, iron, manganese, molybdenum, nickel, silicon, vanadium, and zinc. *J Am Diet Assoc.* 2001;3:294-301.

APPENDIX 2   Dietary Reference Intakes: Recommended Intakes for Elements from the Food and Nutrition Board, Institute of Medicine, National Academy of Sciences

Life Stage Group	Calcium (mg/d)	Chromium (mcg/d)	Copper (mcg/d)	Fluoride (mg/d)	Iodine (mcg/d)	Iron (mg/d)	Magnesium (mg/d)	Manganese (mg/d)	Molybdenum (mcg/d)	Phosphorus (mg/d)	Selenium (mcg/d)	Zinc (mg/d)
Infants												
0-6 mo	210*	0.2*	200	0.01*	110*	0.27*	30*	0.003*	2*	100*	15*	2*
7-12 mo	270*	5.5*	220	0.5*	130*	11	75*	0.6*	3*	275*	20*	3
Children												
1-3 y	500*	11*	340	0.7*	90	7	80	1.2*	17	460	20	3
4-8 y	800*	15*	440	1*	90	10	130	1.5*	22	500	30	5
Males												
9-13 y	1300*	25*	700	2*	120	8	240	1.9*	34	1250	40	8
14-18 y	1300*	35*	890	3*	150	11	410	2.2*	43	1250	55	11
19-30 y	1000*	35*	900	4*	150	8	400	2.3*	45	700	55	11
31-50 y	1000*	35*	900	4*	150	8	420	2.3*	45	700	55	11
51-70 y	1200*	30*	900	4*	150	8	420	2.3*	45	700	55	11
>70 y	1200*	30*	900	4*	150	8	420	2.3*	45	700	55	11
Females												
9-13 y	1300*	21*	700	2*	120	8	240	1.6*	34	1250	40	8
14-18 y	1300*	24*	890	3*	150	15	360	1.6*	43	1250	55	8
19-30 y	1000*	25*	900	3*	150	18	310	1.8*	45	700	55	8
31-50 y	1000*	25*	900	3*	150	18	320	1.8*	45	700	55	8
51-70 y	1200*	20*	900	3*	150	8	320	1.8*	45	700	55	8
>70 y	1200*	20*	900	3*	150	8	320	1.8*	45	700	55	8

Pregnancy												
≤18 y	1300*	29*	3*	**1000**	**220**	**27**	**400**	2.0*	**50**	**1250**	**60**	**13**
19-30 y	1000*	30*	3*	**1000**	**220**	**27**	**350**	2.0*	**50**	**700**	**60**	**11**
31-50 y	1000*	30*	3*	**1000**	**220**	**27**	**360**	2.0*	**50**	**700**	**60**	**11**
Lactation												
≤18 y	1300*	44*	3*	**1300**	**290**	**10**	**360**	2.6*	**50**	**1250**	**70**	**14**
19-30 y	1000*	45*	3*	**1300**	**290**	**9**	**310**	2.6*	**50**	**700**	**70**	**12**
31-50 y	1000*	45*	3*	**1300**	**290**	**9**	**320**	2.6*	**50**	**700**	**70**	**12**

Note: This table presents Recommended Dietary Allowances (RDAs) in **bold type** and adequate intakes (AIs) in ordinary type followed by an asterisk (*). RDAs and AIs may both be used as goals for individual intake. RDAs are set to meet the needs of almost all (97% to 98%) individuals in a group. For healthy breastfed infants, the AI is the mean intake. The AI for other life-stage and gender groups is believed to cover needs of all individuals in the group, but the lack of data or uncertainty in the data prevent being able to specify with confidence the percentage of individuals covered by this intake.

Source: Reference 5, Appendix 5.

Reprinted with permission: Trumbo P, Yates AA, Schlicker S, et al. Dietary reference intakes: vitamin A, vitamin K, arsenic, boron, chromium, copper, iodine, iron, manganese, molybdenum, nickel, silicon, vanadium, and zinc. *J Am Diet Assoc*. 2001;3:294-301.

APPENDIX 3 Dietary Reference Intakes (DRIs): Tolerable Upper Intake Levels (UL[a]) for Vitamins from the Food and Nutrition Board, Institute of Medicine, National Academy of Sciences

Life Stage Group	Vitamin A (mcg/d)[b]	Vitamin C (mg/d)	Vitamin D (mcg/d)	Vitamin E (mg/d)[c,d]	Vitamin K	Thiamin	Riboflavin	Niacin (mg/d)[d]	Vitamin B6 (mg/d)	Folate (mcg/d)[d]	Vitamin B12	Pantothenic Acid	Biotin	Choline (g/d)	Carotenoids[e]
Infants															
0-6 mo	600	ND[f]	25	ND	ND	ND	ND	ND	ND	ND	ND	ND	ND	ND	ND
7-12 mo	600	ND	25	ND	ND	ND	ND	ND	ND	ND	ND	ND	ND	ND	ND
Children															
1-3 y	600	400	50	200	ND	ND	ND	10	30	300	ND	ND	ND	1.0	ND
4-8 y	900	650	50	300	ND	ND	ND	15	40	400	ND	ND	ND	1.0	ND
Males, Females															
9-13 y	1700	1200	50	600	ND	ND	ND	20	60	600	ND	ND	ND	2.0	ND
14-18 y	2800	1800	50	800	ND	ND	ND	30	80	800	ND	ND	ND	3.0	ND
19-70 y	3000	2000	50	1000	ND	ND	ND	35	100	1000	ND	ND	ND	3.5	ND
>70 y	3000	2000	50	1000	ND	ND	ND	35	100	1000	ND	ND	ND	3.5	ND
Pregnancy															
≤18 y	2800	1800	50	800	ND	ND	ND	30	80	800	ND	ND	ND	3.0	ND
19-50 y	3000	2000	50	1000	ND	ND	ND	35	100	1000	ND	ND	ND	3.5	ND
Lactation															
≤18 y	2800	1800	50	800	ND	ND	ND	30	80	800	ND	ND	ND	3.0	ND
19-50 y	3000	2000	50	1000	ND	ND	ND	35	100	1000	ND	ND	ND	3.5	ND

[a] UL = The maximum level of daily nutrient intake that is likely to pose no risk of adverse effects. Unless otherwise specified, the UL represents total intake from food, water, and supplements. Due to lack of suitable data, ULs could not be established for vitamin K, thiamin, riboflavin, vitamin B12, pantothenic acid, biotin, or carotenoids. In the absence of ULs, extra caution may be warranted in consuming levels above recommended intakes.

[b] As preformed vitamin A only.

[c] As α-tocopherol; applies to any form of supplemental α-tocopherol.

[d] The ULs for vitamin E, niacin, and folate apply to synthetic forms obtained from supplements, fortified foods, or a combination of the two.

[e] Beta carotene supplements are advised only to serve as a provitamin A source for individuals at risk of vitamin A deficiency.

[f] ND = not determinable due to lack of data regarding adverse effects in this age group and concern about lack of ability to handle excess amounts. Source of intake should be from food only to prevent high levels of intake.

Source: Reference 5, Appendix 5.

Reprinted with permission: Trumbo P, Yates AA, Schlicker S, et al. Dietary reference intakes: vitamin A, vitamin K, arsenic, boron, chromium, copper, iodine, iron, manganese, molybdenum, nickel, silicon, vanadium, and zinc. J Am Diet Assoc. 2001;3:294-301.

APPENDIX 4 Dietary Reference Intakes (DRIs): Tolerable Upper Intake Levels(UL[a]) for Elements from the Food and Nutrition Board, Institute of Medicine, National Academy of Sciences

Life Stage Group	Arsenic[b] (mg/d)	Boron (mg/d)	Calcium (g/d)	Chromium (mg/d)	Copper (mcg/d)	Fluoride (mg/d)	Iodine (mcg/d)	Iron (mg/d)	Magnesium (mg/d)[c]	Manganese (mg/d)	Molybdenum (mcg/d)	Nickel (mg/d)	Phosphorus (g/d)	Selenium (mcg/d)	Silicon[d]	Vanadium (mg/d)[e]	Zinc (mg/d)
Infants																	
0-6 mo	ND[f]	ND	ND	ND	ND	0.7	ND	40	ND	ND	ND	ND	ND	45	ND	ND	4
7-12 mo	ND	ND	ND	ND	ND	0.9	ND	40	ND	ND	ND	ND	ND	60	ND	ND	5
Children																	
1-3 y	ND	3	2.5	ND	1000	1.3	200	40	65	2	300	0.2	3	90	ND	ND	7
4-8 y	ND	6	2.5	ND	3000	2.2	300	40	110	3	600	0.3	3	150	ND	ND	12
Males, Females																	
9-13 y	ND	11	2.5	ND	5000	10	600	40	350	6	1100	0.6	4	280	ND	ND	23
14-18 y	ND	17	2.5	ND	8000	10	900	45	350	9	1700	1	4	400	ND	ND	34
19-70 y	ND	20	2.5	ND	10000	10	1100	45	350	11	2000	1	4	400	ND	1.8	40
>70 y	ND	20	2.5	ND	10000	10	1100	45	350	11	2000	1	3	400	ND	1.8	40
Pregnancy																	
≤18 y	ND	17	2.5	ND	8000	10	900	45	350	9	1700	1	3.5	400	ND	ND	34
19-50 y	ND	20	2.5	ND	10000	10	1100	45	350	11	2000	1	3.5	400	ND	ND	40
Lactation																	
≤18 y	ND	17	2.5	ND	8000	10	900	45	350	9	1700	1	4	400	ND	ND	34
19-50 y	ND	20	2.5	ND	10000	10	1100	45	350	11	2000	1	4	400	ND	ND	40

[a] UL = The maximum level of daily nutrient intake that is likely to pose no risk of adverse effects. Unless otherwise specified, the UL represents total intake from food, water, and supplements. Due to lack of suitable data, ULs could not be established for arsenic, chromium, and silicon. In the absence of ULs, extra caution may be warranted in consuming levels above recommended intakes.

[b] Although the UL was not determined for arsenic, there is no justification for adding arsenic to food or supplements.

[c] The ULs for magnesium represent intake from a pharmacological agent only and do not include intake from food and water.

[d] Although silicon has not been shown to cause adverse effects in humans, there is no justification for adding silicon to supplements.

[e] Although vanadium has not been shown to cause adverse effects in humans, there is no justification for adding vanadium to food. Vanadium supplements should be used with caution. The UL is based on adverse effects in laboratory animals. These data could be used to set a UL for adults but not for children and adolescents.

[f] ND = Not determinable due to lack of data of adverse effects in this age group and concern about lack of ability to handle excess amounts. Source of intake should be from food only to prevent high levels of intake.

Source: Reference 5, Appendix 5.

Reprinted with permission: Trumbo P, Yates AA, Schlicker S, et al. Dietary reference intakes: vitamin A, vitamin K, arsenic, boron, chromium, copper, iodine, iron, manganese, molybdenum, nickel, silicon, vanadium, and zinc. *J Am Diet Assoc.* 2001;3:294-301.

APPENDIX 5   Selected Nutrition References

1. Bendich A, Deckelbaum RJ. *Preventive Nutrition. The Comprehensive Guide for Health Professionals.* 2nd ed. Totowa, NJ: Humana Press; 2001.
2. Berdanier CD. *CRC Desk Reference for Nutrition.* Boca Raton, FL: CRC Press; 1998.
3. Ensminger AH, Ensminger ME, Konlande JE, et al. *Foods and Nutrition Encyclopedia.* 2nd ed. Boca Raton, FL: CRC Press; 1994.
4. Miller GD, Jarvis JK, McBean LD. *Handbook of Dairy Foods and Nutrition.* 2nd ed. Boca Raton, FL: CRC Press; 2000.
5. National Academy of Sciences, Committee on Dietary Reference Intakes. *Dietary Reference Intakes Series.* Washington, DC: National Academy Press; 1999, 2000, 2001. Available at: http://nap.edu. Accessed July 17, 2002.
6. National Research Council. *Diet and Health Implications for Advancing Chronic Disease Risk.* Washington, DC: National Academy Press; 1989.
7. National Research Council. *Recommended Dietary Allowances.* 10th ed. Washington, DC: National Academy Press; 1989.
8. Pennington JAT. *Bowes and Church's Food Values of Portions Commonly Used.* Philadelphia: Lippincott, Williams & Wilkins; 1998.
9. Rombeau JL, Rolandelli RH. (Eds.) *Clinical Nutrition: Parenteral Nutrition.* 3rd ed. Philadelphia: WB Saunders Co; 2001.
10. Shils ME, Olson JA, Shike M, et al. (Eds.) *Modern Nutrition in Health and Disease.* 9th ed. Philadelphia: Lippincott, Williams & Wilkins; 1999.
11. Wildman REC. *Handbook of Nutraceuticals and Functional Foods.* Boca Raton, FL: CRC Press; 2001.
12. Wildman REC, Medeiros DM. *Advanced Human Nutrition.* Boca Raton, FL: CRC Press; 2000.
13. Wolinsky I. (Ed.) *Nutrition in Exercise and Sport.* Boca Raton, FL: CRC Press; 1998.
14. Wolinsky I, Klimis-Tavantzis D.(Eds.) *Nutritional Concerns of Women.* Boca Raton, FL: CRC Press; 1996.
15. Ziegler EE, Filer LJ Jr. *Present Knowledge in Nutrition.* 7th ed. Washington, DC: ILSI Press; 1996.

APPENDIX 6 Selected Journals and Periodicals

American Journal of Clinical Nutrition
International Journal of Sport Nutrition and Exercise Metabolism
Journal of Nutrition
Journal of Nutrition Education
Journal of Parenteral and Enteral Nutrition
Journal of the American Dietetic Association
Nutrition and the M.D.
Nutrition in Clinical Practice
Nutrition Research
Nutrition Reviews
Nutrition Today

APPENDIX 7   Selected Professional Organizations

American College of Sports Nutrition
401 W. Michigan St.
Indianapolis, IN 46202
(317) 637-9200; fax: (317) 634-7817

American Dietetic Association
216 West Jackson Blvd
Chicago, IL 60606
(800) 877-1600; fax: (312) 899-0040

American Society for Clinical Nutrition
9650 Rockville Pike
Bethesda, MD 20814
(301) 530-7110; fax: (301) 571-1863

American Society for Nutritional Sciences
9650 Rockville Pike (Ste. 4500)
Bethesda, MD 20814
(301) 530-7050; fax: (301) 571-1892

American Society for Parenteral and Enteral Nutrition
8630 Fenton St. (Ste. 412)
Silver Spring, MD 20910
(800) 727-4567; fax: (301) 587-2365

ILSI Human Nutrition Institute
One Thomas Circle, 9th Floor
Washington, DC 20005
(202) 659-0524; fax: (202) 659-3617

Society for Nutrition Education
9202 N. Meridian (Ste. 200)
Indianapolis, IN 46260
(800) 235-6690; fax: (317) 571-5603

APPENDIX 8   Selected Web Sites

Food and Nutrition Information Center
  http://www.nal.usda.gov/fnic/

Food Guide Pyramid
  http://www.ganesa.com/food/index.html

National Library of Medicine: MEDLINE
  http://www.ncbi.nlm.nih.gov/PubMed/

Nutrient Data Laboratory
  http://www.nal.usda.gov/fnic/foodcomp/

The Tufts University Nutrition Navigator
  http://www.navigator.tufts.edu

Index

A

AAAs. *See* amino acids, aromatic (AAAs)
acarbose, 346, 347t
acetoacetic acid, 36
acid-base disturbances
    in parenteral nutrition, 191, 194
    in premature/LBW infants, 191
acidemias, organic, in children, 179–180, 181
acidurias, organic, in children, 179–180, 181
acute care. *See also* enteral nutrition; parenteral
        nutrition
    electrolyte depletion during, 76–77
        drugs causing, 78t
acute renal failure (ARF), 358
    nutritional care of, 359–360
    protein needs in, 236–238, 237t
adenosine, and caffeine, 106
adequate intake (AI), 2
adjusted dosing weight (ADW), 235
adolescents. *See also* children
    anorexia nervosa in, 378
    dieting in, 310, 320
    energy RDAs, 45, 46t, 163t
    enteral nutrition in, 182, 183
    nutrition for, 45–47
    parenteral nutrition in, trace mineral RDAs,
        189t
    physiological changes in, 46
    protein levels in, 160t
    vitamin and mineral needs of, 46–47
adrenergic agents, for weight control, 322, 323,
        332–333
adverse reactions. *See also* drug nutrient
        interactions (DNIs)
    warning patients of, 62–63
ADW (adjusted dosing weight), 235
AI (adequate intake), 2
albumin
    deficiency, 230, 231t
    levels, in nutrition assessment, 160t, 226–227,
        228t–229t, 230
alcohol interactions, 63
    with kava, 63, 64
alcoholism
    and B vitamin malabsorption, 23t
    and folic acid deficiency, 23, 364
    hepatitis associated with, protein needs with,
        238
allergies, food. *See* food allergies
alpha-amylase, 33–34
alpha-tocopherol, 15
aluminum toxicity, in parenteral nutrition

and liver damage, 289
and metabolic bone disease, 196, 290
American Academy of Pediatrics
    dietary recommendations, 45–46
    on hypoallergenic formulas, 177
    on infant formula nutrient content, 164
    on lipid emulsions in hyperbilirubinemia, 186
American Botanical Council, 145
American Cancer Society, guidelines on nutrition
        and cancer prevention, 371
American Dietetic Association, on very-low-calorie
        diets, 318
American Heart Association, on obesity and weight
        control, 308, 310, 320
American Medical Association Nutrition Advisory
        Group (AMA-NAG), on parenteral
        vitamins, 244, 246
American Society for Parenteral and Enteral
        Nutrition (ASPEN), 213–214
    on caloric requirements, 241–242
    on micronutrients, 244
    on nutrition screening, 214
    on parenteral safety, 297
    on protein requirements, 236
amination, 100
amino acid-based formulas
    enteral, 261–263
    for infants, 165t, 167, 177
    parenteral, 184, 185t, 281, 282–283, 287–288
amino acids, 10
    aromatic (AAAs), formulas enriched with, 262,
        281
    branched chain (BCAAs)
        as ergogenic aids, 102–105, 122
        formulas enriched with, 262–263, 270, 281
    in carnitine, 107
    deficient intake of, and nitrogen imbalance, 37
    in enteral formulas, 261–262
    as ergogenic aids, 97–100, 102–105, 122–123
    essential (EAAs), 10
        formulas enriched with, 261, 281
    in infant diet, 45
    in infant formulas, 167
        parenteral, 184, 185t
    in parenteral formulas/nutrition, 281, 284, 290,
        291, 292
        and hepatic dysfunction, 287–288
        for infants and children, 184–186, 185t,
        287–288
    in protein metabolism, 36–37
    in total energy calculation, 184–185
    in vegetarian diet, 11
Aminorex, 322